PRINCIPLES OF MEASUREMENT
AND MONITORING IN ANAESTHESIA
AND INTENSIVE CARE

Principles of Measurement and Monitoring in Anaesthesia and Intensive Care

M. K. SYKES

MA, MB, BChir, DA, FFARCS,
FFARACS(Hon), FFA(SA)(Hon)
Nuffield Professor of Anaesthetics,
University of Oxford, and
Fellow of Pembroke College, Oxford

M. D. VICKERS

MB, BS, DA, FFARCS, FFARACS(Hon)
Professor of Anaesthetics,
University of Wales College
of Medicine, Cardiff

C. J. HULL

MB, BS, FFARCS
Professor of Anaesthesia
University of Newcastle on Tyne

With additional chapters by
P. J. WINTERBURN

BSc, PhD
Lecturer in Biochemistry
University of Wales College, Cardiff

B. J. SHEPSTONE

MA, MSc, DPhil, MD, DSc, FRCR
University Lecturer in Radiology
University of Oxford
Fellow of Wolfson College, Oxford

THIRD EDITION

OXFORD

BLACKWELL SCIENTIFIC PUBLICATIONS

LONDON EDINBURGH BOSTON

MELBOURNE PARIS BERLIN VIENNA

© 1970, 1981, 1991 by
Blackwell Scientific Publications
Editorial Offices:
Osney Mead, Oxford OX2 0EL
25 John Street, London WC1N 2BL
23 Ainslie Place, Edinburgh EH3 6AJ
3 Cambridge Center, Cambridge
  Massachusetts 02142, USA
54 University Street, Carlton
  Victoria 3053, Australia

Other Editorial Offices:
Arnette SA
2, rue Casimir-Delavigne
75006 Paris
France

Blackwell Wissenschaft
Meinekestrasse 4
D-1000 Berlin 15
Germany

Blackwell MZV
Feldgasse 13
A-1238 Wien
Austria

First published 1970 (entitled *Principles of
Measurement for Anaesthetists*)
Reprinted 1973
Second edition 1981 (entitled *Principles of
Clinical Measurement*)
Third edition 1991

Set by Semantic Graphics, Singapore
Printed in Great Britain by
The Alden Press, Oxford
and bound by
Hartnolls Ltd, Bodmin, Cornwall

DISTRIBUTORS

Marston Book Services Ltd
PO Box 87
Oxford OX2 0DT
(*Orders*: Tel. 0865 791155
      Fax: 0865 791927
      Telex: 837515)

USA
Mosby-Year Book, Inc.
11830 Westline Industrial Drive
St Louis, Missouri 63146
(*Orders*: Tel: 800 633-6699)

Canada
Mosby-Year Book, Inc.
5240 Finch Avenue East
Scarborough, Ontario
(*Orders*: Tel: 416 298-1588)

Australia
Blackwell Scientific Publications
(Australia) Pty Ltd
54 University Street
Carlton, Victoria 3053
(*Orders*: Tel: 03 347-0300)

British Library
Cataloguing in Publication Data

Sykes, M. K. (Malcolm Keith)
  Principles of measurement and monitoring in anaesthesia
  and intensive care.—3rd. ed.
  1. Medicine. Anaesthesia 2. Man. Physiology.
  Measurement for anaesthesia
  I. Title II. Vickers, M. D. (Michael Douglas) III. Hull,
  C. J. IV. Sykes, M. K. (Malcolm Keith). *Principles of
  clinical measurement*
  617.96

ISBN 0-632-02408-9

Contents

Preface

The first edition of this book was published in 1970 and was entitled *Principles of Measurement for Anaesthetists*. Its aim was to describe the basic principles of measurement techniques which could be used during anaesthesia. At that time the importance of the subject to anaesthetists had been recognized by its inclusion in the primary FFARCS examination, but the practice of clinical measurement was largely restricted to specialized centres. During the next decade measurement technology improved and sophisticated instruments were developed for use in the operating theatre and in intensive care, premature baby and obstetric units. Techniques which were at one time mainly the province of cardiologists, respiratory physiologists or anaesthetists, became widely available and long-term monitoring on the general wards became a practicable proposition. In the second edition, *Principles of Clinical Measurement* (1981), we therefore broadened the scope of the text to cover the interests of physicians, surgeons, paediatricians and obstetricians as well as anaesthetists.

In this third edition we have made major changes in response to two important developments which have occurred during the past decade. The first was the introduction of microprocessor technology. This has had three major effects. Firstly, it has resulted in a reduction in size and improved performance of the measurement devices; secondly, it has enabled new techniques of measurement to be developed; and thirdly, the development of sophisticated artefact rejection algorithms has resulted in a marked improvement in both the accuracy and reliability of the measurement.

The second factor which has greatly influenced development is the increase in litigation and the widespread demand for monitoring equipment. This has created an enormous market which has not yet stabilized. With these factors in mind we have revised the text to include chapters on the application of the methods of measurement outlined earlier in the book. Again, we have not provided details of the techniques of monitoring but have concentrated on the principles involved in providing a monitoring system which will give adequate warning of apparatus malfunction or a deterioration in the patient's condition. We hope that this simple, if rather dogmatic approach, will help to dispel some of the mysteries associated with clinical measurement apparatus and will provide a sound basis for the development of a comprehensive monitoring system and for the understanding of future developments in the subject.

To accommodate this material without the book becoming too long and expensive, something had to be omitted and we have decided to delete the section on Statistics. This served its purpose at the time, but other texts, the use of statistical packages for microcomputers, and the trend towards the use of non-parametric tests and different kinds of Analysis of Variance, had rendered it obsolete.

M.K. Sykes
M.D. Vickers
C.J. Hull

Acknowledgements

The authors would like to acknowledge the assistance of many colleagues who have helped in the preparation of this edition. First, they are grateful to Dr P.J. Winterburn who wrote Chapter 8 for the second edition (Electromagnetic Radiation and Optical Measurements), and to Dr Basil Shepstone who has contributed a new Chapter 10 on Radionuclides and their Use in Clinical Measurement. Mr Neil Willis, Chief Medical Laboratory Scientific Officer, Department of Medical Biochemistry, University Hospital of Wales, Cardiff, provided invaluable assistance in rewriting Chapter 18 (Blood gas measurements). Dr John Moyle, Consultant Anaesthetist, Milton Keynes, and Dr S.M. Szekely, Lecturer in Anaesthetics, University of Wales College of Medicine, read the text and provided constructive criticism. We should like to thank other authors who kindly gave us permission to use their figures in the text. Needless to say all omissions and errors are the sole responsibility of the three authors.

Part 1
The Physical Basis of
Measurement Systems

1: General Principles of Measurement

Basic components of a measurement system

Successful medical treatment depends on accurate diagnosis. Diagnosis is, in turn, based on the history and on the elicitation of physical signs. Simple instruments, such as the stethoscope, facilitate the detection of physical signs. Other instruments, such as the thermometer, increase the accuracy with which changes can be measured. More complicated instruments, such as the electrocardiograph (ECG), enable changes outside the range of human perception to be charted.

Instruments are therefore used in medicine either to display or record signals which can be appreciated by the human senses, or to detect, display and record signals which are outside the range of human perception. In either event the system must consist of a detector, which senses the signal, and some form of display. The signal may be transferred directly from detector to display or may be altered in some way to make it more suitable for display. Finally the signal may be used to actuate a warning device, or even to set in motion a mechanism which reacts back upon the patient and controls some aspect of function. This plan is summarized in Fig. 1.1.

SENSING DEVICES

The body takes in food and converts the chemical energy contained therein into electrical, mechanical, heat and sound energy. Electrical energy may be sensed by *electrodes* and then processed by standard electronic techniques. Mechanical energy may be sensed directly by connecting the recording devices to the body with a thread or lever but, more commonly, it is transformed into electrical energy in order to facilitate measurement. Heat and sound energy are also usually changed into electrical energy before being measured, although transformations into other types of energy are sometimes used for convenience. Any instrument which is used to change one form of energy to another is known as a *transducer.* Although this term is commonly associated with the measurement of pressure, it will become apparent that it has a more widespread application in the measurement field.

Electrodes

Certain aspects of bodily function (nerve, muscle or sense organ activity) are accompanied by electrical changes which can be sensed by electrodes placed on the active tissue or on the body surface. One of the difficulties in recording from such sites is that electrodes tend to become polarized (i.e. develop a high resistance) when placed in contact with tissues (p. 49). The recording of potentials from the skin surface introduces additional problems because of the very high electrical resistance

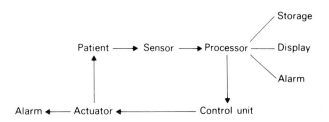

Fig. 1.1. The essential components of a clinical measurement system.

of the skin. Since the changes in electrical potential within the body are usually small (of the order of millivolts) it is important to minimize such resistances if satisfactory recordings are to be obtained.

When the signals are very small, for example in electroencephalography, it may be necessary to place a *pre-amplifier* close to the recording site so that the signal strength is increased to a level which ensures that there is minimal electrical interference during its transmission to the main processing unit.

Transducers

The main types of transducers used in medical applications are listed in Table 1.1. Displacement measurements can be processed to provide signals related to velocity or acceleration, whilst force or weight can be measured by the displacement of the free end of a fixed spring. Similarly the displacement of a flexible diaphragm or a liquid manometer can be used to indicate pressure. Measurements of flow may utilize some property of the liquid or gas (e.g. thermal conductivity, viscosity, density), or may be based on a mechanical device

Table 1.1. Transducers for medical applications

	Quantity measured	Transduction method
1	Displacement (velocity, acceleration) force, weight (spring) pressure (diaphragm)	Resistive, capacitive, inductive,piezo-electric, photoelectric, electromagnetic, ultrasonic
2	Flow (volume)	Electromagnetic, ultrasonic, thermal, optical, mechanical
3	Sound	Piezo-electric, capacitive, resistive, inductive
4	Heat	Thermal expansion, thermochemical, thermoelectric, resistive, thermographic
5	Light	Photoelectric (photovoltaic cell, photodiode, photoconductor, phototransistor)
6	Gases, blood gases, pH	Galvanic cell, electrodes
7	Humidity	Capacitive

which directly meters the volume passing a given point in unit time. Temperature transducers measure a change in some property of a substance induced by heat (e.g. thermal expansion or chemical change), whilst thermographic techniques measure the quantity of heat radiated from the skin. Chemical reactions may also produce electrical energy. A common example is the electrical battery, but similar reactions form the basis of the galvanic cell for oxygen measurement and the various electrode techniques for measuring pH or blood gases.

PROCESSING DEVICES

In a few simple instruments the signal is transmitted directly to the recorder or display unit without intermediate processing. Obvious examples are the measurement and display of temperature by the mercury-in-glass thermometer, or the sensing of pressure by a tambour directly linked by a thread to a pen writing on a rotating drum (Fig. 1.2a). However, if the tambour is connected to the pen by a lever and the fulcrum of the lever is placed closer to the tambour than to the drum, then the amplitude of the pen excursion will exceed that of the tambour so that the signal is *amplified* (Fig. 1.2b). This primitive technique is the simplest example of signal processing.

Amplification is usually required because the signal from the electrode or transducer is inadequate to drive a display or recorder. Amplification is most commonly accomplished by first changing the signal into electrical energy. This energy can then be amplified to a degree which would be quite impossible by the use of mechanical methods.

Most processing units are more complex and modify the signal in some other way. For example, a flow signal from a pneumotachograph may be *integrated* to give a signal proportional to volume or a volume signal *differentiated* to yield flow: impulses from a nerve fibre may be *counted* and their frequency displayed; or a non-linear output from a rapid gas analyser may be *rendered linear* before being displayed or recorded. Many instruments now incorporate much more complicated processing units which may be classified as *micro-*

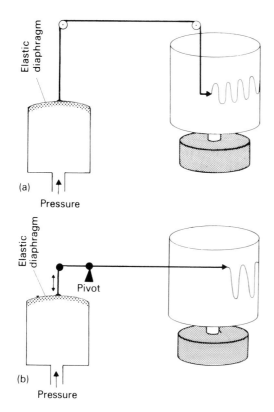

Fig. 1.2. (a) Simple pressure transducer with diaphragm directly connected to a pen writing on a drum. (b) The movement of the diaphragm is amplified by placing the pivot of the writing arm nearer the diaphragm.

computers. For example the processor in an automated blood gas analyser not only controls the whole process of calibrating the electrodes, measuring the electrical output from the electrodes and instigating regular wash and calibration cycles, but also continually checks the functioning of the machine and calculates and prints out the results. A cardiac output computer similarly analyses the indicator-dilution curve, applies calibration factors and displays the results in digital form.

DISPLAY SYSTEMS

The design of data display units has been neglected in the past. As the volume of data increases and the time allowed for digestion of the data decreases (e.g. in avionics), display has been subjected to

closer study. Unfortunately, progress in methods of display has been only slowly assimilated into the medical field.

In some instruments the measurement is displayed directly on a graduated scale as in the gas meter or the mercury thermometer. However, in many measurement systems the processor delivers an *analogue* signal to the display unit. The characteristic of such a signal is that the signal is represented by a continuous output of a voltage or current which varies directly with the magnitude of the input signal. The output may be displayed as a *trace* on a cathode-ray tube (CRT) with the amplitude of the signal on the *y*-axis and time or some other variable on the *x*-axis. Alternatively the magnitude of the signal may be displayed on a graduated *scale*. In some applications the output may be represented by *lights* of varying intensity, colour or size, whilst in diagnostic instruments using ultrasound, radioisotopes or thermography *grey scale* or *colour images* may be produced. In some types of apparatus there is no specific display unit, this being replaced by a trace or image on a recorder, the so-called *hard copy* display.

The increasing use of digital processing has encouraged the use of *digital* forms of display in which the data is presented in the form of alphanumeric characters (alphabetical characters or numbers). This form of display is only suitable for relatively stable signals but such data can often be derived from rapidly changing signals by suitable processing. Thus a microcomputer can be programmed to measure systolic, diastolic and mean blood pressures at each heart beat and then to display the average reading over, say, the preceding ten heart beats.

RECORDERS

These may be divided into those which make an immediate record on paper and those which store the data in some other form for subsequent analysis or display. Direct writing recorders utilize a pen, ink jet or heated stylus to inscribe an analogue trace onto normal or heat-sensitive paper. Photographic or ultraviolet recorders record the movements of a light spot on photographic film or ultraviolet-sensitive paper as it is drawn through the instrument at an appropriate speed, whilst a polaroid camera may be used to photograph the image shown on an oscilloscope screen or video display.

For more prolonged periods of recording, particularly when many channels of information have to be stored, digital techniques are used. The analogue signal is sampled at a frequency which is adequate to characterize the waveform, and the magnitude of the displacement at each sampling point is converted into a digital value. This is then stored either on magnetic tape or in a computer 'store' for subsequent analysis or playback. This type of storage provides immense flexibility because of the facility for data processing. For example, it is possible to subject a 24-hour ECG recording to rapid computer analysis and then to print out only those sections which display an abnormality. Alternatively, the computer can be programmed to provide an analysis of the frequency or duration of various arrhythmias or of S–T depression. Recorders are discussed in more detail in Chapter 7.

CONTROL SYSTEMS

Control systems are widely used in industrial automation but their use in medicine is still limited. Part of the reason has been the high cost of developing safe and reliable systems. However, although the advent of the microprocessor has greatly simplified the instrumental problems there are still major difficulties in securing a reliable patient–sensor interface. These difficulties can, to some extent, be overcome by the use of complicated artefact-rejection systems, alarms and fail-safe mechanisms, but the incorporation of such devices greatly increases the cost of the apparatus, and no control system can function in the absence of a signal from the patient.

Early examples of control systems were the control of the depth of intravenous anaesthesia from electroencephalograph (EEG) signals (Kiersey *et al.* 1954) and the mechanical control of ventilation from the end-tidal $P\text{co}_2$ (Frumin, 1957). The latter technique was even developed to the stage where a further injection of suxamethonium was

given whenever the patient attempted to breathe spontaneously! Other examples of control systems include the demand pacemaker, which is switched on when the heart rate falls below a pre-set level, and the neonatal temperature controller, which regulates the heat supplied by an infrared source to maintain a constant abdominal skin temperature.

Recently systems have been developed to control blood pressure (Reed & Kenny, 1987), the degree of muscular relaxation (Webster & Cohen, 1987) and oxygen, nitrous oxide and end-tidal vapour concentrations during anaesthesia (Westenskow *et al.* 1986; Verkaaik & Erdmann, 1990).

ALARMS

Measurement systems are increasingly fitted with visual or audible alarms which are activated when the measured variable exceeds predetermined limits. Alarms are also fitted to most therapeutic devices to warn of malfunction.

The purpose of an alarm is to attract the operator's attention to the abnormal situation so that corrective action may be initiated. However, because of the inevitable delay between the warning, the diagnosis of the cause of the malfuction and the resultant corrective action it is important to categorize alarms in terms of their urgency: *advisory* creating an awareness of the problem, *caution* requiring a prompt response, and *warning* requiring an immediate response (Schreiber, 1985). Unfortunately there is little agreement between manufacturers and users concerning the alarm limits which define these categories, and there is no uniform system for indicating an alarm status (Kerr, 1985). Most monitoring and therapeutic devices are fitted with their own alarm systems. Since these often generate similar sounds which have poor directional quality, it is often difficult to identify the source of the alarm. These problems, together with the high incidence of false alarms, greatly reduce the value of current alarm systems and result in many alarms being inactivated by doctors or nursing staff (McIntyre, 1985).

The increasing awareness of these deficiences has led some manufacturers to design integrated alarm systems which not only allow a hierarchy to be established (so that attention is directed to the most life-threatening situation when several alarms are activated simultaneously) but also provide a textual or verbal instruction concerning the corrective action to be taken. Attempts are being made to standardize alarm systems so that each type of equipment (ventilator, infusion pump, etc.) will be characterized by a given alarm sound (Kerr, 1985), and a number of manufacturers are providing variable alarm limits with default values to which the machine will revert if alarm limits are not set when the device is switched on. The widespread application of sophisticated microprocessor technology has led to a remarkable improvement in artefact rejection and a consequent decrease in the incidence of false alarms during recent years, so that many devices are now fitted with practical and effective alarm systems. However, the high incidence of false alarms is still a major problem.

MONITORING SYSTEMS

There are still many difficulties in providing effective continuous monitoring of the patient's condition. The major problem is that techniques which provide an accurate continuous measurement of some physiological variable (e.g. arterial pressure) tend to be invasive and therefore carry a risk of complications. This limits their potential duration of use. The second problem is that the variables which can be monitored may not provide the appropriate information. For example, although arterial pressure and arterial oxygen saturation may be measured continuously, what is really needed is a continuous measurement of tissue oxygenation in the vital organs. The third problem is that continuous monitoring generates a vast amount of information which is not easily digested by the attendant. Data compression and trend information thus become important components of any monitoring system.

There are other problems associated with the monitoring of apparatus function. One of the major difficulties is to design a system which can detect all the possible failure modes of any given piece of equipment. This requires the application of sophisticated techniques of hazard analysis which, although commonly used in some industries, have not been widely applied in the medical equipment field. The second major problem is the integration of information provided from a number of devices and the rationalization of alarm systems. This is difficult to achieve when apparatus is purchased from different manufacturers, but a number of firms are now producing integrated monitoring systems which minimize many of these problems.

Essential requirements for a measurement system

A satisfactory measurement system must be capable of isolating the signal of interest from other unwanted signals and then reproducing this signal with consistent accuracy despite normal environmental variations. This requirement can only be satisfied by ensuring that a high signal-to-noise ratio is maintained throughout the system and by using instruments that have good zero and gain stability, minimal amplitude non-linearity and hysteresis, and an adequate frequency response.

SIGNAL-TO-NOISE RATIO

When a biological signal is detected, amplified and recorded, it will be more or less obscured by a variety of unwanted signals, which are collectively described as *noise*. At its source, the signal can be considered to be 'clean', but progressively contaminated by noise as it passes through the various stages in the data pathway.

The most critical stage is the first, since most biological signals are very small, and are therefore easily obscured. For instance, an ECG signal may be mixed with intercostal electromyograph (EMG) signals of equal amplitude, and with wideband noise (i.e. of many frequencies) generated by electrochemical activity at the skin–electrode interface. As the signal travels along a wire to the amplifier, electrostatic and electromagnetic linkage with mains cables and mains-powered devices may add noise which will be predominantly 50 Hz (and its harmonics). Radiofrequency noise may also be added at this stage, from sources such as surgical diathermy, staff-paging systems, or nearby radio-transmitters. Physical disturbance of the cable, by minutely altering its capacitance, may add low frequency noise (microphony) to the signals. As the signal is amplified, it is joined by thermal noise generated within the electronic components themselves. Thermal noise may be a major problem when detecting signals in the microvolt range (such as those recorded by the EEG) so that special 'low noise' input stages are required. As the signal grows larger, thermal noise is still added by each component, but being of relatively constant amplitude, makes very little contribution to the overall noise level. When the signal is transmitted to another location or recorded on magnetic tape, it is often closely associated with other physiological signals undergoing similar treatment. Each signal is usually referred to as a *channel*, and may acquire some signal from an adjacent channel (cross-talk) which must now be considered to be noise.

Successful recording of a signal therefore depends upon isolating the signal, not only from unwanted biological signals, but also from electronic noise sources. The efficiency with which a signal can be isolated is thus defined by the signal-to-noise ratio. Since signal-to-noise ratios may vary widely, the logarithmic bel scale is often used to define them. Thus 1 bel is a ratio of 10:1, whilst 2 bels represents a ratio of 100:1. For convenience bels are usually multiplied by 10 to yield decibels, so that 10:1 = 10 dB whilst 100:1 = 20 dB. If, therefore an instrument claims a signal-to-noise ratio of 45 dB a ratio of 31 623:1 is implied.

A low signal-to-noise ratio can often be improved by selective *filtering* (rejecting unwanted frequencies), by employing amplifiers with a *high common mode rejection* ratio (CMRR; p. 39) and by the use of special techniques such as *signal averaging*.

ACCURATE REPRODUCTION OF
THE INPUT SIGNAL

The second requirement of any system of instrumentation is that it should provide an accurate display or record of the input signal. Most instrumentation systems are inherently unstable, their

performance being affected by temperature, mains voltage and frequency, ageing of components, etc. When considering the accuracy of any system one must consider the zero stability, the gain stability, the linearity and the frequency response. The latter includes a consideration of damping and phase shift.

Zero stability

The first aspect to be assessed is zero stability i.e. the ability to maintain a zero reading on the display unit or recorder when the input signal is zero. A certain amount of zero instability can usually be tolerated but obviously, the degree of stability required will vary with the application. For example, slight zero instability will prove less of a disadvantage when recording blood pressures during cardiac catheterization than when recording blood pressures over prolonged periods of days or weeks.

Zero drift may vary around a mean or the signal may drift progressively in one direction. In either case it may be regarded as noise of very low frequency. Progressive drift is extremely important in long-term measurements because of its inherently cumulative nature. Furthermore, in some types of apparatus, zero drift may be amplified or integrated thus affecting the gain stability.

Gain stability

The sensitivity of the processing device can usually be adjusted to vary the ratio between input and output signals by means of one or more 'gain' controls. There should always be ample reserve gain in the instrument and, once set, the degree of gain should remain constant over a period which is adequate for the purpose in hand.

Amplitude linearity

The degree of amplification of the signal should be equal throughout the whole range of signal strengths likely to be encountered. If it is not, the system is said to be non-linear. Figure 1.3 illustrates non-linearity in a blood pressure transducer–

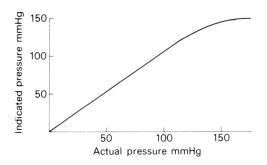

Fig. 1.3. Non-linearity in a blood pressure measuring system in the higher ranges of pressure.

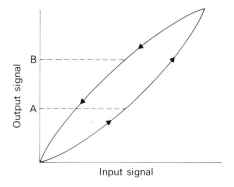

Fig. 1.4. A hysteresis loop. A given input signal produces an output signal 'A' when the signal is rising, and an output signal 'B' when it is falling.

amplifier–recorder system which occurred only in the higher range of pressure.

Normally the linearity of an instrument or system is specified in such terms as 'better than ±1%'. This means that the reading on the display unit should never be in error by more than ±1% of the actual reading throughout the range of the instrument. Unfortunately, this statement sometimes only applies to part of the range and this may not be made clear in the literature provided by the manufacturer. It is most important to assess the linearity of the complete system, since minimal nonlinearity in each component may prove additive and so lead to a greater error in the recorded signal.

Certain instruments such as thermistors and humidity sensors may display *hysteresis*. This means that the signal produced by a given temperature or humidity is different when the input is rising than when it is falling. A hysteresis loop is thus produced (Fig. 1.4). This is another cause of non-linearity.

Frequency response

Most signals follow a complicated pattern or waveform. Fourier showed mathematically that any complex waveform could be constructed by taking a simple sine wave of the same frequency as the slowest component (called the fundamental frequency) and adding to it a number of sine waves, the frequencies of which bore simple whole-number relationships to the fundamental

(Fig. 1.5). These higher-frequency components are called harmonics of the fundamental frequency. Electrical and mechanical systems which transmit waveforms behave as though all the components of a complex wave are really separate. To reproduce a complex wave accurately, therefore, the system must be able to handle all the component frequencies in the waveform in a similar manner. This implies equal amplification of each frequency (i.e. no *amplitude* distortion), and, if any delay occurs in the system, there must be no alteration in the relative postions of the various components of the wave (i.e. no *phase* distortion). Although this is the ideal solution, for many purposes it is sufficient if the system reproduces accurately up to the 10th harmonic, that is up to 10 times the fundamental frequency. However, if one is particularly concerned with the high-frequency components, then a higher frequency response is necessary.

Matching

A complete instrumentation system consists of a number of units each of which has special characteristics. The efficiency of the complete system depends, not only on the behaviour of the components, but also on the way they are matched to each other. Such matching must take account, not only of the strength and character of the signals fed from one unit to another, but of the way in which each part interacts with the other.

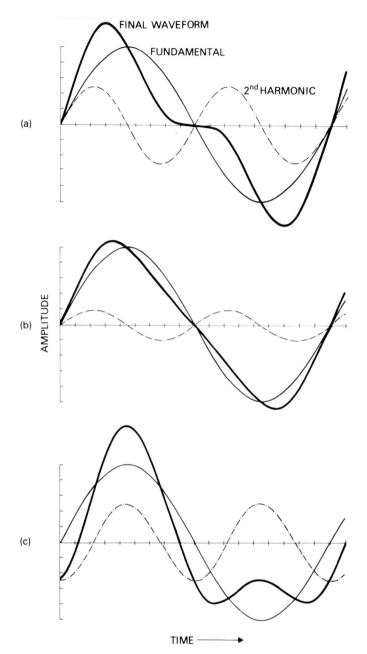

(a)

(b)

(c)

AMPLITUDE

TIME ⟶

Fig. 1.5. Fourier analysis. A complex waveform can be resolved into the fundamental waveform and a series of harmonics. Variations in the shape of a complex wave (bold line) are due to differences in amplitude and phase of the harmonics present.
(a) Fundamental (first harmonic) plus second harmonic. (b) Effect of reducing amplitude of harmonic. (c) Effect of changing phase of harmonic.

In complete systems this is properly taken care of by the maker, but when systems are constructed of separate 'black boxes' it is necessary to match both the current or voltage and the input and output impedances (see Chapter 3). If this is not done the characteristics of one part of the system may be considerably altered by the other. A false record may also be obtained by adding a recorder to a device which normally only feeds a meter. A recorder may create a shunt across the meter and provide a path for part of the signal. Both the recorder and the meter will then give a lower reading from a standard signal than would have been shown on the meter with the recorder unconnected.

It will be apparent from the above discussion that a large number of factors have to be taken into account when considering any system of measurement. Before a choice of instrumentation is made it is necessary to consider the degree of accuracy required and the manner in which the system is to be used. When these fundamentals have been decided, detailed planning of the complete system becomes possible. If they are ignored the system may prove inadequate or unnecessarily expensive.

References

Frumin, M.J. (1957) Clinical use of physiological respirator producing N_2O amnesia-analgesia. *Anesthesiology* **18**, 290–299.

Kerr, J.H. (1985) Warning devices. *British Journal of Anaesthesia* **57**, 696–708.

Kiersey, D.K., Faulconer, A. & Bickford, R.G. (1954) Automatic electro-encephalographic control of thiopental anesthesia. *Anesthesiology* **15**, 356–364.

McIntyre, J.W.R. (1985) Ergonomics: anaesthetists' use of auditory alarms in the operating room. *International Journal of Clinical Monitoring and Computing* **2**, 47–55.

Reed, J.A. & Kenny, G.N.C. (1987) Evaluation of closed-loop control of arterial pressure after cardiopulmonary bypass. *British Journal of Anaesthesia* **59**, 247–255.

Schreiber, P. (1985) *Safety guidelines for anesthesia systems.* North American Drager, Telford, PA.

Verkaaik, A.P.K. & Erdmann, W. (1990) Respiratory diagnostic possibilities using closed circuit anesthesia. *Acta Anaesthesiologica Belgica* **41**, 177–188.

Webster, N.R. & Cohen, A.T. (1987) Closed loop control of atracurium. *Anaesthesia* **42**, 1085–91.

Westenskow, D.R., Zbinden, A.M., Thomson, D.A. & Kohler, B. (1986) Control of end-tidal halothane concentration. *British Journal of Anaesthesia* **58**, 555–562.

Further reading

Blitt, C.M. (1990) *Monitoring in anesthesia and critical care medicine*, 2nd edn. Churchill Livingstone, London.

Gravenstein, J.S. & Paulus, D.A. (1987) *Clinical monitoring practice*, 2nd edn. J.B. Lippincott Company, Philadelphia.

Lake, C.L. (1990) *Clinical monitoring.* W.B. Saunders Co., Philadelphia.

2: Units of Measurement and Basic Mathematical Concepts

Units of measurement

Measurement became necessary when human beings began to exchange one commodity for another. Initially, measurements were related to commonly available objects. Thus in early Egyptian times length was related to the width of the finger (the digit) or to the distance from the elbow to the fingertips (the cubit). The fathom, equivalent to the 6 ft span of the arms, is still used to measure the depth of the sea, and the hand (4 in) is still used to measure the height of a horse. Later, an attempt was made to rationalize the measurements so that individual variation did not affect the comparisons. For example, the Egyptians standardized on the cubit and ordered that all other measurements should be fractions or multiples of a cubit. Thus the digit became 1/28 of a cubit, and the fathom 4 cubits.

Even greater exactitude became possible when standards were adopted. Thus, even in Anglo-Saxon times, there was a standard yard, in the form of an iron bar kept at Winchester. A similar standard was maintained at Westminster until 1959, but after that date both the pound and the yard were related to the kilogram (kg) and the metre (m).

Metric standards were first developed in France at the end of the 18th century. Initially the metre was supposed to be a distance equal to 1/10 000 000 of the distance along the Earth's surface between the pole and equator, and the litre and kilogram were defined from this primary standard. In 1875 an International Bureau of Weights and Measures was established at Sèvres, a suburb of Paris, and new standards for the metre and kilogram were set up and sent to a number of countries. Later on, this International Bureau concerned itself with other standards. As the need for greater and greater accuracy has become apparent, the Bureau has increasingly turned towards standards present in natural phenomena, since these can be measured by scientists anywhere in the world. Thus the standard metre (a bar made of platinum and iridium and kept at Sèvres) was discarded in 1960 in favour of a standard related to the wavelength of the orange light emitted by krypton-86 and, in 1967, time was related to atomic vibrational frequency.

Because of its decimal basis the metric system has always been more attractive for scientific use. The metric system based on the centimetre, gram and second (CGS) was initially replaced by the MKS system (metre, kilogram, second). Further refinement and extension of this became the Système Internationale d'Unités (SI), the principle difference being the creation of a non-gravitationally-derived unit for force.

The replacement of the imperial by the metric system has proceeded at different rates for different applications and in different countries. European trade ministers decided in 1989 to phase out most imperial units within ten years. The pint may be retained for milk and beer but other drinks will have to be sold by the litre by 1995. For loose goods, such as vegetables, imperial measures may be retained until 1999 but grams and kilograms will have to be used for all packaged items by 1995. It has been left to the government to decide the fate of the mile, acre and troy ounce (used for weighing bullion), and the government has decided that the mile, at least, will be retained indefinitely in the UK.

All units relevant to medical practice have been metric for nearly 20 years but the specific change to SI has been patchy and scientists in many countries around the world have not uniformly adopted SI units. Since the principal difference relates to the definition of force, it is pressure measurements (force per unit area) which show the greatest diversity. There are in routine use at present, units of pressure based on non-gravitational definitions in the CGS system (e.g. the bar) as well as the SI system (the pascal) and gravitationally-based definitions in metric terms (kilograms and kiloponds per square metre, Torr, standard atmosphere, mmHg, cmH$_2$O) and in imperial terms (inch of water, pound per square inch). SI units are used throughout this book, conversion factors and explanations being provided where necessary.

SI UNITS

SI is an extension of the traditional metric system. There are seven base units from which most of the other units are derived (Table 2.1). The exact definition of these units is set out in Table 2.2 but the physical basis for the standards is as follows.

The *metre* (m) is defined in terms of the wavelength in a vacuum of a specified emission from the krypton-86 atom. The vacuum wavelengths of specified emissions from other atoms, such as ^{198}Hg and ^{144}Cd, are precisely related to the primary standard and can therefore be used as secondary standards.

The *second* (s) is defined in terms of the frequency of structure transitions in the atoms of caesium-133. With present instruments the time

Table 2.1 SI base units and supplementary units

Quantity	Unit	
	Name	Symbol
Base units		
Length	metre	m
Mass	kilogram	kg
Time	second	s
Electric current	ampère	A
Thermodynamic temperature	kelvin	K
Amount of substance	mole	mol
Luminous intensity	candela	cd
Supplementary units		
Plane angle	radian	rad
Solid angle	steradian	sr

Table 2.2 Definition of SI base units

The metre is the length equal to 1 650 763.73 wavelengths in vacuum of the radiation corresponding to the transition between the levels 2p$_{10}$ and 5d$_5$ of the krypton-86 atom.

The kilogram is the unit of mass; it is equal to the mass of the international prototype of the kilogram.

The second is the duration of 9 192 631 770 periods of the radiation corresponding to the transition between the two hyperfine levels of the ground state of the caesium-133 atom.

The ampère is that constant current which, if maintained in two straight parallel conductors of infinite length, of negligible circular cross-section and placed one metre apart in a vacuum, would produce between these conductors a force equal to 2×10^{-7} newtons per metre of length.

The kelvin, the unit of thermodynamic temperature, is the fraction 1/273.16 of the thermodynamic temperature of the triple point of water.

The mole is the amount of substance of a system which contains as many elementary entities as there are atoms in 0.012 kg of carbon 12. When the mole is used the elementary entities must be specified and may be atoms, molecules, ions, electrons, and other particles or specified groups of such particles.

The candela is the luminous intensity, in the perpendicular direction, of a surface of 1/600 000 m^2 of a black body at the temperature of freezing platinum under a pressure of 101 325 newtons per square metre.

difference between two caesium atomic clocks amounts to less than 1s in 30 000 years.

The *kilogram* (kg), the unit of mass, is equal to the mass of the international prototype kilogram, a platinum–iridium cylinder preserved at the International Bureau of Weights and Measures at Sèvres, France. The platinum–iridium alloy is used because it has a thermal coefficient of expansion close to zero.

The *ampère* (A) is the unit of electric current and is defined as the amount of current which would have to flow down each of two parallel conductors of infinite length and negligible circular cross-section in a vacuum to generate a given force between them.

The *kelvin* (K), the unit of temperature, is 1/273.16 of the temperature of the triple point of water (the point at which solid, liquid and gaseous phases are in equilibrium). A difference in temper-

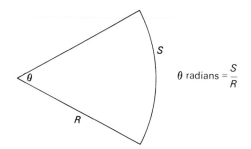

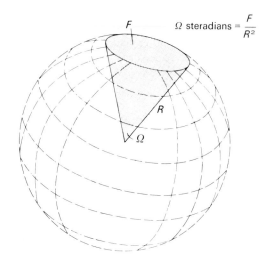

Fig. 2.1. An angle of 1 radian (rad) is subtended by an arc of a circle (S) equal in length to the length to the radius (R). Hence θ rad = S/R and 2π rad = 360°.

ature may be expressed in kelvins or degrees Celsius (°C) for 1 K = 1 °C.

The *candela* is the unit of luminous intensity and is defined in terms of the brightness (looked at perpendicularly) of a small area of molten platinum at a given temperature and pressure (see p. 16).

SUPPLEMENTARY SI UNITS

These are used in the definition of derived units, but are not regarded as base units since they have no dimensions. They are the unit of plane angle (radian) and solid angle (steradian) and are defined as follows.

The *radian* (rad) is the plane angle between two radii which, on the circumference of a circle, cut an arc equal in length to the radius. (Since 2π radians = 360°, 1 radian = 57.296°. See Fig. 2.1.)

The *steradian* (sr) is the solid angle which has its apex at the centre of a sphere, and which describes, on the surface of the sphere, an area equal to that of a square having its side as the radius of the sphere (see Fig. 2.2)

DECIMAL MULTIPLES AND SUBMULTIPLES

The approved prefixes and their symbols are given in Table 2.3. These are normally attached to the appropriate unit as in millisecond (ms or s × 10^{-3}), and kilometre (km or m × 10^3). In the case of mass, however, the adoption of the kilogram as the base unit would lead to millikilogram to indicate a gram. Accordingly in the case of mass,

Fig. 2.2. One steradian (sr) is subtended at the centre of a sphere of radius R by a portion of its surface of area R^2. Hence Ω sr = F/R^2 and 1 sphere = 4π sr.

the prefixes are attached to gram and to the symbol 'g', e.g. mg (milligram) and μg (microgram).

When a derived unit is expressed as a function (e.g. 1000 ohms per metre) it is permissible to apply the prefix to the numerator (1 kilohm per metre), to the denominator (1 ohm per millimetre) or to both if appropriate (1 megohm per kilometre). Compound prefixes such as millimicrometre are not permitted.

Note that some prefixes use the same letter as some units: thus 'm' is used for both milli and metre. To clarify the meaning it is necessary to observe the convention that the prefix precedes the unit symbol without space or punctuation. Thus ms indicated millisecond, mm millimetre and

Table 2.3 Prefixes and their symbols used to designate certain decimal multiples and submultiples

Factor	Prefix	Symbol	Factor	Prefix	Symbol
10^{18}	exa	E	10^{-1}	deci	d
10^{15}	peta	P	10^{-2}	centi	c
10^{12}	tera	T	10^{-3}	milli	m
10^{9}	giga	G	10^{-6}	micro	μ
10^{6}	mega	M	10^{-9}	nano	n
10^{3}	kilo	k	10^{-12}	pico	p
10^{2}	hecto	h	10^{-15}	femto	f
10^{1}	deca	da	10^{-18}	atto	a

MHz megahertz. To denote the product of two symbols the symbols are separated by a space or by a central point. Thus metre × second is m s or m·s whilst metre per second is m s^{-1} or m·s^{-1}.

DERIVED SI UNITS

Almost all of the units required in scientific work can be derived from the seven base and two supplementary units listed in Table 2.1. Derived units are expressed in algebraic form as the products of powers of the base and supplementary units. For example, the unit of force is the newton (N). This is the force required to accelerate a mass of 1 kg at a rate of 1 metre per second per second and is expressed in terms of m·kg·s^{-2}. The unit of pressure, the pascal (Pa), can be represented in base units as m^{-1}·kg·s^{-2}, and electric resistance (Ω) by m^2·kg·s^{-3}·A^{-2}. This representational system may not strike the reader as self-evident

until one recalls that 1/10 can also be expressed as 0.1 which in turn can be represented as 10^{-1}. Using minus powers such as 10^{-1} is therefore a convenient way of expressing fractions or ratios and 10^{-1} can be regarded as 1 per 10. In the same way, m^{-1} means 'per metre', s^{-1} means 'per second' and kg^{-1} means 'per kilogram'. A speed of 25 metres per second can therefore be simply expressed as 25 m·s^{-1}. An acceleration of 6 metres per second per second is likewise 6 m·s^{-2}.

In Table 2.4 are listed those derived SI units which have officially been accorded special names (eponyms): the third column expresses each quantity by reference to others from which it is most simply derived. For example, a pascal is a newton per square metre (N·m^{-2}), a joule is a newton metre (N·m) a watt is a joule per second (J·s^{-1}), a volt is a watt per ampere (watts = volts × amps, therefore V = W/A or W·A^{-1}), an ohm is a volt per ampere (V·A^{-1}), and so on. In the fourth column

Table 2.4 Derived SI units having names and symbols

Quantity	Unit		Expression	
	Name	Symbol	In other SI units	In terms of base or supplementary SI units
Frequency	hertz	Hz		s^{-1}
Force	newton	N		m·kg·s^{-2}
Pressure, stress	pascal	Pa	N·m^{-2}	m^{-1}·kg·s^{-2}
Energy, work, quantity of heat	joule	J	N·m	m^2·kg·s^{-2}
Power	watt	W	J·s^{-1}	m^2·kg·s^{-3}
Quantity of electricity, electric charge	coulomb	C		s·A
Electric tension, electric potential, electromotive force	volt	V	W·A^{-1}	m^2·kg·s^{-3}·A^{-1}
Electric resistance	ohm	Ω	V·A^{-1}	m^2·kg·s^{-3}·A^{-2}
Electric conductance	siemens	S	A·V^{-1}	m^{-2}·kg^{-1}·s^3·A^2
Electric capacitance	farad	F	C·V^{-1}	m^{-2}·kg^{-1}·s^4·A^2
Magnetic flux	weber	Wb	V·s	m^2·kg·s^{-2}·A^{-1}
Magnetic flux density	tesla	T	Wb·m^{-2}	kg·s^{-2}·A^{-1}
Electric inductance	henry	H	Wb·A^{-1}	m^2·kg·s^{-2}·A^{-2}
Luminous flux	lumen	lm		cd·sr
Illuminance	lux	lx	lm·m^{-2}	m^{-2}·cd·sr
Activity	becquerel	Bq		s^{-1}
Absorbed dose*	gray	Gy	J·kg^{-1}	m^2·s^{-2}

* And other quantities of ionizing radiations of the same dimensions.

the dimensions are given in their most fundamental form in terms of the base and supplementary units.

Many other quantities can be derived directly from the base and supplementary units, but have not yet been given a special name. Some common ones are listed in Table 2.5.

A special word of explanation may be helpful concerning luminous flux and illuminance which invoke the steradian. The base unit of luminous intensity, the candela (cd), is defined in terms of brightness in the perpendicular direction of an emitting surface, slightly larger than a square millimetre. The luminous flux in lumens (lm) which is being emitted depends on the brightness and the angle in space through which the light is distributed. The unit of angle in space, the steradian, is the angle at the point of a cone whose apex is at the centre of a sphere and whose base has an area equal to the square of the radius of that sphere (see Fig. 2.2). Luminous flux therefore has the dimensions of cd·sr. The amount of light actually shining on a surface, illuminance (lx), is further dependent on the area of the surface. Illuminance therefore has the dimensions of $lm \cdot m^{-2}$, or $cd \cdot sr \cdot m^{-2}$.

Radioactivity

The amount of radioactivity in a substance is defined in terms of the rate at which that substance is disintegrating. The SI unit is the becquerel (Bq) which is one disintegration per second (s^{-1}). The curie (Ci), which is now obsolete, is 3.7×10^{10} Bq.

A measure of X-ray or gamma-ray emissions is given by the quantity known as *exposure*. This defines the intensity of X-rays or gamma-rays in terms of the amount of ionization they produce in the air. The unit is the *roentgen*: this is the exposure of X- or gamma-radiation which produces 2.58×10^{-4} coulombs per kilogram of air (1.61×10^{15} ion pairs per kilogram of air). This unit is used for the calibration of instruments which measure X-ray or gamma-ray intensity.

Of greater clinical importance is the unit of *absorbed dose*. This is a measure of the energy transferred to a substance by beta and other radiation, as well as by X-ray or gamma-ray radiation. The SI unit of absorbed dose is the *Gray* (Gy) which is equal to 1 joule per kilogram ($= 10^7$ ergs per kilogram). The old unit of absorbed dose was the *rad*: this was equal to 100 ergs per gram of material and so 1 Gy = 100 rad. Note that the absorbed dose due to an exposure of 1 roentgen depends on the energy of X-ray or gamma-ray radiation and on the type of material being irradiated. In body tissue 1 roentgen produces about 0.85–0.95 rad.

The biological effects produced by different types of ionizing radiation such as X-rays, neutrons or alpha particles differ from one another quantitatively rather than qualitatively. For example, a

Table 2.5 Examples of other derived SI units

Physical quantity	SI unit	Symbol for unit
Area	square metre	m^2
Volume	cubic metre	m^3
Density	kilogram per cubic metre	$kg \cdot m^{-3}$
Velocity	metre per second	$m \cdot s^{-1}$
Angular velocity	radian per second	$rad \cdot s^{-1}$
Acceleration	metre per second squared	$m \cdot s^{-2}$
Kinematic viscosity diffusion coefficient	square metre per second	$m^2 \cdot s^{-1}$
Dynamic viscosity	newton second per square metre, i.e. (pascal second)	$N \cdot s \cdot m^{-2}$ or Pa·s
Surface tension	newton per metre	$N \cdot m^{-1}$

given amount of chromosome damage may result from an absorbed dose of 1 rad given by neutrons or, say, 10 rads given by X-rays. When persons are liable to be exposed to a mixture of different radiations it is convenient to use units which will sum up the overall effect of the radiation exposure on the organism. Such *equivalent doses* used to be expressed in *rems* (roentgen equivalent for man). The SI unit is now the sievert (Sv) which is equal to 1 joule per kilogram.

This method of expressing radiation dosage is less rigorous than the other units already referred to, for it depends on a somewhat arbitrary choice of quality factors for different types of radiation. However, it is a convenient method of expressing dosage when dealing with problems of radiation protection.

Another aspect of radiation dosage which must be considered is the distribution of radioactivity within the body. Some isotopes are distributed throughout the body (for example, in the blood-stream) so that the distribution of radiation mirrors the distribution of blood flow. Other isotopes may be localized in a particular organ such as its kidney or the thyroid. This is then called the *critical organ* for that isotope.

The energy of any radiation is defined in terms of the electron volt (eV): this is equal to the energy of an electron accelerated through 1 volt ($= 1.6 \times 10^{-19}$ joules). Most radiations used in medical work have energies between a few keV (thousand electron volts) and 1 MeV (million electron volts).

SPECIALLY-AUTHORIZED NAMES AND SYMBOLS

SI allows the retention of some quantities which, although they can be defined in terms of the base units, are not decimal multiples or submultiples of them (see Table 2.6). The *litre* is a necessary convenience, particularly in medicine, or we would find ourselves measuring cardiac output, for example, in cubic metres per second. Because of the potential confusion in print between 1 and l, both l and L may be used as contractions for the litre, although it has been agreed that at some future date one of these alternatives will have to be abandoned. Some texts have extended the use of this optional alternative by writing mL rather than ml for millilitre, despite the fact that in this situation there is no comparable confusion with ml, which would have no meaning. This usage is not, therefore, in the spirit of the Directive and should be avoided. The *bar* (100 kPa) is a pressure close to atmospheric pressure and is useful in meteorology and in the gas industry. The unified *atomic mass* unit is 1/12 of the mass of an atom of ^{12}C. It is approximately equivalent to $1.660\ 565\ 5 \times 10^{-27}$ kg.

NON-SI UNITS TEMPORARILY RETAINED

Several non-SI units have been retained, but will be reconsidered in the future. Of interest in medicine are the millimetre of mercury (1 mmHg = 133.322 Pa) for blood pressure, the standard atmosphere (1 atm = 101.325 Pa) and the wavelength unit, the ångstrom (Å = 10^{-10} m). Also temporarily retained are some CGS units which are familiar in medicine such as the *poise* (P) for dynamic viscosity (1 P = 10^{-1} Pa·s) and the *stokes* (St) for kinematic viscosity (1 St = 10^{-4} m^2·s^{-1}).

Table 2.6 Special authorized names and symbols

Quantity	Name	Symbol	Value
Volume	litre	L	$1\ L = 1\ dm^3 = 10^{-3}\ m^3$
Mass	metric ton	t	$1\ t = 1\ Mg = 10^3\ kg$
Pressure	bar	bar	$1\ bar = 10^5\ Pa$

Definitions and standards

With some quantities, the standard can be 'defined' in a way which is reproducible. For such quantities, definitions have been developed which involve substances which are universally available. For example, time and length are now defined in terms of physical phenomena which are reproducible anywhere in the world. In practice, of course, an acknowledged authority provides a secondary standard, such as Greenwich for time or the National Physical Laboratory for temperature, and this is trusted to be as accurate as is humanly possible.

With regard to mass, however, such an approach is not at present possible. The definition of mass (p. 13) is quite circular; a kilogram is equal to the mass of a lump of metal which we have chosen to say has a mass of a kilogram. If a lighter piece of metal were to be secretly substituted, all other masses would, by *definition*, now be greater than they were! There is no external reference which would prove that the earth and all its works had not got more massive, although commonsense could be invoked in favour of the alternative explanation.

Several important quantities involve mass in their definition, in particular the newton and pascal. The newton is the force which would give a frictionless mass of 1 kilogram an acceleration of 1 metre per second per second, in a vacuum. It is impossible to create such conditions terrestrially and quite difficult even in an orbiting satellite. The pascal is derived from the definition of the newton. Such definitions cannot, therefore, be used as standards for calibration.

For such purposes, the gravitational effect of the earth on mass has to be invoked so that columns of fluids of known density are still needed as standards for calibration even though they do not serve as a definition. Thus for the calibration of blood pressure manometers, columns of mercury will always be required. It can be argued that if blood pressure is being both calibrated and measured in millimetres of mercury it is only logical to express it in these units. (The fact that the marks on a sphygmomanometer are not exactly millimetres apart, due to the need to compensate for the change in level in the reservoir, is not relevant to this argument: although the marks are not millimetres apart, the pressure *is* in millimetres of mercury).

The case for abandoning such units and adopting pascals is not, therefore, related to a more universally available standard or to a more precise definition, but is concerned with providing a single measurement quantity for *all* pressure measurements. This is of particular importance to anaesthetists who may meet pressure in a cylinder (labelled in atmospheres, $lb \cdot in^{-2}$, kPa × 100, or $kg \cdot m^{-2}$), pressure in pipelines (labelled in kPa, bars, atmospheres or $lb \cdot in^{-2}$), airway or ventilator pressure (in cmH_2O or pascals), blood pressure (in mmHg), central venous pressures (in mmHg with transducers or cmH_2O with U-tube manometers), pneumotachograph pressure manometers (in mmH_2O) and blood gases in kPa or mmHg. The universal adoption of SI would clarify the magnitude of these pressures in relation to one another and prevent a great deal of confusion. Until then it is necessary to use the greatest care when converting one unit of measurement into another. This is particularly important in pressure measurement. Not only is it very easy to confuse the factor for conversion from old to new and vice versa, but a small error in a conversion factor when applied to a large number may result in a considerable absolute error. Suitable conversion factors for respiratory, cardiovascular and biochemical measurements are given in Tables 2.7 and 2.8.

Basic mathematical concepts

Clinical measurement systems can normally be satisfactorily operated by persons who have no special mathematical knowledge. However, the principles on which measurement techniques are based can only be understood by those with some grasp of basic concepts such as differentiation, integration, exponential and trigonometrical functions, and logarithms. This section attempts to provide a simple introduction to these concepts.

SYMBOLS AND FUNCTIONS

Mathematical statements are expressed as equations which are abbreviated by the use of symbols.

Table 2.7. Conversion factors for units used in respiratory and cardiac physiology

Quantity	Traditional units (x)	SI unit or multiple (y) Name	Symbol or units	Conversion factors (f) Old to SI $y = fx$	SI to old $x = fy$
Force	dyne	newton	N	1×10^{-5}	1×10^{5}
	kilopond / kilogram-force	newton	N	9.806	0.102
Pressure	mmHg or Torr			0.133	7.501
	cmH$_2$O	kilopascal	kPa	0.098	10.197
	atmosphere			101.325	0.010
	lb/square inch			6.895	0.145
Energy	kilocalorie	joule	J	4.187	0.239
Work	kilopond metre/min	watt	W	9.806	0.102
Flow	litres/min	L/sec	$L \cdot s^{-1}$	0.017	60.0
Resistance—gas	cmH$_2$O/L/s	kPa/L/s	$kPa \cdot L^{-1} \cdot s$	0.098	10.197
—liquid	mmHg/L/min	kPa/L/s	$kPa \cdot L^{-1} \cdot s$	7.999	0.125
Conductance	L/s/cmH$_2$O	L/sec/kPa	$L \cdot s^{-1} kPa^{-1}$	10.197	0.098
Compliance	L/cmH$_2$O	L/kPa	$L \cdot kPa^{-1}$	10.197	0.098
Elastance	cmH$_2$O/L	kPa/L	$kPa \cdot L^{-1}$	0.098	10.197
O$_2$ consumption	ml/min STPD	mmol/min	$mmol \cdot min^{-1}$	0.045	22.40
CO$_2$ output	ml/min STPD	mmol/min	$mmol \cdot min^{-1}$	0.045	22.26*
O$_2$ concentration	vol. %	mmol/L	$mmol \cdot mL^{-1}$	0.446	2.240
CO$_2$ concentration	vol. %	mmol/L	$mmol \cdot L^{-1}$	0.449	2.226*
Transfer coefficient	ml/min/mmHg	mmol/min/kPa	$mmol \cdot min^{-1} \cdot kPa^{-1}$	0.335	2.985

* Non-ideal gas.

Table 2.8. Conversion factors for blood chemistry and haematology

Measurement	Traditional unit (x)	SI unit (y)	Conversion factors Old to SI $y = fx$	SI to old $x = fy$
Blood gases	mmHg, Torr	kPa	0.133	7.501
Standard bicarbonate / Base excess	mEq/L	mmol/L	1.0	1.0
Calcium	mg/100 ml	mmol/L	0.25	4.0
Chloride	mEq/L	mmol/L	1.0	1.0
Cholesterol	mg/100 ml	mmol/L	0.026	38.7
Cortisol	μg/100 ml	nmol/L	27.6	0.036
Creatinine	mg/100 ml	μmol/L	88.4	0.011
Glucose	mg/100 ml	mmol/L	0.056	18.0
Magnesium	mg/100 ml	mmol/L	0.411	2.43
Potassium	mEq/L	mmol/L	1.0	1.0
Sodium	mEq/L	mmol/L	1.0	1.0
Urea	mg/100 ml	mmol/L	0.167	6.0
Hb	g/100 ml	g/dl	1.0	1.0
RBC / WBC / Platelets	cells/mm^3	cells/L	10^{6}	10^{-6}

These symbols may confuse those with a non-mathematical mind but can usually be rendered clearer by translating the statement into English. Thus $P \times V = k$ (Boyle's law) means that pressure (P) multiplied by volume (V) always equals a constant value (k) so that pressure must be inversely proportional to volume. In this equation P and V are *variables* and k is a *constant*.

If two variables are related in such a way that the value of one of them can only be determined when the other is known, one variable is said to be a *function* of the other. The mathematical statement of this is that $y = f(x)$. The values of x and y which correspond with each other can be regarded as the *coordinates* of a point on an ordinary two-dimensional graph and the shape of the graph is characteristic of f.

In many cases, plotting $y = f(x)$ yields a straight line. In such a case, it is the slope which is determined by f (Fig. 2.3). The line passes through zero on both x and y axes for if x is zero, $f(x)$ is also zero. A slightly more complicated relationship is $y = f(x) + b$. In this case the slope of the line is the same but there is an intercept on the y axis: when x is zero $y = (f \times 0) + b$, or $y = b$. More complex equations yield graphs with different

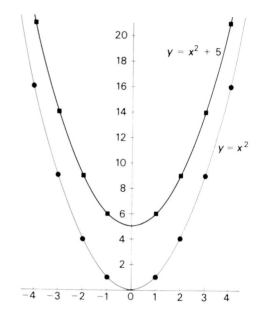

Fig. 2.4. Graphs of the two functions $y = x^2$ and $y = x^2 + 5$.

shapes. For example, the equation $y = x^2$ yields a parabola which passes through zero (since zero squared is zero) whilst $y = x^2 + 5$ produces a similar parabola which has a y intercept at $+5$ (Fig. 2.4).

In these examples y varies in a manner which is related to the change of x. Therefore y is said to be the *dependent* variable and x the *independent* variable: f and b are *constants* which are fixed for a particular set of conditions but may have a different value if conditions change. They are therefore called *parameters*.

SIMPLE TRIGONOMETRY

A knowledge of this topic is essential in order to understand wave motion and biological signals. The functions to be considered are those relating to any triangle which contains one right angle (90°). It does not matter how large or small such a triangle is: when the size of one angle has been specified, the ratios of the lengths of the sides to each other are constant for all triangles in which that angle is the same. There are three pairs of sides and therefore three primary ratios (Fig. 2.5a). The side opposite the right angle is called the hypotenuse.

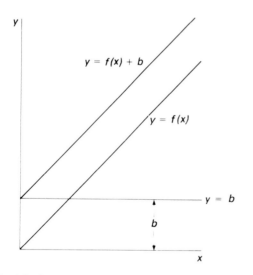

Fig. 2.3. Graphs of three functions $y = b$, $y = f(x)$ and $y = f(x) + b$, x is the independent variable, y is the dependent variable, f is a parameter (the slope of the line) and b is a parameter (the y intercept).

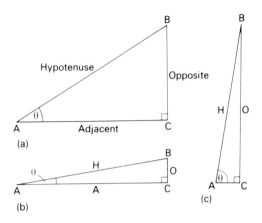

Fig. 2.5. (a) A right-angled triangle. (b) The sine of the angle is very small when θ is small. (c) The sine approaches 1 when θ approaches 90°.

The ratio of the length of the side opposite the defined angle (θ) to the length of the hypotenuse (BC ÷ AB) is called the *sine* of the angle θ. When the angle is very small the sine of the angle is itself very small (Fig. 2.5b). When the angle is close to 90° (Fig. 2.5c) the ratio approaches unity. The ratio of the adjacent side to the hypotenuse is called the *cosine*, so named because the cosine of the angle added to the sine of the complementary

angle opposite must add up to unity. The remaining ratio 'opposite divided by adjacent' is called the *tangent*.

The sine wave

Figure 2.6a represents a point (A) rotating around the circumference of a circle at constant velocity in the direction shown by the arrow. If the *amplitude* of displacement of point (A) from the axis (B–C) is plotted on the y co-ordinate, and time on the x co-ordinate, the graph shown in Fig. 2.6b is obtained. At each point in the cycle (A, A', A'') the displacement is given by sin θ, sin θ' and sin θ'', so that the resultant shape is called a *sine wave*. Since the point is moving at constant velocity, the time axis can be calibrated in degrees, radians or *cycles*, the term used for a complete revolution. The number of complete cycles per second is the *frequency* of the wave in hertz (Hz). The use of angular displacement as a measure of time is particularly valuable when comparing phase differences between waves. Thus a second sine wave of identical characteristics starting at point X in Fig. 2.6b would be 90° *out of phase* with the original wave.

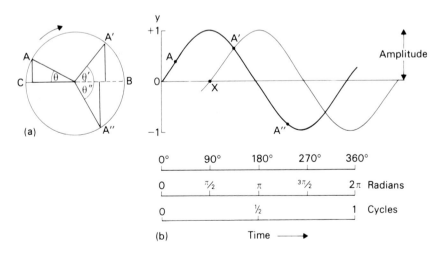

Fig. 2.6 (a) The relationship of the sine wave to uniform motion in a circle. As the point (A) rotates at constant velocity its projection moves as in the graph on the right. (b) Points A, A', A'' correspond with the points in the circle A, A', A''. The y value on the graph is equal to sin θ and time can be measured in degrees of rotation or in cycles.

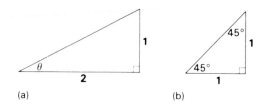

Fig. 2.7. Two right-angled triangles:
(a) tan θ = 1/2 = 0.5. (b) tan 45° = 1.

Physical quantities which vary in such a sinus-oidal fashion are legion. The generation of mains electricity is accomplished by rotating a coil in a magnetic field. The voltage generated is therefore sinusoidal in character. Oscillating systems oscil-late in a sinusoidal fashion: the position of a weight, moving up and down on the end of a spring describes such a motion. Wave motion, e.g. light, is also sinusoidal. The important relationship to appreciate is that the relative magnitude of the y-axis at any particular instant can be derived by knowing the x value solely in terms of an angle.

The tangent

The tangent (opposite ÷ adjacent) is another trigonometrical ratio which is often involved in measurement. The tangent is a number which expresses the commonly understood notion of slope. A hill which rises 1 m in a horizontal distance of 2 m has a slope of one in two (1/2 or 0.5). Drawn on paper (Fig. 2.7a) such a slope is found when the angle is approximately 26.6°.

Tan 26.6° is therefore 0.5. (If the slope rises 1 m for a distance of 2 m measured *up the hill* the angle is 30°.) Tan 45° can be seen to equal one when both the opposite and adjacent sides equal one. (Fig. 2.7b). In fact, between 0° and 90° the value of the tangent goes from zero to infinity.

The slope of a line can equally be viewed in terms of an increase in the value of y for a given change of x when the line is plotted on a traditional graph, i.e.

$$\text{slope} = \frac{y'' - y'}{x'' - x'},$$

where x', y', and x'', y'' are the co-ordinates of two points which lie on the line in Fig. 2.8. When $y'' - y' = 1$ and $x'' - x' = 2$, the relationship can equally be described by the equation $2y = x$ or $y = 0.5\,x$. Thus the value which multiplies x in the straight line relationship between x and y is the value of the *slope*. In statistics the quantity mea-suring the slope is called the *regression coefficient*.

In the first example, slope must have its natural meaning of a change of vertical distance per change of horizontal distance. Obviously, any such relation-ship when plotted has a slope even though the quan-tities themselves are unrelated to the notion of slope. For example, velocity (loosely equated with speed in common parlance), can be thought of as the slope of a line relating distance travelled to time. Thus, a graph showing the progress of a person walk-ing 1 mile in 2 h would look exactly the same as Fig. 2.8, the y axis representing distance and x-axis rep-resenting time. Distance divided by time, i.e. miles

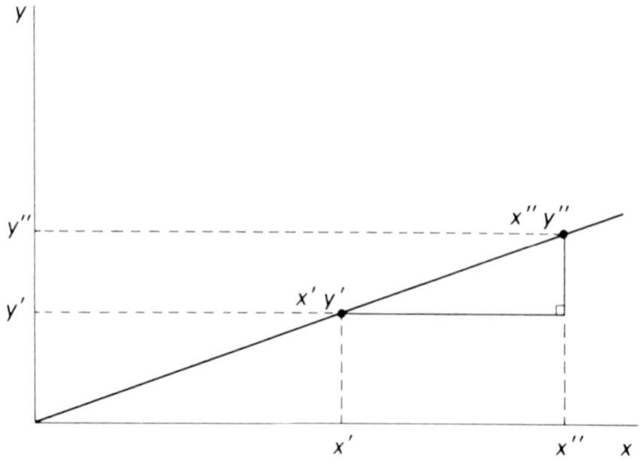

Fig. 2.8. A slope of 1 in 2. This corresponds with the straight line equation $y = 0.5x$.

per hour, is velocity; this is represented on the graph by the slope, tan 26.6°. If this idea is extended so that y represents velocity and x represents time, the graph will show how velocity increases with time. The rate of change of velocity with time is now represented by the slope and so indicates acceleration.

DIFFERENTIALS

There are, of course, numerous situations in which quantities do not change linearly with respect to another variable. When a relationship between y and x is a complex function the result is a curve of some kind. For example, the trigonometric function $y = \sin x$ results in an oscillating wave, the slope of which is constantly changing (Fig. 2.6). At the height of the peak and the bottom of the trough y is, for an instant, *not* changing, and at these points the slope is zero. Likewise one can see that the slope is steepest as the line passes through the x-axis. There is no easy way of seeing, from the formula, what the slope is at any other given moment. However, if one imagines that one could greatly enlarge a very, very short segment of the line (Fig. 2.9) at the point of interest, it would *seem*

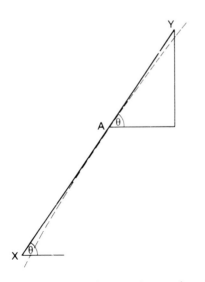

Fig. 2.9. An enlargement of a very short section of the curve of $y = \sin(x)$ from Fig. 2.6. θ is the angle between the straight line X–Y and the horizontal, and instantaneously also between the curve and the horizontal at the point (A).

to be almost straight. The slope would still be change of y for change in x, i.e the tangent of the angle θ at point (A). The solid line, which is straight, just touches the curve at one point only; because the tangent of the angle at that point is the slope, it is not surprising that the solid line is said to touch the curve 'tangentially'. Such graphical solutions are neither sufficiently accurate nor efficient. By using *calculus* (a form of mathematical manipulation which considers what the situation will be when one takes curves in infinitely small bits), one can calculate the slope at any required value of x. This is done by the mathematical process of *differentiating* the equation of the slope and substituting the required value of x. The differential of y which is thus obtained is the slope: in consequence, velocity is often said to be the differential of distance with respect to time, and acceleration is the differential of velocity with respect to time. Acceleration may therefore be called the second differential of distance with respect to time. The word differential indicates the underlying concept: it is the actual difference in y for an infinitely small change in x.

INTEGRALS

The slope is not the only secondary function of a curve which may be of interest in measurement. The area between the curve and the x-axis between defined values of x is often required because of the quantity it represents. Again, it is simplest to start with a straight line example. Figure 2.10a represents the record which would be obtained when a flow of gas is turned on, allowed to flow at a constant rate for a given time, and then switched off. The record shows that a flow of $5\ \text{L}\cdot\text{min}^{-1}$ flowed for 6 minutes. It is intuitively obvious that the total volume that passed was 30 L. This answer can be obtained by multiplying the y and x values and is thus represented by the area between the line and the x-axis. (In dimensional terms, we have: L^3T^{-1}(flow) $\times$ T(time) $= L^3$(volume).

Even if the volume had changed from minute-to-minute as in Fig. 2.10b the same principle could be applied by adding up the separate columns. In this example the total volume would be 21 L.

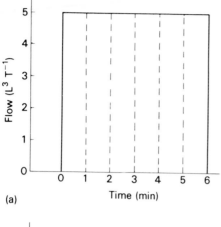

(a)

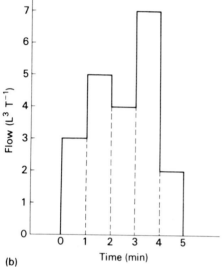

(b)

Fig. 2.10. Representation of (a) a constant flow of 5 L·min⁻¹ running for 6 min. (b) An irregular flow varying between 2 and 7 L·min⁻¹ and changing each minute. Total volume: (a) 30 L, (b) 21 L.

However, when the line varies rapidly the application of this method is not so easy. Under such circumstances the total area could only be obtained by dividing the area under the curve into an infinite number of small strips and adding their areas (see Fig. 2.11). This technique is employed by the calculus and is termed *integration*.

The area under a curve is usually related to the total quantity of a substance. The area under a flow-time curve is a volume; an equation relating

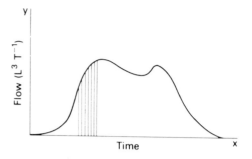

Fig. 2.11. A varying flow plotted against time. Again the area can be derived by summating columns under the curve to give the total area.

flow and time can therefore be integrated to give volume. The area under a concentration curve plotted against time gives quantity and is used in the calculation of cardiac output by the dye-dilution method (see p. 215). Similarly the area under the peak of a gas chromatogram represents the total quantity of the substance present. Both differentiation and integration are easily performed by electronic means. Integration may also be performed mechanically, if rather inelegantly, either by cutting out the area of the curve and relating the weight of the paper to the weight of a known area of paper or by using an instrument such as a *planimeter* which mechanically integrates the area as a small wheel is moved around the line delineating the curve.

POWER FUNCTIONS AND LOGARITHMS

The notion of powers is a commonplace one and, in its simplest form, easily comprehended. The notation 10^2, may be read as '10 squared' or '10 to (the power of) 2'. The arithmetic solution is the number 10, multiplied by itself, i.e: 10×10, or 100. At the practical level, it gives the area of the square, the length of whose sides is 10 units. In the same way it is easy to visualize the practical meaning of 10^3, i.e. 10 cubed or 1000, which is the volume of a cube whose sides are each 10 units long. However, such a concrete view is not helpful when one considers 10^4 and higher powers, even though the mathematical answer ($10^4 = 10\,000$, $10^5 = 100\,000$) is but a simple extension of the same idea.

The figure 5 in 10^5 is an *exponent* and signifies that five 10s are to be multiplied together to get 100 000, or that 10 is to be raised to the power of five. The five may also be referred to as the logarithm of 100 000 to the base 10. In mathematical notation this is written $\log_{10} 100\,000 = 5$. Thus the logarithmic notation is another way of expressing exponential relationships.

It will be apparent that all the numbers between 10 and 100, or between 10 000 and 100 000 can be characterized by exponents between 1 and 2, or between 4 and 5. These can be derived from tables of common logarithms or from an electronic calculator. Thus the logarithm of 10 is 1, and the logarithm of 20 is 1.301; whilst the logarithms of 10 000 and 20 000 are 4 and 4.301. Logarithms can be converted back to ordinary numbers by *exponentiation*, referred to in base 10 logarithms as *anti-logarithms*. A logarithm, then, is the power to which a fixed number (the base) must be raised to produce a given number. Note that since $\log 1 = 0$ the logarithm of any number below 1 must be a negative quantity. It is not possible to have a logarithm of a negative number.

Logarithms have several useful properties. Thus two large numbers may be multiplied together very simply. Because $10^n \times 10^m = 10^{n+m}$, the logarithms of the two numbers are added together. The anti-logarithm of the sum is the answer to the problem. While this might seem a rather complicated approach, it is in fact very simple because tables of logarithms and anti-logarithms reduce the calculation to a single addition. Division is achieved by subtracting one logarithm from another and a number can be raised to a given power by multiplying the logarithm of the number by that power. In all these manipulations the answer is obtained by taking the anti-log of the result. Table 2.9 summarizes these calculations in both logarithmic and exponential notation.

Logarithms are also used to compress a numerical scale. Thus the normal hydrogen ion concentration is 0.00000004 grams per litre (i.e. 4 out of 100 000 000) or $4 \times 10^{-8} \, g \cdot L^{-1}$. Since $pH = -\log [H^+]$ we may rewrite this as:

$$-pH = \log(4) + \log(10^{-8})$$
$$= 0.6 - 8 = -7.4$$

or

$$pH = 7.4.$$

It should be noted that because of logarithmic scale compression, 1 pH unit represents a 10-fold change in $[H^+]$.

Logarithmic changes are of importance in biology because many input–output functions are related logarithmically. Thus a 10-fold increase in drug concentration is often required to double the effect, whilst a 10-fold increase in energy input is required to make a light appear twice as bright. Logarithmic units are also used when comparing amounts of power. The relevant unit is the bel (B), two amounts of power P_1 and P_2 differing by N bels when:

$$N = \log \left(\frac{P_2}{P_1} \right).$$

For example if $P_2 = 1000 \, W$ and $P_1 = 10 \, W$, then $P_2/P_1 = 100$, $\log 100 = 2$, so that the ratio is 2 bels. Thus 1 bel represents a 10-fold alteration in power, 2 bels a 100-fold alteration and so on. In electronic apparatus power comparisons are

Table 2.9 Methods of calculation using logarithmic and exponential notations

Logarithmic	Exponential
$\log (M \cdot N) = \log(M) + \log (N)$	$B^m \cdot B^n = B^{m+n}$
$\log \dfrac{M}{N} = \log (M) - \log (N)$	$\dfrac{B^m}{B^n} = B^{m-n}$
$\log (M^n) = n \cdot \log (M)$	$(B^m)^n = B^{m \cdot n}$
$\log \sqrt[n]{M} = \log (M^{1/n}) = \dfrac{1}{n} \log (M)$	$\sqrt[n]{B^m} = (B^m)^{1/n} = B^{m/n}$

usually made in decibels (dB). These units are 1/10 of a bel so that:

$$N = 10 \cdot \log \frac{P_2}{P_1} \text{ dB.}$$

One decibel represents an alteration in sound intensity of about 26%, which is about the smallest change that the ear can detect.

Other bases

Logarithms to the base 10 are termed ordinary, *common* or *Briggsian* logarithms after the Englishman who invented them nearly four centuries ago. Their convenience lies in the fact that common logarithms of numbers with the same significant figures differ by a whole number, the difference depending on the relative positions of the decimal point in the numbers. Thus log 3.65 = 0.5623, whilst log 365 = 2.5623. However, there is no reason why we should not use some other base such as 2. Then, since $2^2 = 4$, 2 is the logarithm (to the base 2) of 4. This base is used in binary arithmetic (p. 60).

Strangely enough the most common base other than 10 is an *irrational* number, a non-terminating decimal denoted by the symbol e. It has a value of 2.71828 . . . . This number and the constant π (= 3.14159 . . .) are the two most widely-used constants in mathematics.

Logarithms to the base e are variously known as *natural*, *Naperian* or, less commonly, as *hyperbolic* logarithms. They offer none of the computational conveniences of common logarithms, their importance being related to the function e^x, which is fundamental to many growth and decay processes in biology and medicine. In modern terminology $\log_e x$ is usually written $\ln x$ (the natural logarithm of x), whereas $\log_{10} x$ is often written log x.

It is important to realize that the special characteristics of a logarithmic pattern of change are not affected by the base used, since the logarithms simply differ by a proportionality factor. Conversions between common and natural logarithms are calculated easily by using the following equations:

$$\ln y = 2.302585 \times \log y$$

$$\log y = 0.434294 \times \ln y.$$

In order to grasp the significance of e it is now necessary to consider the exponential function.

THE EXPONENTIAL FUNCTION

This is a function which arises so often in physics and in physiology that it requires a special mention. A number of processes increase or decrease in a way in which the rate at which the process is proceeding, is proportional either to how far it has gone, or to how far it still has to go. These processes are said to change exponentially, and the mathematical formulae which describe them are termed exponential functions. Compound interest is an example of a process in which an invested sum of money grows at a progressively faster rate if the interest is continuously reinvested. The passive emptying of the lung is a process in which the rate slows down as it approaches a final figure because the difference between the recoil pressure of the lung and the atmospheric pressure becomes progressively smaller as the lung empties. The filling of the lungs in response to the application of a constant positive pressure to the airway is an example of the same process in reverse. These phenomena are typified by the three curves shown in Figs 2.12, 2.13 and 2.14; known respectively as as tear-away, washout and wash-in curves. Why is e the basis of such curves? It is easiest to grasp the concept by considering compound interest, which follows the simple tear-away function $y = e^x$. Suppose one was lucky enough to invest £100 at 100% per annum (or expressed as a fraction, $\times$ 1 per annum). If the interest were calculated and paid at the end of every complete year one would possess £200 at the end of the first year. Suppose, however, that the interest were calculated every 6 months and immediately reinvested. At the end of the first 6 months one's investment would be worth £150. During the second 6 months the interest would be calculated on £150 rather than the original sum, so that £75 would be earned instead of £50. The total at the end of the year would now be £225, which is £25 more than with the single calculation day. One would need to be an inept investor not to suggest even more frequent calculation points! If the interest were calculated and then reinvested three, four, five . . . eight . . . ten times a year, the year end sum would be respectively, £237, £244, £248 . . . £259. Clearly the gain from more and more frequent calculations is not getting very much greater. Ultimately if one calculated daily, hourly or even by the minute, the 'best' one can ever do is to realise £271.83. The original sum has thus been increased by a factor of 2.7183 which is an approximation to the value of e. Expressed mathematically:

$$\frac{\text{final sum}}{\text{starting sum}} = 2.7183 = e$$

Now we can define e in simple functional terms. If a variable y were to increase by a factor of 1 in unit time, the outcome would be $2y$. However, if the rate of growth were not 1 but adjusted continuously to y itself, the outcome would be e^y. Thus e can be regarded as the universal proportionality constant.

Returning to the compound interest example, if the interest rate were set at 200% or $\times 2$, the effect of compound growth would be even more startling, for the investment would not yield £300 (simple interest) but £739. The above equation can now be written

$$\frac{\text{final sum starting}}{\text{starting sum}} = 7.39 = e^2.$$

It can now be seen that raising e to the power of the interest rate (expressed as a fraction), yields the growth of the starting sum over a single time period. To calculate for several years, the exponent (2 in this case) is simply multiplied by the number of time periods. Thus $y = e^{kt}$ where k is the rate, and t the number of periods (Fig. 2.12a). After 5 years at 50% interest, the investor would therefore have:

$$100 \times e^{0.5 \times 5} = 100 \times e^{2.5} = £1218.25.$$

Now if we take natural logarithms of both sides of the equation $y = e^{kt}$, the result is $\ln y = kt$ because the natural logarithm of a number is the power to which e must be raised to yield that number.

A graph of $\ln y$ against t will therefore be a straight line of gradient k (Fig. 2.12b).

From this graph a fundamental property of exponential change can be deduced. The time taken for any value of y to increase by a factor of 2.718 (i.e., 1 on the natural log scale since $\ln 2.713 = 1$) is constant and is the reciprocal of

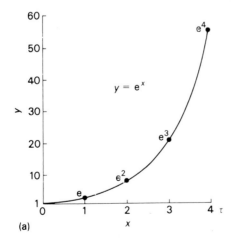
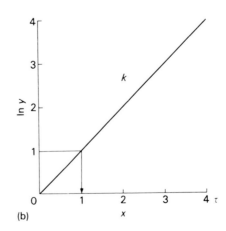

Fig. 2.12. (a) The break-away function $y = e^x$. This would describe the pattern of growth associated with compound interest. (b) The logarithmic replot of (a). k = constant, τ = time constant.

the rate k. Thus if it takes 1 year the slope is 1, but if it takes 2 years it is 0.5. Since kt is the exponent in the equation $y = e^{kt}$, the ratio of final to starting value can be solved for any value of t.

For example, if the accrued sum were found to be £271.83 after 0.5 years, $k = 1/0.5 = 2$, or 200%. If, on the other hand, it took 10 years to accrue, $k = 1/10 = 0.1$, or 10% interest. The time to rise by a factor of $2.718\ldots$ is called the time constant, and given the greek letter τ (tau). k is termed the rate constant, and since it is $1/\tau$, has the dimension of reciprocal time, i.e. s^{-1} or, in this example, years^{-1}. It will now be evident that given a starting value and either τ or k, the value at any time can easily be calculated.

If a process is thought to be exponential and some values at different times are known, then a plot of $\ln y$ against time will be most useful. A straight line confirms that the process *is* exponential, and the rate constant can be determined by simply measuring the gradient.

If logarithms are not readily available, a less precise alternative is to plot the values of y on graph paper whose vertical axis is printed at logarithmic intervals. This method demonstrates the linear relationship, but does not help us to calculate k. The log of one variable plotted against a second variable is called a semi-logarithmic or log–linear plot, as opposed to a log–log plot in which both axes are on logarithmic scales. Semi-log plots are very useful in that they both demonstrate the exponential relationship and enable extrapolation or interpolation to other parts of the time scale (e.g. computation of cardiac output from part of the dilution curve).

The *washout*, or *exponential decay function* is mathematically very similar to the breakaway function, except that the rate constant is negative. Thus the ratio of 'new' to 'starting value' (y) in an exponentially decaying system is characterized by $y = e^{-kt}$ (see Fig. 2.13). This yields a straight line on a semi-log plot of gradient $-k$. The decay of charge as a capacitor discharges through a resistor is a simple example of washout exponential decay. It is also exemplified by the change in concentration of a gas in the lung when replaced by a second gas, by the change of lung volume during a passive expiration, or by the down-slope of a dye-dilution curve. In all these circumstances, the quantity under consideration decreases at a rate which is proportional to the amount still present. (The similarity with the breakaway function should now be clear since in both cases the rate of growth or decay is directly proportional to the amount

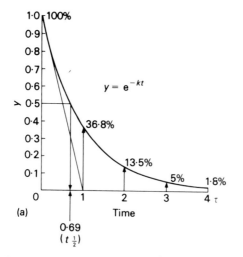
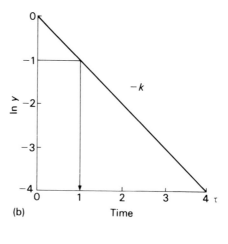

Fig. 2.13. (a) The washout curve $y = e^{-kt}$. This would describe the discharging of a capacitor or the passive emptying of the lungs. Time expressed in terms of time constants. $t_{1/2}$, is seen to be 0.69 of a time constant. (b) The logarithmic replot of (a). k = rate constant.

present.) If the initial decay rate is extrapolated (Fig. 2.13) it reaches zero after one time constant (τ). During one time constant, the value in fact decays to $1/e$ of its initial value (i.e. $1/2.718 = 36.8\%$).

In a second similar period, the value will again fall by the same proportion, but during the decay over two time constants, it will fall to $1/e^2 = 1/7.389 = 13.54\%$. Over four time constants it decays to $1/e^4 = 1/54.60 = 1.83\%$ of the original value. As the decay proceeds, it approaches zero at an ever decreasing rate, and theoretically reaches it at time infinity.

Exponential decays are often characterized by a parameter known as the half-life ($t_{1/2}$). This is the time taken for the value to diminish by half, and is, of course, constant throughout the decay. Since $\tau = 1/k$, the value of t when $y/y_0 = 0.5$ will be: $\ln 0.5 = -t/\tau$, so $t = 0.689\tau$. The half-life is thus a simple fraction of the time constant.

The time constant is determined by the characteristics of the system. For example, the rate of emptying of the lungs depends on the compliance of the lungs (C) and the resistance of the airways (R) so that $\tau = CR$. Hence if compliance is increased (i.e. there is a smaller recoil pressure for a given volume) or resistance is increased, the rate of

emptying will be reduced because of the increased time constant.

The wash-in exponential function is different from the other two, in that the variable rises to a final value (called the asymptote) at an ever-decreasing rate (Fig. 2.14). The ratio of present to final volume (y) is characterized by the expression $y = 1 - e^{-kt}$. The rate constant is negative since this is really an exponential decay although the function is rising. The wash-in function is exemplified by the increase in volume of the lung resulting from the application of a constant pressure to the airway, by the change in gas concentration in a lung after it is suddenly switched to a new gas mixture or by the increase in blood P_{CO_2} after a step reduction in ventilation.

As in the other functions, it is possible to obtain a straight line by a logarithmic transform, but not directly, since taking logarithms in $y = 1 - e^{-kt}$ does not yield a linear function. Instead, the equation is rearranged to $1 - y = e^{-kt}$. Now taking logarithms we obtain the simple linear equation: $\ln(1 - y) = -kt$.

The recognition that there is a logarithmic relationship between two variables greatly facilitates data handling in many measurement applications. For example, the down-slope of the dye-

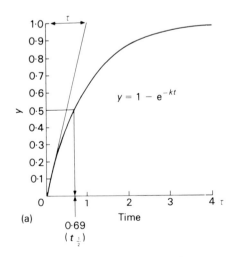
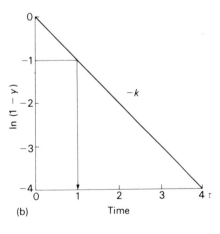

Fig. 2.14. (a) The wash-in curve $y = 1 - e^{-kt}$. This would describe the pattern of charging of a capacitor or the filling of the lungs in response to the application of a constant pressure to the airway. τ = time constant. (b) The logarithmic replot of (a). k = rate constant.

dilution curve in cardiac output measurement is known to be exponential, but the lower part of this curve is altered by the occurrence of recirculation of the indicator. By establishing the rate constant from a semi-log plot of the early part of the downslope it is possible to predict the shape of the lower part of the curve and so establish the area under the curve (p. 216). Another example is provided by the analysis of washout curves which represent a composite of two or more exponential processes (e.g. the washout of slow and fast compartments in the lung, or the washout of a radioactive tracer from the grey and white matter in the brain). Replotting of the washout data on semi-log paper permits the two processes to be separated by manual exponential stripping of the curves (p. 210) so that the contribution of each process can be defined. Many biological mechanisms respond logarithmically to a stimulus. Thus the output of biological receptor systems such as touch, hearing and sight varies as the logarithm of the stimulus whilst many responses to drugs are also related to the logarithm of drug concentration. Thus if the intensity of pharmacological effect is plotted against the logarithm of the dose of a drug, a straight line may be obtained. This greatly facilitates subsequent statistical processing of the results.

The breakaway curve of compound growth is commonly encountered in biology and medicine but has little application in measurement. The wash-in and washout curves are, however, ubiquitous. Light decreases exponentially in intensity as it passes through a coloured solution: voltages build up and discharge from capacitors exponentially: lungs empty, drip rates fall, drug concentrations fall, radioactivity decreases, all exponentially.

It is unlikely that a doctor undertaking clinical measurement will need to be able to work out any particular exponential function from first principles. However, it is not difficult, and anyone wishing to acquire the simple mathematical skills involved is recommended to read Waters and Mapleson (1964), Franklin and Newman (1973), Duffin (1976), Nunn (1987), and Hogben (1989).

References

Duffin, J. (1976) *Physics for anaesthetists*. C.C. Thomas, Springfield, Illinois.

Franklin, D.A. & Newman, G.B. (1973) *A guide to medical mathematics*. Blackwell Scientific Publications, Oxford.

Hogben, L. (1989) *Mathematics for the million*. Allen & Unwin Ltd., London.

Nunn, J.F. (1987) *Applied respiratory physiology*, 3rd edn. Butterworth, London.

Waters, D.J. & Mapleson, W.W. (1964) Exponentials and the anaesthetist. *Anaesthesia* **19**, 274–293.

Further reading

Baron, D.N. (1988) *Units, symbols and abbreviations. A guide for biological and medical editors and authors*, 4th edn. Royal Society of Medicine Services.

Mushin, W.W. & Jones, P. (1987) *Physics for the anaesthetist*. 4th edn. Blackwell Scientific Publications, Oxford.

Her Majesty's Stationery Office (1988) *SI. the international system of units*, National Physical Laboratory, London. HMSO, London.

3: Simple Electronics

Although most clinical measurement devices can be operated without any knowledge of electronics, some understanding of this subject is necessary for those who wish to use their equipment to fullest advantage. This chapter deals with some fundamental concepts which are referred to in later sections of the text.

Direct current

When a potential difference exists between two points on a conductor, a current will flow. The relationship between the current and potential difference is expressed by Ohm's law:

The current flowing through a conductor is proportional to the electromotive force (e.m.f.) causing that current.

This relationship can be expressed in terms of a proportionality constant R. Thus:

$$\frac{E}{I} = R$$

where E is the potential difference in volts (V), I is the current in amperes (A) and R is the resistance expressed in ohms (Ω). By rearrangement, $E = IR$ and $I = E/R$. The use of this relationship is illustrated in Fig. 3.1a.

If two resistors are connected in series the total resistance presented by the combination is simply the sum of the two (Fig. 3.1b). If, on the other hand, the same two resistors are connected in parallel (Fig. 3.2), the combined resistance is determined by the expression:

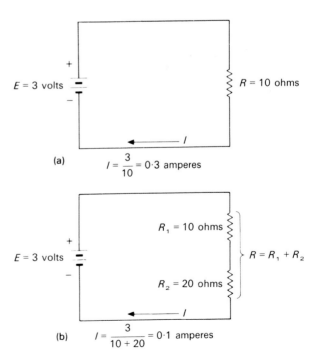

$E = 3$ volts $R = 10$ ohms

(a) $I = \dfrac{3}{10} = 0.3$ amperes

$E = 3$ volts

$R_1 = 10$ ohms

$R = R_1 + R_2$

$R_2 = 20$ ohms

(b) $I = \dfrac{3}{10 + 20} = 0.1$ amperes

Fig. 3.1. Ohm's law is used to calculate the current (I) (a) in a simple resistive circuit and (b) in a circuit with two resistances in series.

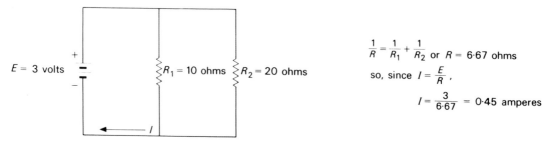

$$\frac{1}{R} = \frac{1}{R_1} + \frac{1}{R_2} \text{ or } R = 6\cdot67 \text{ ohms}$$

so, since $I = \frac{E}{R}$,

$$I = \frac{3}{6\cdot67} = 0\cdot45 \text{ amperes}$$

Fig. 3.2. Ohm's law applied to two resistances (R_1 and R_2) in parallel.

$$\frac{1}{R} = \frac{1}{R_1} + \frac{1}{R_2}.$$

When current passes through a conductor, work is done and heat generated. The rate at which work is done is power. Thus if 1 joule (J) of work is done in 1 s, 1 watt (W) of power is dissipated. Power dissipation in the conductor can be calculated as the product of current flowing and the potential difference (volts) across it. Thus in Fig. 3.1a, 0.3 A and 3 V dissipate 0.9 W, or 900 mW.

Note we can derive expressions for power for all three variables in Ohm's law. For example:

$$W = EI, \quad \text{so } W = \frac{E^2}{R} \quad \text{and } W = I^2R.$$

Power calculations are basic to even the simplest circuit design, since all electronic components must be capable of dissipating the heat generated. For example, if we take a 100 Ω resistor rated at 5 W, and pass 0.5 A through it, the power dissipation will be $0.5^2 \times 100 = 25$ W, so that it will promptly explode!

Alternating current

In simple terms, Faraday's Law of electromagnetic induction states that when the flux-linkage between a coil and a magnetic field is varying, an electromotive force (e.m.f.) proportional to the rate of change of flux-linkage is induced in the coil. If a loop of wire is rotated between the poles of a permanent magnet, the flux-linkage will change continuously, inducing an e.m.f. which reverses in polarity after every 180° of rotation. The rate of change of flux-linkage is proportional to the sine of the angle through which the loop has turned, and so produces an e.m.f. whose magnitude is also proportional to the sine of the angle (Fig. 3.3).

Thus if we designate peak current as I_{max} and the rotational angle of the coil θ, the current I at any time will be $I_{max} \sin \theta$, a simple sinusoidal function. When an alternating current (a.c.) passes through a resistor, the potential across it obeys Ohms law, and therefore has a sinusoidal waveform $E = E_{max} \sin \theta$ in phase with the current. The

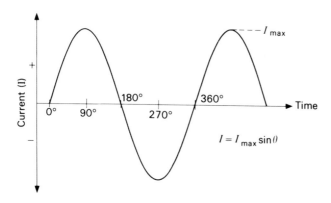

$$I = I_{max} \sin \theta$$

Fig. 3.3. Alternating current produced by the rotation of a coil in a magnetic field. The horizontal axis represents *time* and is therefore related to the angular position of the coil (θ) as it turns.

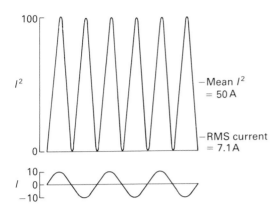

Fig. 3.4. Current I alternates between $+10$ and -10 A (lower trace). The upper trace shows I^2 drawn as a continuous function. This alternates between 0 and 100 A, about a mean value of 50 A. The r.m.s. current is 7.1 A. If this current were passed through a 10 Ω resistor, 71 W of heat would be dissipated.

frequency of the a.c. is the number of complete cycles per second, and is expressed in hertz (Hz). Mains electricity is supplied at 50 Hz in the UK but at 60 Hz in the USA.

If an a.c. current is passed through a resistor, work will be done and heat generated. Since both current and voltage are constantly changing, there is no convenient static way of calculating power, so that we must go back to first principles. Since power dissipation (in watts) is expressed by: $W = I^2R$, it is evident that we need a value for I^2.

Figure 3.4 shows the sinusoidal current, and a continuously computed line representing I^2. This is always positive, and the mean value of I^2 can be inserted directly into $W = I^2R$. The square root of

this 'mean I^2' value, known as the root mean squared (r.m.s.) current, is the form in which amperes are expressed in a.c. circuits, and can be used in Ohm's law equations.

Voltages can be treated similarly, and are often expressed in r.m.s. terms. Thus the 50 Hz domestic mains supply r.m.s. voltage of 240 V has a sinusoidal waveform with peak values of ± 339 V.

Capacitance

If two conductors are separated by an insulator, known as the dielectric, a capacitor is formed. In its simplest form, this consists of two metal plates separated by a thin layer of air. When connected to a battery as in Fig. 3.5a (with S_1 closed) a current flows.

This current cannot escape from the other plate, but is stored as a static charge in the dielectric. If the potential of this charge were measured, it would be seen to rise progressively to the same voltage (E) as the source (Fig. 3.5b). As the difference between the battery potential and the potential of the capacitor decreases, the current also decreases.

The size of a capacitor determines the quantity of electricity it can absorb for a given charge potential, and depends upon the surface area of the plates, the thickness of the dielectric, and its ability to store charge (permittivity). The unit of capacitance is the Farad (F). One coulomb of electricity (which passes when 1 A flows for 1 s) will charge a 1 Farad capacitor to a potential of 1 V. Thus if Q coulombs charge C Farads to E volts, $E = Q/C$. It

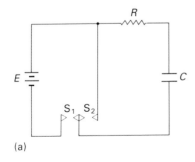

(a)

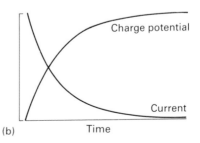

(b)

Fig. 3.5. (a) Circuit containing resistance (R) and capacitance (C). If S_1 is closed, the capacitor charges; if S_2 is closed it discharges. (b) The current and voltage waveforms following closure of the switch (S_1).

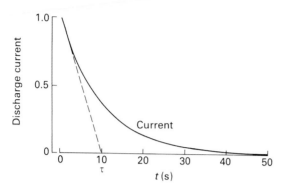

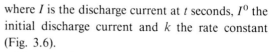

Fig. 3.6. Exponential decay of current during the discharge of a capacitor through a resistor, τ is the time constant, during which the current falls to 1/e of its initial value (i.e. 37%).

follows that if a capacitor is charged by a constant current, the potential will rise at a constant rate.

If the capacitor in Fig. 3.5a is charged to 10 V (by closing S_1 for a few seconds) and then allowed to discharge through the resistor (by closing S_2) the initial current will be E/R = 10/10 = 1 A. As soon as this initial current flows the charge on the capacitor is reduced. When it is reduced to, say 9 V, the discharge current will fall to 0.9 A; when 5 V to 0.5 A and so on. Thus as the capacitor discharges, the current decreases progressively according to the simple exponential expression:

$$\frac{I}{I^0} = e^{-kt}$$

where I is the discharge current at t seconds, I^0 the initial discharge current and k the rate constant (Fig. 3.6).

If a capacitor is placed in an a.c. circuit (Fig. 3.7a) a more complex situation arises.

When a direct voltage is applied to a capacitor the current rapidly falls to zero, and the charge potential rapidly rises to that of the source (Fig. 3.5b). In an a.c. circuit, the applied voltage is constantly changing directions, so that current and voltage never reach steady-state conditions, but follow sinusoidal waveforms of the same frequency as the source. Figure 3.5b shows that the voltage on the capacitor and the current do not change in direct proportion (as would be the case for a resistor), and Fig. 3.7b shows that they are, in fact, 90° out of phase, because the current is maximal when the voltage is changing fastest (i.e. passing through zero), and minimal when the voltage is not changing at all (i.e. at peak values). The phase difference is such that the current waveform leads the voltage by 90°. Figure 3.7b shows that when the current reaches its peak at 360°, the voltage has risen only to zero.

The current 'through' a capacitor is proportional to the rate of change of the applied voltage. Thus a rise in frequency, increasing the rate of change of current, results in an increased current, and vice versa. Variation in current with frequency suggests that 'opposition to current flow' by the capacitor also changes. Since this 'opposition' varies with

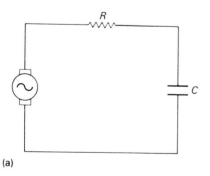

(a)

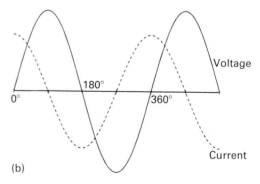

(b)

Fig. 3.7. (a) An a.c. circuit containing resistance (R) and capacitance (C) in series. (b) Current through and voltage across the capacitor.

frequency, it cannot be termed resistance, and so is given the special term 'reactance'. The reactance of a capacitor (X_c) may be calculated from the formula:

$$X_c = \frac{1}{2\pi f C} \text{ ohms}$$

where f is the frequency (Hz). Although the units of reactance are ohms they cannot be inserted directly into Ohm's law equations because of the phase difference between current and voltage in a capacitative circuit. We must instead consider both resistive and reactive 'ohms' present in the circuit, and calculate the overall opposition to current flow (the impedance) at the frequency required, taking the phase differences into account. Only then can Ohm's law be used to compute current, etc.

The resulting 'impedance ohms' can be used directly in Ohm's law equations, but cannot be added directly to other resistances or reactances, because both resistance and capacitance in the circuit must be taken into account when calculating impedance.

Inductance

An inductor consists of a number of turns of wire wound as a coil. The centre space of the coil may contain air or a core of magnetic material. When a steady current flows through the inductor, it is impeded only by the relatively small resistance of the wire forming the coil. However, a change in current produces a change in the magnetic field around the coil, which in turn induces an e.m.f. in the coil. This induced e.m.f. opposes the change in current which produced it (the so-called back-e.m.f.). An inductor acts like a brake, since it slows down any *change* of current, irrespective of whether the current is increasing or decreasing. When, in Fig. 3.8a, the switch is closed the current rises rapidly, but is 'braked' by the back-e.m.f. so that it approaches its final value quite slowly (Fig. 3.8b).

The voltage across the inductor is maximal when the switch is first closed, and the rate of change of current maximal; it then decays to zero as the current settles to a steady value. Current and

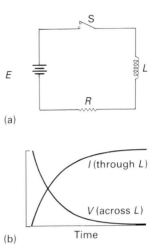

Fig. 3.8. (a) A circuit containing a resistance (R) and inductance (L) in series. (b) Voltage and current waveforms following closure of switch S.

voltage are 90° out of phase, but in a different manner to that of a capacitor. In the capacitor, the charge potential is maximal and current zero when a steady e.m.f. is applied, whereas in the inductor, the current is maximal and the voltage across it zero under the same conditions.

The unit of inductance is the henry (H). When the current through a coil changes at the rate of $1 \text{ A} \cdot \text{s}^{-1}$, a 1 H coil will induce a back-e.m.f. of 1 V. The voltage across the inductor in Fig. 3.8a decays exponentially. Thus:

$$\frac{V}{E} = e^{-tR/L}$$

where the time constant is now L/R seconds. If, at steady state, the switch is suddenly opened, a reverse situation exists, in that the current now tends to stop, but the collapsing magnetic field induces an e.m.f. which attempts to maintain the current. Since the 'resistance' of the circuit is now infinite, the continuing current raises the voltage until the current sparks across the switch contacts. Switches controlling heavy inductive loads have to be protected against this eventuality, which may lead to the switch contacts welding together.

There is always some resistance in an inductive circuit, due to the resistance of the wire from which

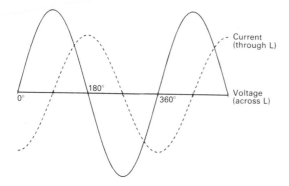

Fig. 3.9. Voltage and current waveforms in an inductive circuit.

the coil is wound, so that a perfect inductor is unattainable (this is not strictly true, perfect inductors *can* exist under cryogenic conditions, where superconductivity reduces electrical resistance to a negligible level). The efficiency of an inductor is indicated by the ratio of the inductance to its resistance, and is greatly increased by the presence of a magnetically permeable core.

In an inductor in an a.c. circuit the current and voltage follow sinusoidal waveforms. Since the current changes constantly so does the back-e.m.f. which is related to the rate of change of the applied current. Thus the voltage across the inductor is greatest when the current is changing most rapidly.

Consider Fig. 3.9. At 90° the voltage has reached its peak, but the current has only just risen to zero, so that the current lags by 90°. The inductive reactance increases linearly with frequency, according to the expression:

$$X_L = 2\pi f L$$

where L is the inductance in henrys.

The circuit in fig. 3.10 contains inductance, capacitance and resistance. The combined reactance of the capacitor and inductor is $X_L - X_C$, because as we have just shown, the voltages across the two are 180° out of phase and tend to cancel out. Consider then the variation of capacitative (X_C) and inductive (X_L) reactance with frequency (Fig. 3.10b). There is a resonant frequency (f_r) at which X_C and X_L are identical and they cancel out, with resistance providing the only opposition to the current.

Figure 3.11 shows that since the reactance at f_r is zero, the circuit current will be at a maximum at

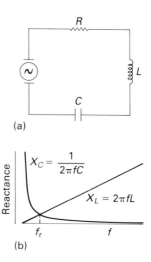

Fig. 3.10. (a) An a.c. circuit containing resistance (R), inductance (L) and capacitance (C) in series. (b) Variation of reactance (X) with frequency (f).

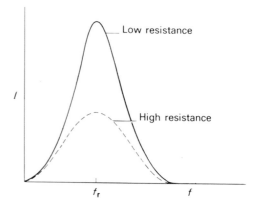

Fig. 3.11. The selectivity of the circuit in Fig. 3.10 depends upon the series resistance.

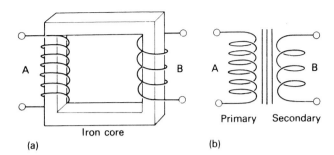

Fig. 3.12. (a) Mutual inductance: the transformer. (b) Symbolic representation of a step-down transformer.

(a)   Iron core   (b)

this point. At all other frequencies the impedance will be higher, hindering current flow. This is the basis of a passive 'band-pass' filter. The selectivity of such a filter increases as circuit resistance is reduced.

If an inductor and a capacitor are arranged in parallel, circuit impedance is maximal at f_r, so that circuit current is minimal at that frequency. This forms the basis of a selective 'band-reject' filter. Filters are widely used in measuring equipment to select frequencies of interest and to reject those, such as 50 Hz mains interference, which are considered undesirable.

Mutual inductance

If two coils A and B are placed close together and a current is passed through coil A, then the changing magnetic field will induce an e.m.f. in coil B. This flux-linkage with B due to current in A is called mutual inductance, and is measured in henrys. The flux-linkage, and therefore the mutual inductance, depends upon:

1 The size and number of turns of the two coils.
2 The proximity and orientation of the coils.
3 The magnetic permeability of the material within the coils. (If they are wound onto an iron core, the mutual inductance will be many times greater than if on a plastic former.)

The a.c. transformer is a good example of the application of mutual inductance. In Fig. 3.12a two coils are wound onto an iron core and an alternating current passed through A. Mutual inductance will induce an alternating e.m.f. in B, whose voltage will relate to that in A by the ratio of

the number of turns in each coil. Thus if A = 100 turns and B = 10 turns the voltage across B will be 10 times smaller than that across A.

Transformers are widely used in modern electronics, but appear most frequently in power supplies, where the mains voltage is stepped down to low voltages for transistor circuits. The low voltage output from the secondary winding is rectified and smoothed using a large capacitor to produce a relatively steady direct current (d.c.) voltage. The power supplies for instrumentation circuits need very precise voltage regulators, which are both complex and expensive.

The semiconductor diode

Currents will pass equally well through resistors, capacitors and inductors regardless of direction. The diode is a uni-directional device, since it will pass current in one direction, but not the other.

Figure 3.13 shows two diodes connected in a resistive circuit. The 'point' in the diode symbol

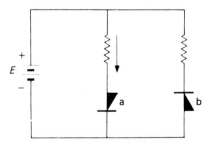

Fig. 3.13. Diode (a) allows current to flow, but diode (b) does not.

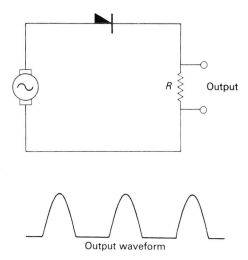

Fig. 3.14. The diode rectifies the generated sine wave.

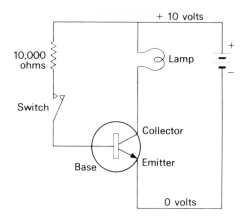

Fig. 3.15. Transistor operating as a switch.

indicates the direction in which conventional current (+ to −) will flow so that diode (a) conducts but diode (b) does not. Diodes are frequently used as rectifiers, which allow signals of one polarity to flow, but reject signals of the opposite polarity. In Fig. 3.14 the diode rectifies an a.c. signal, such that only positive half-cycles appear at the output.

Amplifiers

The passive components considered so far are of limited use, since their function is always to reduce the size of the signal. In order to detect and 'condition' biological signals, some means of amplification must be available. Today, this is almost invariably achieved by means of transistor technology, and every electronic instrument contains these devices in large numbers.

TRANSISTOR ACTION

The transistor is a three-terminal device, in which a very small change of current at one terminal (the base) may induce a large change of current between two others (emitter and collector).

Figure 3.15 shows a transistor operating as a current switch. When the switch in the base lead is open, no current flows from collector to emitter, the transistor is said to be off, and so is the light

bulb. When the base switch is closed, a small current flows through the 10-kΩ resistor to the base and through the transistor to the emitter. This has the effect of turning on the transistor, so that current now flows from collector to emitter, and the bulb lights up. The important point to appreciate is that the lamp current, which might be 80 mA, has been controlled by the base current of less than 1 mA.

It is possible to choose a base current which causes the transistor to be turned partly on. Now, any small change in base current will cause a much larger change in collector current, and the device operates as a crude amplifier.

There are all manner of limitations to such a simple circuit, so that it is very rarely used in practice. The modern amplifier designer uses circuits in which large numbers of transistors are combined in a single package to yield a device which is virtually devoid of non-linearity, temperature instability, frequency restriction, etc. Such a multi-transistor device is known as an operational amplifier, and can be used as a 'black box' amplifier with no knowledge whatever of its internal structure.

The operational amplifier

The operational amplifier can, for a moment, be considered to be an ideal device represented by the

symbols in Fig. 3.16, with the following characteristics:

1 The amplification of input signals is infinite.
This implies that to produce a full-scale positive
output, an infinitesimally small positive signal is
required at the non-inverting input, or an infinitesimally small negative signal is required at the
inverting input.

2 Neither input takes current from its source. Both
inputs therefore have an infinitely high input
resistance.

3 The output can drive any load, irrespective of
the current required. Therefore the output must
have an infinitely low output resistance.

4 If the same input signal is applied to both inputs
simultaneously, the positive and negative amplifi-
cations cancel out, so that no output appears. The
ability to reject such signals is called the 'common
mode rejection ratio' (CMRR) and is infinite for an
ideal device.

5 All frequencies (including d.c.) will be amplified
to exactly the same degree. It therefore has an
infinitely wide bandwidth.

All practical amplifiers fail to reach these ideals,
in some or all respects. Generally speaking, the
more expensive the amplifier, the nearer to 'ideal'
it will be. Operational amplifiers have increased in
performance and decreased in cost in recent years
(i.e. 50p will now buy a better amplifier than would
£25 in 1965).

The reader might wonder as to the usefulness of
an amplifier having infinite gain. The answer lies in
the principle of negative feedback.

Consider Fig. 3.17 where two resistors are added

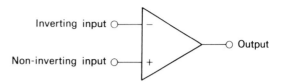

Fig. 3.16. The operational amplifier.

to the basic amplifier. R_2, connecting the 'inverting' input to the output is called the 'feedback'
resistor, and going to the negative input, carries a
negative feedback current. If no input signal is
applied (i.e. input terminals joined together), the
output will settle at 0 V. (If the output went
positive, it would make the inverting input go
positive, which would make the output go negative!
The effect of this is a balance at which both the
non-inverting and inverting inputs are at the same
voltage (0 V), so that the output does not swing in
either direction.) If + 1 V is applied to the input,
the output will swing negative until the feedback
current exactly balances the input current. Since by
definition no current enters the amplifier itself, it
will be evident that when the inverting input is at
0 V, 1 mA must be flowing along R_1, and then
along R_2. The output will therefore settle at that
voltage which takes precisely 1 mA from R_2.

By Ohm's law $E = IR = 0.001 \times 2000 = 2$ V.
The output therefore settles at -2 V; precisely
double the input voltage. It should now be clear
why the gain (amplification factor) is the ratio of
$R_2:R_1$, with the amplifier itself simply acting as a
sort of electronic lever. Thus the output voltage

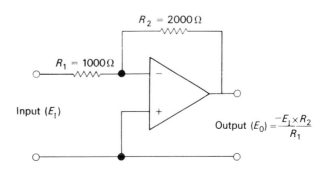

Fig. 3.17. An inverting amplifier, with a gain
of 2.

$$E_0 = \frac{-E_1 \times R_2}{R_1}$$

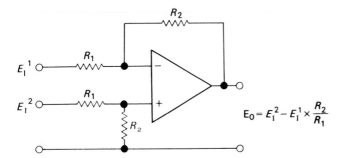

$$E_0 = E_I^2 - E_I^1 \times \frac{R_2}{R_1}$$

Fig. 3.18. A differential amplifier.

$E_0 = -E_1 \times R_2/R_1$. By choosing appropriate values for R_1 and R_2, any desired gain can be achieved, to an accuracy limited only by errors in the resistor values.

In a more complex configuration (Fig. 3.18) the amplifier operates in differential mode. Here the device amplifies the *difference* between the two inputs, but rejects any signal which is common to both of them. This type of circuit is widely used in amplifiers of biological signals, where considerable interference by common mode signals may be encountered (see Chapter 4).

Figure 3.19 shows another refinement. This circuit is a straightforward inverting amplifier, but has a capacitor providing additional negative feedback. Since a capacitor passes more current at high than at low frequency there will be more feedback at high frequency. This means that the gain will be reduced at high frequencies, but will, under d.c. conditions, adhere to the simple $R_2:R_1$ ratio. The circuit is, in effect a simple low-pass filter and the range of frequencies rejected can be selected by the choice of capacitor.

Capacitors can be used in operational amplifier circuits to perform special functions such as differentiation and integration.

Figure 3.20 shows how, by placing a capacitor in the feedback pathway, an integrator can be constructed. In this configuration, all the current passed down R_1 is stored by C, the output voltage showing the charge potential. The effect is to integrate the input voltage with respect to time. Such a device may be used, for example, to convert the flow signal from a pneumotachograph to volume.

In Fig. 3.21 the converse arrangement is seen, with a capacitor in the input pathway. In this case,

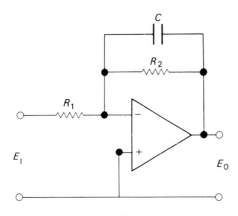

Fig. 3.19. An inverting amplifier with 'low-pass' filter characteristics.

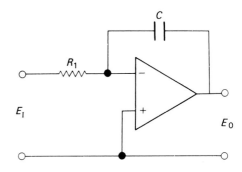

Fig. 3.20. Replacing R_2 with a capacitor creates an integrator.

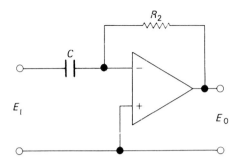

Fig. 3.21. Replacing R_1 with a capacitor creates a differentiator.

current passing through the capacitor is amplified and appears at the output. Since the current through the capacitor is proportional to the rate of change of voltage (see Fig. 3.7b), the output will also have this function. The output is therefore the first derivative of the input. The values of R and C are chosen so as to provide a rate constant ($R \cdot C$ seconds) which will give a suitable output range for the range of rate of change signals likely to be experienced at the input.

The differentiator so produced may be used to derive the rate of change of left ventricular pressure as an index of myocardial contractility (see p. 58).

It should not have escaped the reader that this circuit is also a high-pass filter.

Figure 3.22 shows the functions of integration and differentiation on various input signals.

Operational amplifier circuits are ubiquitous in modern instrumentation and may be very complex, since the ingenious designer is often able to build circuits which perform several functions simultaneously. However, most circuits are based on those described here, so that by application of first principles the functions of most operational amplifier circuits may be deduced.

Gain measurement

In specifying the performance of a practical amplifier circuit, the signal gain at different frequencies must be considered. The unit by which the ratio of output to input can be directly stated is the decibel (db).

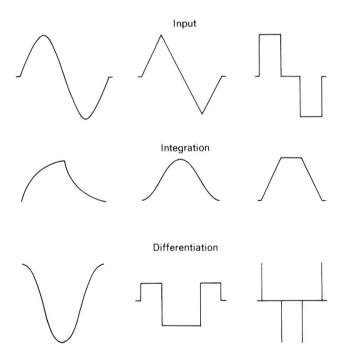

Fig. 3.22. Integration and differentiation of sine, triangular and square waveforms.

If the power dissipated by a resistor is increased from P_1 watts to P_2 watts, then the common logarithm of the ratio $P_2:P_1$ expresses the power gain in bels. Therefore, 1 bel represents a power gain of $\times 10$, 2 bels a gain of $\times 100$, and so on. Since the bel is rather a large unit, it is more conveniently expressed as 10dB. Thus a gain of $\times 10$ is 10 dB; $\times 100$, 20 dB; $\times 1000$, 30 dB; and so on.

Bridge circuits

Circuits based on the Wheatstone bridge are to be found throughout medical electronics, but may be disguised by a number of other components. However, the principles of the bridge circuit are universally applicable, so that time taken in their study is amply rewarded.

Consider the circuit in Fig. 3.23. The object is to measure resistance R_B. The circuit consists of two resistive limbs, R_A–R_B and R_C–R_D, and current passes through both. Some current will also flow through the galvanometer (X→Y or X←Y) unless points X and Y are exactly equipotential. A state of balance, indicated by a 'null' indication on the galvanometer, will exist when the ratio of resistors $R_A:R_B$ is the same as the ratio of $R_C:R_D$, since the supply voltage will in each case be divided by the same fraction. Thus if $R_C = R_D$, and R_B is the unknown, we can substitute known resistances into

position A until balance occurs. At that point, $R_A = R_B$.

If we put a known voltage across resistor R_B and measured the current with an ammeter, we could, knowing Ohm's law, compute the resistance rather more simply than using the Wheatstone bridge. Consider then, the effect of increasing R_B by 1%. This will reduce the current by 1% and the meter deflection by 1% — a barely discernible decrement. In the bridge circuit, however, a 1% increase in R_B will raise the potential at 'X' by 1% while 'Y' remains constant. Since the galvanometer current reflects the potential difference between X and Y, it will rise from 'null' to a small indicated current which is in percentage terms, an infinitely large increase! The sensitivity of the bridge is therefore limited only by that of the galvanometer itself. Since the galvanometer does not have to carry the energizing current (as in the simple Ohm's law circuit) it can be made very sensitive, and therefore able to detect very small changes in resistance. It should now be clear that the bridge has effectively isolated the change in resistance (ΔR_B) from the original value (R_B). Many transducers are resistive elements which change by a small fraction, so that, by using a bridge circuit which is initially set at balance, only ΔR_B is indicated. There is, however, a complication. The current through the galvanometer is not linearly related to R_B, so that it would appear that a bridge is only accurate at balance.

The output from a bridge circuit will, however, be linear if points X and Y in Fig. 3.23 are led to a differential amplifier whose input resistance is very high compared with the resistances in the bridge. Under these conditions an altered value for R_B does not cause current to flow from X to Y, so that the output is directly proportional to R_B.

Bridge circuits may feature reactive elements as well as, or instead of, resistors. For instance, the active elements of some pressure transducers are variable capacitors, so that an a.c.-energized bridge is used to measure the very small change in capacitance (see p. 16).

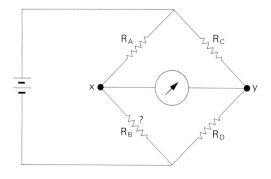

Fig. 3.23. The Wheatstone bridge.

Mixing and modulation

Signals of different frequencies can be combined together to form complex waveforms (Fig. 3.24). If signal B (high frequency, f_B) is simply added to signal A (low frequency, f_A), they are said to be mixed.

Passing the mixed signal through a low-pass filter will block the high frequency 'B' component, so that signal A will appear alone at the output. Similarly, a high-pass filter will block the 'A' component, so that signal B appears alone at the output.

If signal B (the carrier frequency) is made to fluctuate in amplitude according to the waveform of signal A, it is said to be amplitude modulated (AM). The modulated signal consists of three signals mixed together; the carrier (signal B) and the upper and lower side-band frequencies (upper SB frequency $= f_B + f_A$; lower SB frequency $= f_B - f_A$). Since frequency A is not present in the mixture of carrier and side-band signals, the modulated signal cannot be separated into signals A and B by filtering. Separation can only be achieved by demodulation. If the modulated signal is fed to the circuit of Fig. 3.14 it will be rectified, and the half-cycles appearing at the output will fluctuate at frequency A. Since the fluctuations of the upper side-band are no longer balanced by those of the lower side-band, a capacitor placed across resistor R will act as a low-pass filter and remove the carrier frequency. The output will be signal A added to a d.c. voltage corresponding to the rectified carrier signal.

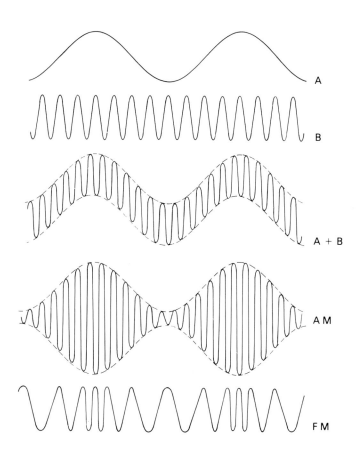

Fig. 3.24. Mixing and modulation. Signals A and B are simply added together to form the mixture A + B. In amplitude modulation (AM), the carrier signal (B) is modulated by A. In frequency modulation (FM) the carrier (B) remains constant in amplitude, but fluctuates in frequency according to the modulating signal A.

If signal B (carrier) is made to fluctuate in frequency according to the wave form of signal A, it is said to be frequency modulated (FM). Signal B is said to be the centre frequency and the degree of frequency shift depends upon the amplitude of signal A. An FM signal can be separated into its original components only by frequency demodulation. In its simplest possible form, a demodulator is a rate meter. Practical demodulators are usually constructed using devices known as phase-locked loops, which are complex integrated circuits beyond the scope of this text.

Modulators and demodulators are ubiquitous in modern instrumentation and will be discussed further in later chapters.

4: The Detection and Amplification of Biological Potentials

This chapter is concerned with the detection and amplification of electrical potentials on (or in) the body. These potentials are as follows:

1 Spontaneously occurring potentials of physiological origin.

2 Physiological potentials evoked by external stimuli.

3 Passive signals caused by externally applied electrical currents.

Spontaneous potentials

Activity in a nerve or muscle cell is accompanied by depolarization of the cell membrane. This temporarily reduces the potential difference which normally exists between the inside and the outside of the cell and creates a potential difference between the active cell and its surroundings. These single-cell action potentials can be sensed with either intracellular or extracellular electrodes.

Intracellular potentials can be recorded by inserting an extremely fine, saline-filled glass pipette directly into the cell. The technique demands a high degree of technical skill and is only used in physiological research. Extracellular recording is effected with needle or wire electrodes, and is increasingly used in clinical measurement. For example, needle electrodes can be inserted into muscles to record muscle action potentials (the electromyogram or EMG) and may be used to determine conduction velocities in nerves. Electrodes can be placed directly onto the heart surface at operation so that complex conduction patterns may be defined by epicardial mapping of the electrocardiogram (ECG).

The potentials arising from single cells summate with those arising from adjacent cells. Synchronous depolarization of a large number of cells leads to the formation of an electrical field, so that changes in potential can be detected at points far distant from the primary event. For instance, electrical events in the heart can be followed by means of electrodes on the body surface; these may be simple conductive plates, complex multilayer devices or percutaneous needles. Surface electrodes are most frequently used for monitoring the ECG, EMG and electroencephalogram (EEG). Electro-oculogram (EOG) signals can also be acquired in this way.

SIGNAL AMPLITUDE

When detected by surface electrodes, the signal amplitude depends upon a number of factors. In the case of the ECG signal, the main deflection is caused by depolarization of the large ventricular tissue mass. Furthermore, the process is highly coherent, with various zones depolarizing in a strict sequence controlled by the conducting mechanism. Since a great proportion of depolarizing cells act in concert, it follows that the potentials of many such cells summate to generate a well-recognizable signal at the body surface. Thus the larger the mass of synchronously depolarizing tissue, the greater the measured potential. With random depolarization and non-coherent propagation (as in ventricular fibrillation) the potentials are averaged so that the voltages detected by chest wall electrodes are of small amplitude.

Electroencephalogram signals arise from the largely asynchronous activity within the brain (or at least, the simultaneous activity of many organized activities), whereas EMG signals from an actively contracting muscle detect the electrical activity in a very large tissue mass.

45

The nature of the tissue between signal source and electrodes is also important. Whereas EEG electrodes are separated from the brain by an all-enveloping, poorly conducting box, EMG electrodes can be placed directly adjacent to, or even in, the muscle itself. It is not surprising that the EEG signal rarely exceeds 200 μV in amplitude, the ECG R-wave amplitude is usually 1–2 mV, while the EMG signal recorded by needle electrodes may easily reach 1 mV (see Table 7.1).

SIGNAL FREQUENCY

Any repetitive signal waveform may be seen as the algebraic sum of a number of sine waves. These comprise a *fundamental*, which is the repetition frequency, and a series of *harmonics*, whose frequencies are multiples of the fundamental. If the signal is to be reproduced faithfully by detection, amplification and display systems, all the constituent harmonics must be treated similarly; failure to do so may lead to gross distortion of the waveform. In the case of a clearly repetitive signal such as the ECG, the fundamental frequency is the pulse rate, but in more complex situations, such as the EEG, it may be less obvious. The fundamental frequency and the amplitudes of the harmonics in an epoch of any complex signal may be determined by a mathematical technique known as Fourier analysis. This is the method used by spectrum analysers, which display the EEG signal in terms of relative power over a range of frequencies. The various spontaneously arising signals vary widely in frequency content (Table 7.1). When considering the very different signal amplitudes involved, it is not surprising that each of these signal types requires a specially designed amplifier whose characteristics match those of the signal (see below).

Evoked potentials

There is growing interest in the measurement of potentials which arise as a result of specific external stimuli. For instance, a series of 'clicks' may be presented to the subject through headphones, and the evoked EEG responses detected by means of electrodes placed on the scalp overlying the audi-

tory cortical area. Similarly, repetitive visual stimuli can be applied using a strobe lamp, and the evoked visual responses detected by electrodes overlying the visual cortex. Somatosensory responses can be recorded by application of electrical stimuli to a peripheral nerve (such as ulnar or radial) with signal detection by electrodes overlying the appropriate sensory area. Since the evoked EEG signals are mixed with 'background' EEG activity, they cannot be identified without the use of a special instrument known as a transient averager or correlator (Fig. 4.1). This instrument takes a consecutive series of evoked responses, each 'saved' waveform starting at the exact moment of the stimulus. Then all the responses are added together, so that events which were synchronized with the stimulus will summate while asynchronous

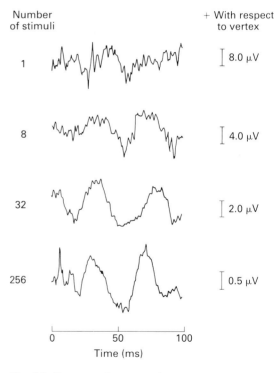

Fig. 4.1. By summating successive responses to an auditory stimulus, the evoked response (bottom) can be extracted from the background of general EEG activity (top). The recordings show 100 ms of EEG activity after the stimulus. The number of stimuli averaged is shown at the left. (From Thornton & Newton, 1989.)

events (such as random EEG activity) will average out to zero. Over a series of several hundred stimuli, the evoked response then emerges as a clear, uncluttered signal.

Evoked EEG techniques have been used intensively in the search for some method to determine 'depth of anaesthesia'. While it has been shown that the latency of the evoked cortical auditory response *is* increased with deepening planes of anaesthesia, the technique requires further development before it is suitable for clinical application (see p. 338).

Passive potentials: the measurement of tissue impedance

The electrical impedance of tissues depends on their constitution. When a small alternating current (a.c.) is applied across a portion of tissue, changes in its impedance can be detected as a change of a.c. voltage between the electrodes (Fig. 4.2). Changes in impedance occur when the average composition of the tissue between the electrodes changes. For example, this can occur in a limb which, because of vasodilatation, contains a greater amount of blood, or across the thorax when the intake of air causes a change in thoracic contents and dimensions.

Absolute calibration, based on the actual values of impedance, is virtually impossible, for so much depends on the position of the electrodes, the frequency or current employed, and the tissue structure of the individual. However, changes in impedance can often be shown to have a reasonably linear approximation to the substance (air, blood, etc.) under examination, and the voltage changes can thus be calibrated empirically in each individual case (Geddes & Baker, 1989).

The frequencies employed in impedance measurements are high enough to prevent polarization of the electrodes; for impedance spirometry frequencies in excess of 10 kHz are used. At these frequencies, the threshold for sensation is very much higher than at 50 Hz so that a 1–2 mA current can be used safely and without discomfort.

For impedance spirometry the electrodes are placed on either side of the chest in the mid-

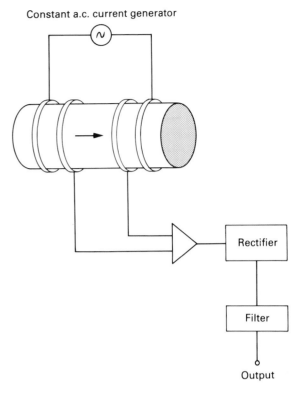

Fig. 4.2. If four circumferential electrodes are attached to a block of tissue, such as a limb, and a constant a.c. current is passed between the outer pair, the signal detected by the inner pair reflects the potential gradient across the tissue and therefore the impedance. The impedance signal, proportional to tissue volume, is extracted by rectification and filtering.

axillary line, and the amplifier gain is adjusted to give an adequate change of signal during the respiratory cycle. If a semi-quantitative display is the only requirement, this may be sufficient. If accurate calibration is required, the actual impedance of the patient at end-expiration can be determined by substituting a variable known resistance between the electrodes. A complete volume–impedance calibration curve can be derived by having the patient breathe (actively or passively) in and out of a spirometer while simultaneously measuring thoracic impedance. Then, any change in impedance can be read in terms of volume. This technique provides a non-invasive means of measuring successive tidal volumes without involving the airway, so long as the subject's posture remains unchanged; any such change is likely to alter the calibration.

The same technique, using circumferential electrodes around neck and abdomen can demonstrate the changes in thoracic blood volume associated with each cardiac cycle (see Chapter 16), and a number of algorithms have been proposed for the determination of stroke volume. Impedance techniques have also been used to monitor changes in lung water (Severinghaus, 1971).

Impedance techniques can be applied to limb plethysmography, using volumetric or strain-gauge plethysmographs as calibrators. However, given the availability of such a calibration device, there can be few applications where the less precise impedance technique could be shown to offer any real advantage. Consequently, impedance measurements are usually employed when absolute values are of less interest than relative changes.

Noise and interference

Since the design of suitable amplifiers for these applications is largely related to the prevention of noise and interference, the sources of these unwanted signals will precede an account of desirable amplifier characteristics.

As was pointed out in Chapter 1, the first essential in any instrumentation system is that the signal-to-noise ratio should be high. Noise may originate in the patient, his surroundings or even the instruments used for recording, amplification and display. Instrumental noise can be reduced by good design, the use of high-grade components and careful screening. However, noise arising from the patient or his surroundings is often more difficult to eradicate and requires an understanding of the underlying causes.

NOISE ORIGINATING FROM THE PATIENT

The electrical changes associated with cardiac activity produce potential differences of about 0.5–2 mV on the surface of the body, whilst the EEG signal on the scalp has a magnitude of only 50 μV. Since EMG signals can be much larger than

either, muscular activity (especially shivering) can lead to gross interference.

Although the ECG signal is much larger than the EEG it is rarely a troublesome source of interference, since the ECG potentials are substantially in phase at all points on the head and can therefore be eliminated by using an amplifier which is able to attenuate the in-phase signals and amplify those which are out of phase. It operates by amplifying the difference between two input signals, but attenuating their sum. A differential amplifier of this type is said to have high common mode rejection. The interference caused by muscular activity is generally composed of higher frequencies than those in the EEG signal, and can often be eliminated by attenuating the high frequency response of the amplifier to a level which does not interfere greatly with the characteristics of the EEG.

When monitoring the fetal ECG during labour, the maternal ECG creates an interfering signal. In this application, signals from the maternal abdomen are very difficult to separate, and the signal-to-noise ratio can be improved dramatically by placing electrodes on the fetus itself (usually on the presenting scalp).

Clearly, the choice of electrode and electrode site is important, and amplifiers with high common mode rejection are essential.

NOISE ORIGINATING FROM THE PATIENT–ELECTRODE INTERFACE

Unfortunately, recording electrodes do not behave as passive connectors. When a metal surface is brought into contact with an electrolyte solution, as occurs with a simple skin–metal electrode system, an electrochemical half-cell is produced. This will generate an electromotive force (e.m.f.).

If a differential amplifier is connected to a pair of such electrodes with the two half-cells in opposition, their output potentials can be compared. If the cells are identical the potentials will be self-cancelling, yielding zero output. If not, the difference in potential between the two cells will be amplified. Furthermore, the small current produced by the offset potential may change the characteristics of the electrodes themselves by electrolytic action. This phenomenon is known as polarization.

A polarized electrode (as may occur with platinum : saline) will seriously distort any signal applied to it, since the signal affects the current through the cell, and this in turn alters the cell potential. An electrode which comprises a metal plated with one of its own salts, e.g. silver : silver chloride (Ag : AgCl) does not behave in this way. Because current in either direction leaves the composition of the electrode unchanged, the cell potential remains constant. Such an electrode is said to be reversible.

If a material such as iron were to be used as a skin electrode, corrosion would occur, so developing a highly irregular electrochemical potential. These corrosion potentials would superimpose on any recorded biological potential and, having a wide range of frequency components, would seriously reduce the signal-to-noise ratio. Modern recording electrodes are almost invariably provided with Ag : AgCl surfaces, so that polarization and corrosion potentials should never be a practical problem.

Mechanical movement of recording electrodes may also result in large potential changes. These are due to an alteration of the physical dimensions of the electrode–skin half-cell, thus modifying the cell potential, and also to changes in skin–electrode impedance, which may impair the common mode rejection ratio (CMRR) of the recording amplifier (see p. 52).

NOISE ORIGINATING FROM SOURCES OUTSIDE THE PATIENT

Interference from outside sources is due principally to electrostatic or electromagnetic induction from mains or radiofrequency sources.

Electrostatic sources

When a charged body is brought close to an uncharged one, an equal and opposite charge develops on the uncharged body. If an unearthed patient is close to any object such as a cable or lamp element which is connected to the mains supply, he will develop a surface charge of equal and opposite potential even though no current is actually flowing between them. Since the mains potential is a sinusoidal function, fluctuating between ± 339 V at a frequency of 50 Hz, the induced potential will have the same characteristics. In effect, the patient acts as one plate of a capacitor. If the patient could be electrically isolated from all his other surroundings, his surface potential would be the same at all points but fluctuating at 50 Hz. In practice, however, there are always other stray capacitances between the patient and such objects as the bed or operating table, the floor, nearby staff and electronic instruments. Many of these bodies (including the patient) may be earthed, so that the patient becomes part of a potential gradient between the source potential and ground, along which a very small a.c. current flows. It follows, therefore, that his body surface is no longer at a single potential, but shows considerable spatial variation depending upon the relative positions of all the bodies to which he is electrostatically coupled and the pathway to earth. This is illustrated by considering the surface potentials detected by a simple electronic amplifier, which measures electrical potentials with reference to ground (Fig. 4.3). The patient is subjected to stray capacitance from an a.c. source close to his head. Electrode B is at ground potential, so that an alternating potential gradient is established along the patient. Electrode A is at a point on that gradient, and so will detect and amplify the a.c. potential at that point.

Since the surface a.c. potential may be as large as 1 V (root mean squared (r.m.s.)) the amplifier would be swamped with 50 Hz interference. Moreover, the electrode lead itself is also likely to be affected by the source and will add to the 50 Hz signal which is detected. This effect will be intensified if there is a high electrode contact resistance.

Electromagnetic induction

This form of interference occurs in the vicinity of wires carrying alternating currents (Fig. 4.3). As with stray capacitance the result is 50 Hz interference mixed with the output signal, but the causa-

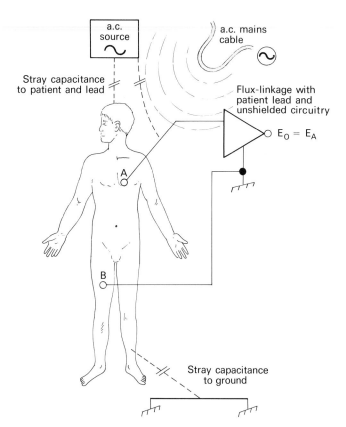

Fig. 4.3. A simple 'single input' amplifier is subject to gross interference from electrostatic (broken lines) and electromagnetic sources.

tion is quite different. When a current flows it generates a magnetic field: with an a.c. current the field is constantly growing and collapsing with successive half-cycles, so that any conductor within the field will have constantly changing flux-linkage, and therefore an electromagnetically-induced current will flow at the same frequency as the source. All conductors carrying mains currents are surrounded by electromagnetic fields, with the flux density depending upon the current.

Since simple electrostatic cable screens are readily penetrated by electromagnetic fields, electromagnetic interference would appear to be a major problem. Fortunately, the mains supply is usually arranged so that for every live cable carrying current to a device, there is a neutral cable carrying an exactly equal current away from it (or vice versa), these two wires lying either immediately adjacent to each other, or even better, twisted

around one another. The electromagnetic fields are thus equal and opposite, and to a large extent self-cancelling.

If at some point in the building the neutral cable is accidentally connected to ground, the supply will work perfectly well. However, the live–neutral current mismatch will generate a large magnetic field. Similarly, when a machine or instrument develops a high leakage current, live and neutral currents are no longer equal and self-cancelling, so that an electromagnetic field is generated. Such a field induces an e.m.f. in all the wires within its vicinity, the effect being multiplied if the wires are coiled. Leads connecting patient electrodes to sensitive amplifiers are most frequently affected, but inadequate protection of amplifier circuitry from electromagnetic fields may also result in inductive interference.

High electrode impedance

Among the factors leading to electrical interference, high electrode impedance is arguably the most important. Consider an ECG electrode placed on the skin surface and connected to an amplifier by means of an imperfectly screened lead. The skin–electrode resistance can be represented (Fig. 4.4) by an equivalent resistor R_e. The amplifier is assumed to take no current from the lead (i.e. has infinite input impedance).

An external source of interference, such as a nearby mains power cable, induces (by mutual inductance) a very small a.c. current in the patient lead. If the electrode impedance is very low, the potential at the amplifier input must remain close to that of the skin surface, so that minimal interference results. If, however, electrode impedance is high, the small induced current may set up a significant potential difference across that imped-

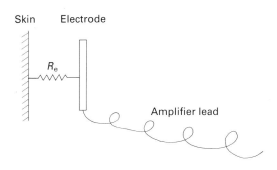

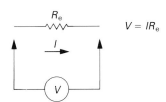

Fig. 4.4. The resistance of an electrode may be seen as the equivalent resistor R_e. Any induced current I in the lead to the amplifier must set up a potential difference $R_e I$ across the electrode. This will be amplified and appears at the output.

ance. This, when applied to the amplifier input, may lead to massive 50 Hz interference at the output.

It will be evident that any effort to minimize interference which is not preceded by close attention to electrode impedance is unlikely to be effective.

Earth-loop interference

If a patient is connected to two electrical devices, each of which is separately earthed, interference may arise due to the earth-loop effect. The mechanism is very simple and depends upon the two earth points having slightly different potentials (Fig. 4.5).

This usually occurs in old installations where the earth connections have deteriorated, so that any leakage current flowing along the earth (often from some quite separate, and even distant device) will set up a potential difference between two earth points in the same room.

If, under these conditions, a patient is connected to the earthed plate of a diathermy machine and also to the leads of an ECG in which one lead is earthed, there will be an a.c. potential gradient across the patient equal to the difference between earth potentials. Unless the ECG has good common mode rejection and the electrodes are correctly orientated to the potential gradient, 50 Hz interference will result. In modern devices, all circuits making contact with the patient must be isolated from ground (see Chapter 11), so that earth loops are now uncommon.

Radiofrequency interference (RFI)

Radiofrequency (>100 kHz) noise can enter a recording system by three possible routes:
1 It may enter through the mains distribution system, mixed with the 50 Hz current. (Sources are diathermy machines, and unsuppressed sparking contacts as may be found in switch-gear and electric motors.)
2 It may be applied directly, as when a patient is touched by the active electrode of a surgical diathermy and coagulation performed. (In this case the noise behaves as if it were coming from the patient, and is detected by the recording electrodes.)

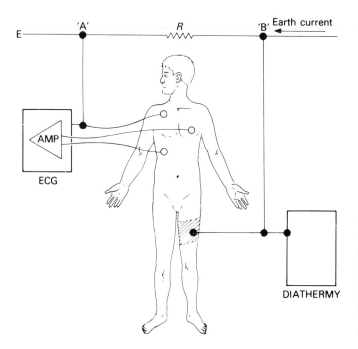

Fig. 4.5. Interference due to an earth loop. An earth current (usually due to a leakage from some other device attached to the earth) sets up a potential difference across the small resistance R. This potential now exists between the earth connections of two devices, and so appears across the patient. The potential gradient across the patient is detected by the amplifier (AMP) and appears as interference.

3 It may be transmitted by radiopropagation. If the diathermy probe is simply held in the air and the circuit activated, a nearby ECG system will show gross interference. Here the active diathermy electrode and its lead acts as a radiotransmitting aerial, and the patient lead as a receiving aerial.

Radiofrequency potentials detected by the recording electrodes and patient leads present the greatest problem, since they are likely to be rectified by the input stages of the amplifier. Then, any low-frequency signal with which the radiofrequency carrier was modulated will be demodulated and amplified with the ECG signal itself. If this demodulated signal is large, the amplifier may 'block' altogether, so that no signal appears at the output. More often a large 50 Hz signal appears which obscures the ECG mixed with it. Newer diathermy machines (whose output waveforms are modulated at higher frequencies) may produce somewhat less interference, due to the limited bandwidth of the ECG amplifier.

Amplifiers for biological signals

Once detected by electrodes, a signal must be amplified. As already discussed (Chapter 3), am-

plification involves an increase in amplitude (current or voltage) and also a decrease in impedance. Other amplifier characteristics are chosen so as to minimize the effect of unwanted noise and interference.

INPUT IMPEDANCE AND COMMON MODE
REJECTION

It has already been established that amplifiers for biological signals require high common mode rejection and high input impedance. High input impedance minimizes current flow through the electrodes, which themselves have significant impedance which tends to vary with time. If the amplifier had a low input impedance, some current would flow between electrode and amplifier. Then the electrode and input impedances would act as a potential divider with consequent attenuation of the signal. This is especially important where the augmented ECG leads are concerned, since here the signals from two limb leads are summed and then compared with the third. If one of the two signals to be summed is attenuated due to high electrode impedance, the mean signal will be biased towards the other, with a resulting error in the geometry of the lead. To a much lesser extent, the bipolar leads are subject to the same type of distortion.

In the detection of physiological potentials such as ECG, EEG, etc., the amplifier CMRR should always exceed 1000:1, and is generally much higher. Input impedance must exceed 5 MΩ if the above problems are to be avoided (10 MΩ is a common value in modern ECGs). If small, high impedance electrodes are to be used (as in the EEG), a high input impedance amplifier is especially important.

FREQUENCY RESPONSE

The bandwidth of the amplifier must cover the range of frequencies that are of importance in the signal. The American Heart Association (1967) standard for ECG machines specifies a flat response from 0.14 up to 50 Hz and allows up to 30 dB attenuation at 0.05 and 100 Hz (30 dB is a 1000-fold attenuation). EEGs can be recorded satisfactorily using an amplifier with a similar bandwidth but more voltage amplification, although purpose built machines usually have a bandwidth extending from 0.5 Hz up to nearly 100 Hz. EMGs or nerve action potential recordings require a flat response from about 20 Hz up to at least 2 kHz and preferably up to 10 kHz, if the high frequencies contained in the signal are to be reproduced faithfully.

Direct current (d.c.) amplifiers have a bandwidth down to 0 Hz, but are unsuitable for ECG recording because the signal is subject to slowly changing offset potentials which, if amplified, would drive the trace right off the screen or recording paper. They are largely due to fluctuating differences between electrode half-cell potentials, and should be seen as a very low-frequency component of the noise spectrum.

These problems may be overcome by employing a first-stage amplifier with high common mode rejection but low gain, thus ensuring that offset signals do not exceed the output voltage range. This is coupled to a second, higher gain amplifier by means of a resistor-capacitor network which operates as a simple high-pass filter which allows the ECG signal to pass, but blocks out offset or slow drift signals. In commercial amplifiers, active baseline control circuits are able to restore the visible waveform following an artefact much more quickly than could be achieved by this simple circuit.

The choice of time constant for an ECG amplifier involves a compromise between trace fidelity and stability. A long time constant (>2 s) gives optimal reproduction of the waveform, but at the expense of some baseline instability, especially in the case of a moving or ambulant patient. On the other hand, a short time constant (<0.5 s) ensures good baseline stability at the expense of waveform reproduction. In particular, slow elements such as the T-wave are likely to be differentiated and may even appear to be biphasic. Thus amplifiers designed for diagnostic electrocardiography may have time constants as long as 3 s, but for those designed for monitoring applications (where trace continuity is more important than minor distortions) the time constant may be 1.5 s or even less. Diagnostic EEG amplifiers usually allow the user to select a suitable time constant.

Special filters may be incorporated, which introduce additional attenuation at particular frequencies. For example, a highly selective band-reject filter is usually incorporated to remove 50 Hz interference from the signal, and a low-pass filter may be used to eliminate muscle artefacts from an EEG signal.

Calibration voltages may be incorporated so that the gain of the amplifiers can be correctly adjusted. It is customary to calibrate the ECG so that a 1 mV input will produce a 1 cm pen deflection on a direct-writing recorder. Similarly, 100 μV calibration signals are provided on EEG amplifiers. With the increasing use of oscilloscope screens, the 1 cm standard is often abandoned in favour of arbitrary graticule scales.

ELIMINATION OF INTERFERENCE

Mains-frequency interference can, to a large extent, be prevented by good amplifier design, but the user must be aware that noise-free recording is unlikely to be achieved in an environment littered with a.c. potential sources, stray capacitance, electromagnetic fields and radiofrequency radiations, however well the amplifier is designed.

An ECG amplifier should be of the differential type with high input impedance and high CMRR.

High CMRR means that the amplifier strongly attenuates signals (such as those due to inductive or capacitative coupling) which are common to both inputs, but amplifies the difference between the two signals. The efficiency of common mode rejection is also related to the amplitude of the common, in-phase signal to be rejected. Earthing the patient with a right-leg electrode is undesirable for safety reasons (see Chapter 11), but it also intensifies the potential gradients on the patient's surface. By allowing the whole amplifier to 'float' at the same potential as the patient, these gradients are minimized so that common mode voltages are reduced, and therefore become less difficult to reject.

Electrostatic induction in the leads is prevented by surrounding each lead with braided copper screen (connected to the amplifier reference voltage) so that stray capacitances couple with the screen instead of the lead.

When EEG monitoring is disturbed by electromagnetic fields, a cure can be very elusive since ordinary electrostatic screens are not effective. The circuitry itself can be protected by surrounding it with a copper or aluminium enclosure, in whose walls eddy currents are induced. These produce opposing fields which at least partially cancel the effect of the original field, so that circuits within the enclosure remain free of interference. Materials with high magnetic permeability, such as mu-metal or iron, which concentrate the field within themselves can also be used for electromagnetic screens. Unfortunately, it is the patient leads which are most susceptible to this form of interference, and screening them with sheets of iron is just not practicable! The only effective method of screening is to enclose the entire patient in an iron box (or room) together with the low-level stages of signal detection and amplification. Although this approach is widely used for low-level measurements (such as the EEG) it is not really suitable for clinical monitoring.

The effects of electromagnetic fields can be mitigated by ensuring that all the patient leads are the same length, and are closely bound together, or even better, twisted together, until very close to the electrodes. This ensures that, as far as possible, the induced signals are identical and therefore susceptible to common mode rejection. The only real cure is to eliminate the sources of the unwanted electromagnetic fields.

In critical applications where very small signals are to be detected in a normal clinical environment (EEG recording in the intensive therapy unit is a good example), it is good practice to keep the signal leads as short as possible. Thus a mobile EEG system will usually feature a 'head box'. This is a pre-amplifier unit, attached to the main system by a screened cable, which may be mounted *very* close to the patient's head, thus reducing lead lengths to a few inches only.

For many years, RFI from surgical diathermy (300 kHz to 3MHz) presented insuperable problems, especially with spark-gap and valve-modulated generators. In a simple ECG system, large radiofrequency signals enter the amplifier as both common mode and differential signals which tend to saturate the input stages. Furthermore, the entire input circuit and associated metal work may act as an aerial, radiating radiofrequency signals throughout the instrument to such an extent that conventional screening appears to be ineffective. To make matters worse the sensitive input stages, floating at radiofrequency, 'see' nearby earthed metal work as a source of RFI. Finally, diathermy generators may add radiofrequency signals to the mains supply itself, to be picked up by the ECG instrument power cable. The total effect is catastrophic, and all these sources of interference must be eradicated before a clean signal can be obtained. Figure 4.6 shows the basic structure of a diathermy-immune ECG amplifier. The ECG signal passes through a filter before entering the isolated input circuit, which is surrounded by a double screen. When combined with a simple filter in the power supply to block mains-borne radiofrequencies, these simple measures can result in total freedom from diathermy interference.

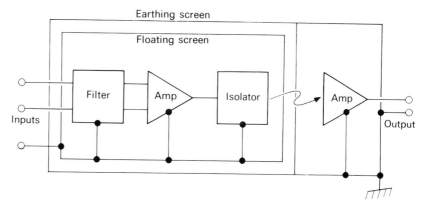

Fig. 4.6. The principles of a diathermy-immune ECG amplifier (AMP = amplifier)

Electrode requirements

The importance of having an amplifier input impedance significantly greater than the electrode skin resistance has already been emphasized. At one time, biological signals could only be displayed using string galvanometers, and since these inevitably had a low input impedance it was vital to lower the electrode–skin resistance as much as possible. Originally, this was achieved by placing the hands and feet in saline baths, but later the electrodes were refined to large surface plates coated with electrically-conductive jelly, applied to skin which had been abraded with the purpose of removing the high-resistance cornified layer.

With the introduction of modern amplifiers with high input impedance, smaller electrodes with higher impedances could be used without compromising signal quality. However, excessive electrode impedance is undesirable because mains interference may be accentuated and differences between electrode impedances may lead to geometric errors. Signal distortion is also produced by polarized electrodes and can be a major problem when the measured potentials are small, as in electroencephalography. Low-noise, reversible electrodes are best constructed of silver, coated electrolytically with silver chloride.

The silver chloride layer is very thin, and after a few uses becomes imperfect. However, the best modern disposable electrodes have Ag : AgCl surfaces, which will not deteriorate during single-use.

It has been found that movement artefacts are greatly reduced if the electrode surface is separated

from the skin by a relatively thick layer of electrolyte. This ensures that mechanical distortion of the skin under the electrode does not significantly alter the electrode potential or resistance. This characteristic is often achieved by separating the electrode surface from the skin by a foam pad impregnated with electrolyte gel (Fig. 4.7).

The electrolyte gel does not require specially conductive properties but should be non-abrasive, non-allergenic, soap-free and, ideally, sterile if the skin is not to be damaged during long-term use. Although it is not necessary to abrade the skin to achieve ultra-low impedances, it is a good idea to de-grease it with ether before applying an electrode. This reduces the resistance and ensures satisfactory adhesion. Because of their poor electrical performance and greatly increased danger of diathermy burns (Chapter 11), needle electrodes are to be avoided unless strictly necessary.

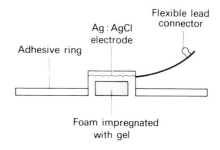

Fig. 4.7. Diagrammatic section through a disposable ECG electrode. The signal reaches the Ag : AgCl after passage through an electrolyte-impregnated contact pad.

ELECTRODES FOR FETAL ELECTROCARDIOGRAPHY

Fetal electrocardiography has an established role in perinatal care. The fetal ECG can be recorded from abdominal skin electrodes on the mother, but the signal will be mixed with a much larger maternal ECG signal. If the maternal ECG is also recorded from chest leads, it will contain no fetal signals, so that with very careful waveform matching the maternal signal can be subtracted, leaving the fetal signal alone at the output. In the clinical environment, this is not a practical proposition, as the equipment is complex and requires very careful setting-up procedures. The fetal ECG can be more readily obtained by means of a scalp electrode. This usually takes the form of a stainless steel spiral, rather like a very small double corkscrew, which can be attached to the scalp through the cervix using a special applicator.

A second electrode is attached to the mother's skin (usually on the inside surface of the thigh) and acts as a common connection to the fetus through the uterus and liquor. Using this technique, a good quality fetal ECG, free from maternal artefacts, can be obtained early in labour. As may be expected, a high impedance amplifier is needed if signal distortion is to be avoided.

References

American Heart Association (1967) Report of a committee on electrocardiography. *Circulation* **35**, 583–610.

Geddes, L.A. & Baker, L.E. (1989) *Principles of applied biomedical instrumentation*, 3rd edn. John Wiley & Sons, New York.

Severinghaus, J.W. (1971). Electrical measurement of pulmonary oedema with a focusing conductivity bridge. *Journal of Physiology (London)*, **215**, 53p–55p.

Thornton, C. & Newton, D.E.F. (1989). The auditory evoked response: a measure of depth of anaesthesia. In Jones, J.C. (ed.) *Baillière's clinical anaesthesiology, 3.3, Depth of anaesthesia*, pp. 559–585. Baillière Tindall, London.

5: Data Processing and Storage

Signal acquisition is but the beginning of the process of measurement. In some instances we may simply feed the signal into an oscilloscope or pen recorder and then interpret it intuitively, as we are accustomed to do with the ECG. However, some signals (such as pressure waveforms) require accurate measurements of maximum, minimum and mean values, and therefore must be calibrated against some standard. Of course, it is essential that such signals are free of noise which might be falsely interpreted as part of the waveform. Calibration enables a displayed waveform to be compared with the scale on a cathode-ray tube (CRT) graticule or recording paper, and ensures that numerical information (such as a displayed pressure value) is, in fact, accurate.

It is now commonplace for raw signals to be processed extensively before they are used to make clinical decisions. Indeed, if the required information has to be derived from one or more data sources it is often necessary to extract data from several recordings before calculating the result. This process is laborious and open to both bias and error. Therefore, it is preferable to have a system that performs the calculations by direct processing of the original data. Such a device is not only faster, and usually more reliable than manual computation, but also remains independent of subjective influences. An example of signal processing is provided by the simple ratemeter.

Ratemeters

If a signal (such as the ECG) occurs at more or less regular intervals it is possible to measure the repetition rate, which can then be displayed in analogue or digital form. Ratemeters are of two basic types; integrating and instantaneous. An integrating ratemeter determines the average rate over a period, whereas an instantaneous ratemeter determines the reciprocal of the period between successive pulses to yield a value for rate (i.e. it measures in the time domain, and then converts to frequency).

Clinical ratemeters are usually of the integrating type, since the information is more useful to determine trends, even over short periods. In fact, the instantaneous ratemeter gives more information about rhythm than it does about rate; thus an instantaneous rate record from a patient with atrial fibrillation will show a wide scatter of rates corresponding to the inherent cardiac irregularity.

Derivation of a variable such as heart rate lends itself to further data processing, such that audible and visible warning devices are activated when the rate lies outside preset values (high and low limits). Needless to say the usefulness of such a warning system is dependent upon the quality of the signal whose rate is being measured. Early ratemeters were notoriously unreliable, since the trigger circuits were unable to distinguish QRS complexes from small artefacts, and patient movement often led to 'amplifier-blocking' and consequent signal loss for short periods. These difficulties led to erroneous estimates of heart rate which, only too often, caused alarm circuits to be activated. It is hardly surprising that alarm systems acquired a reputation for unreliability and were rarely used. Modern systems have largely overcome these shortcomings, since trigger circuits are commonly preceded by sophisticated filters and signal recognition algorithms which both remove noise and stabilize the trace.

Analogue computation

Rate determination is an example of simple analogue processing, and in its most basic form may be achieved by very simple electronic circuits. More complex functions can be solved by use of operational amplifiers which are, of course, the building blocks of the analogue computer (see below). For example, continuous integration of a pneumotachograph signal yields a volume waveform, while differentiation of the intraventricular pressure waveform gives a continuous value for 'rate of change of pressure'.

The function dP/dt_{max}, the maximum positive rate of change of pressure in the left ventricle, has been shown to be a useful index of cardiac contractility. By using a high fidelity pressure transducer and amplifier, a voltage may be obtained which is a faithful reproduction of the changing pressure in the left ventricle. This voltage could be recorded and the function dP/dt_{max} derived by repeatedly measuring the slope of the pressure trace and taking the maximum value. However, derivation of the slope by manual methods is very inaccurate and open to subjective error. By feeding the voltage representing the pressure into a suitable electronic circuit, differentiation can be performed continuously with a high degree of accuracy. The record of the electrical output from such a circuit (Fig. 5.1) shows both positive and negative peaks. Since left ventricular pressure both increases and decreases during the cardiac cycle, it is a simple matter to read the peak value of dP/dt from the ordinate, providing this scale has been previously calibrated.

One way of calibrating this scale is to apply a triangular input of known amplitude and frequency. Since this signal rises at a constant rate, the rate of change is constant. Therefore, the output signal is a square-wave whose amplitude is proportional to the rate of change of the triangular input (Fig. 5.2).

Given a properly calibrated pressure signal, and a known rate of change of voltage from the calibrator, it is easy to calibrate the output in terms of dP/dt. It will be appreciated that the power of the analogue method lies in its ability to perform continuous differentiation upon a rapidly changing input waveform. In mathematical terms the task is formidable, but to the analogue differentiator, very simple.

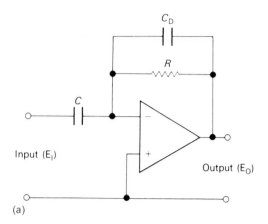

(a)

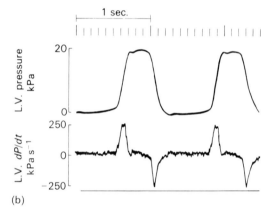

(b)

Fig. 5.1. Analogue differentiation of left ventricular pressure, to derive dP/dt_{max}. (a) Circuit diagram of simple analogue differentiometer. (b) Record of left ventricular pressure and left ventricular dP/dt showing that maximum deflections of the dP/dt trace occur when left ventricular pressure is rising or falling at maximal rate.

APPLICATIONS FOR ANALOGUE COMPUTERS

Although digital methods of computation have largely replaced analogue computers (see below) there are certain applications for which analogue methods are ideally suited.

They can perform a wide range of mathematical functions including addition, subtraction, multiplication and division, but their most powerful (and useful) function is that of continuous integration and differentiation. Indeed, despite the rapid advances in digital processing (see below), analogue devices continue to be used widely in these applications by virtue of low cost and technical simplicity.

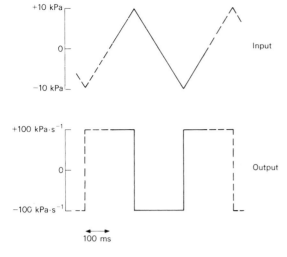

Fig. 5.2. Calibration of an analogue differentiator. A 'triangular' input waveform produces a 'square wave' first derivative. Since the rate of rise is 10 kPa in 100 ms the calibration is $100 \, \text{kPa} \cdot \text{s}^{-1}$.

They can be used to provide a continuous indication of the volume entering or leaving the lung by integration of the flow signal; body displacement can be differentiated to give acceleration in the ballistocardiogram; or the area under a dye-dilution curve can be obtained by integrating the area under the curve (Chapter 16). A large analogue computer might have 50 or more operational amplifiers which can be arranged to solve many complex equations simultaneously. For example, it is possible to study the uptake and distribution of drugs by modelling a series of body compartments with different blood flows and different capacities for the drug, and then to study how regional variations in blood flow might affect drug disposition. Since each constant is controlled by a potentiometer controllable from the operator's panel, it is a simple matter to produce some perturbation and then observe its effect on the remainder of the system. In all these applications the amplitude of the input voltage is scaled to match the variable under observation while the time scale is adjusted to provide a reasonable duration for the computation. Amplitude and time scaling add greatly to the versatility of the instrument for they enable processes with very long or very short time scales to be stimulated at a rate

which can be adjusted to provide the most information in the available time. For examples of analogue computer applications see Hull and McLeod (1976) and Fukui and Smith (1981a,b).

Digital computation

An alternative method of determining $\text{d}P/\text{d}t_{\text{max}}$ is to use digital processing. The first step is to convert the electrical signal from the pressure transducer into digital form (analogue-to-digital conversion or ADC). This is done by measuring the pressure signal at regular intervals with an electronic voltmeter circuit (available as a single integrated circuit) which expresses the results in digital form. The value for $\text{d}P/\text{d}t_{\text{max}}$ is then calculated from the large number of pressure measurements within a single cardiac cycle. Finally, the result can either be displayed in digital form or stored in digital memory for comparison with previous values.

The overwhelming advantage of the digital approach is that the processor can easily be programmed to perform much more sophisticated tasks at no extra cost. For example, the processor might take $\text{d}P/\text{d}t_{\text{max}}$ for successive cardiac cycles and after each cycle, print out the running mean of the last ten values, so as to minimize beat-to-beat variations and show underlying trends. Whilst this task is technically possible in an analogue computer, it would be extremely complicated.

In some cases, it may be useful to convert digital information back to analogue form. This can be achieved by use of a digital-to-analogue converter (DAC), which generates a voltage proportional to the digital value at the input.

THE BINARY NUMBER SYSTEM

Most electronic devices used in processors are capable of assuming one of two stable states. Thus a switch can be on or off, or a transistor can be conducting or non-conducting. For this reason, computers use binary arithmetic rather than the more familiar decimal notation which would require devices able to assume ten different stable states. To illustrate the use of this system let us take the binary number 10011001. It is eight digits or bits long, and the value of each bit is always either

'1' or '0'. The least significant 'bit' is on the right (as in a decimal number), and represents either 1 or 0. The next bit is twice as significant again, so that a '1' represents 2, and a '0' nothing. The next bit is twice as significant again, so that a '1' represents 4. Successively significant bits therefore double in value, so that the '1' in the most significant bit (far left), represents 128. The decimal equivalent of the number 10011001 is the sum of the values of the four 1s in the binary number, i.e. $128 + 16 + 8 + 1 = 153$.

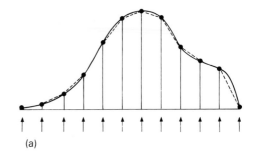

(a)

ANALOGUE-TO-DIGITAL CONVERSION (ADC)

The converter samples the input signal at regular intervals, each sample yielding a number whose magnitude is proportional to that of the signal. The resolution of the converter depends upon the number of bits in the binary number produced. An 8-bit number (properly called a byte) can resolve a given analogue signal with an accuracy of one part in $1 + 2 + 4 + 8 + 16 + 32 + 64 + 128 = 255$. This is an accuracy of 0.4% of full scale. For more accurate applications a 12-bit byte resolving to one part in 4095 or 0.02% of full scale may be required. However, this is not the only factor governing the accuracy of ADC, because sampling frequency must also be considered. Whilst a relatively low sampling frequency may provide a representative sample of values for a slowly-changing waveform it may prove quite inadequate for one containing higher frequency components (Fig. 5.3).

The detail with which the input voltage is digitized thus depends upon the length of the data byte and the sampling frequency, a frequency of 100 bytes per second (or correctly 100 baud) being adequate to capture the fastest likely rate of change of a physiological pressure signal.

THE DIGITAL PROCESSOR

After ADC each 12-bit byte can be led in parallel to a processor (parallel connection means that information is carried by 12 interconnecting wires, each carrying a yes/no bit of information corresponding to one of the 12 bits in the byte). Not many years ago this processor would have been a large, slow, device which generated more heat than

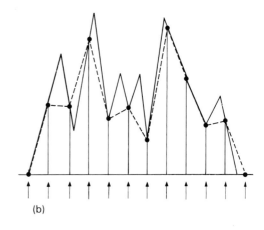

(b)

Fig. 5.3. Analogue-to-digital conversion. The sampling rate indicated by the arrows would provide a reasonably accurate reproduction of the slow variations in waveform a, but would not provide an accurate representation of waveform b. The waveform which would be reconstructed from digital data is shown as a dotted line.

information. Today, powerful processing devices with large associated memory circuits can be mounted in single integrated circuits, and are generally known as microprocessors. Indeed, complete computers can now be placed within single integrated circuits.

In its most basic form, a microprocessor consists of three essential parts:
1 An arithmetic logic unit (ALU) which can perform simple arithmetic operations, and has several temporary storage locations (registers) for single bytes.
2 Binary data storage areas. Some of these contain low-level programming instructions, while others

are used by the processor for both storage and recall of data bytes during computation. These memory devices may take one of several forms. Random Access Memory (RAM) areas consist of large numbers of minute binary storage devices mounted on a silicon wafer, and may be either volatile or non-volatile. Volatile memory devices (often called 'Dynamic RAM') 'remember' binary information for as long as the device is connected to a power supply, but lose it as soon as the power supply is switched off. Their advantage lies in the speed and low power consumption which can be achieved, and arrays of such wafers can be arranged to form very large memories with low power consumption. Non-volatile memories do not lose their information when the power supply is turned off, but retain it in the form of electrical charges on a great number of minute capacitors. They are, however, less compact and have greater power requirements than dynamic memories. Information can be stored in RAM arrays, and read from it or over-written when required. Read Only Memories (ROM) are binary data storage arrays which can be programmed with information during construction, but cannot easily be re-programmed. This information can then be read very quickly by the processor. Read Only Memory devices are used to hold basic information such as program sequences or 'look-up' tables which may be needed repeatedly during use.

COMPUTER PROGRAMMING

Micro-instructions in the form of binary numbers tell the processor how to perform each basic task. (Thus the instructions 'take a number from location A, multiply it by 2, and put the answer in location B' might well require more than 10 micro-instructions). Since programming in micro-instructions would be very tedious, most micro-computers have a set of built-in, higher-level instructions called machine code, each of which performs some specific task by executing a number of micro-instructions. These instructions are very powerful, but still in the form of binary numbers. They can be handled more conveniently by using mnemonics, which simply substitute two or three-character abbreviations (such as ADD, DIV, etc.)

for the rather unpalatable binary numbers. This is called assembly level programming. To facilitate programming still further, a number of high level 'languages' have been developed. Such a language uses 'words' which are similar in form and function to the same words in English and has a highly structured syntax. However, it should be appreciated that the similarity is often more apparent than real, and that the inventor of a computer language is equally likely to 'borrow' an English word and then give it some quite different meaning. For instance, the word FIELD, common to several languages, refers to a memory area into which a patient's name or some numeric value can be placed.

While BASIC is widely used by novices, PASCAL is preferred by experts and the difficult but very flexible 'C' is increasingly used for programming instrumentation applications.

A single high level language command can often perform a very complex task. For example, the BASIC language includes the statement: $y = \text{LOG}(x)$. When executed, this will perform all the manipulations necessary to compute the natural logarithm of a variable x and assign the answer to variable y. This requires many machine code instructions, and literally thousands of micro-instructions, but would occupy but a single step of a written program.

First, the program is prepared in the form of a flow diagram which states what is to be done and in what order. The flow diagram is then used to help the programmer in writing the actual program in a selected language. Many small computers have a built-in language, such as BASIC, which is available whenever the machine is turned on. Other languages must be loaded from some external storage device (such as a disk) before they can be used. Many languages can be used as interpreters, whereby the program is loaded into memory and then executed step by step. At each step the language interpreter converts the command into a sequence of machine code instructions which are themselves executed in sequence. A language compiler translates the entire program into machine code before any execution is possible. Although compilation may be tedious the program will then run much more rapidly than would have been the case with an interpreter.

THE DEDICATED MICROPROCESSOR

A wide range of monitoring instruments contain dedicated microprocessors which perform a wide variety of tasks, ranging from signal processing and self-diagnostic programs to formatting the display and overall management of the instrument. In many cases the user remains unaware that a microprocessor is involved, except that switches and knobs have given way to simple keyboards. Frequently, these make extensive use of the 'soft-key' principle, by which a key may have many functions depending upon the options offered on a screen at any time. This technique allows an instrument to be programmed in many different ways and to offer a wide variety of options to suit individual applications (and clinicians), while having a front panel limited to a screen and four or five keys. Were such a range of options offered on a traditional control panel, it would require literally hundreds of switches, knobs and selectors.

Dedicated processors are used to calculate acid base variables from the outputs of P_{O_2}, P_{CO_2} and pH electrodes (Chapter 18), to calculate cardiac output from indicator dilution curves (Chapter 16) or from the arterial pressure waveform (Wesseling *et al.* 1974). Digital processing is also used for automated ECG analysis, in both off-line diagnostics and real-time, on-line arrhythmia and S–T level monitoring. Several commercial monitoring systems now offer these facilities as standard options.

Electroencephalogram (EEG) signal analysis has been revolutionized by dedicated, real-time digital processing (Simons & Pronk, 1983), and a number of sophisticated systems are now available. They are discussed in more detail in the concluding section of this chapter.

On-line computation is now standard in many pulmonary function analysers, some of which are designed to monitor patients on mechanical ventilators. An entirely new field is that of computed trend analysis in which the analysis of monitored data is used to predict the likelihood of an impending complication.

MICRO- AND MINICOMPUTERS

Bigger problems require bigger processors which can be programmed to perform many functions. Several years ago the term minicomputer was coined to describe all machines smaller than the large mainframe devices. The average minicomputer might have possessed 8–56 kilobyte (kb) storage capacity. The term microcomputer was used to describe the tidal wave of very small (and almost useless) machines which flooded the domestic market. All that has changed. Today, a 'personal' microcomputer is likely to have a storage capacity of some 640 kb with ample capacity for further expansion. Such devices find widespread applications in medical instrumentation. Some systems (such as that required for a cardiac catheterization laboratory) are available complete with a computer already programmed for all the operations required, together with a sophisticated data management system.

The basic architecture of a small computer system is shown in Fig. 5.4. The computer has a

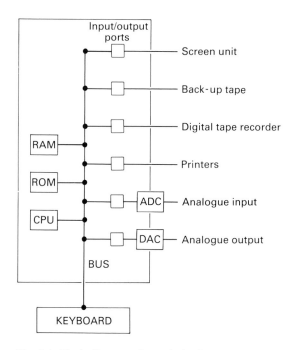

Fig. 5.4. Block diagram of a typical microcomputer with peripherals.

number of integral devices such as keyboard, screen and magnetic disk data storage, as well as peripheral units such as external disk drives and a magnetic tape back-up recorder (often known as a 'tape streamer').

A number of internal 'slots' allow the system to be extended with, for instance, more memory or additional disk drives. External sockets permit access to various types of interface circuit, by which the machine can communicate with other devices (such as measuring instruments)

The heart of the computer is the central processing unit (CPU) which executes all the program instructions. It is connected to other parts of the computer by a parallel 'data bus' which consists of eight, 16 or even 32 parallel data lines, which can transmit information at very high speed. The CPU operates under the control of the instructions held in RAM or ROM.

The CPU is supported by a number of back-up data stores. Random access memory is rapidly accessible but of limited size (the most generally used operating system is only able to address 560 kb of memory) and is used to store both programs and binary data during processing. Information which does not need to be retrieved quite so quickly can be stored in a magnetic disk system. A fixed, or 'hard' disk may contain many megabytes of information any of which can be retrieved within a few milliseconds, but is fixed permanently within its drive and cannot be exchanged for another containing different information. Less urgent data and duplicate backup copies of the program files are recorded on flexible disk or magnetic tape. Flexible disks have the advantage that they can be removed from the drive for storage, and a large library of material may be held in this way. They are, however, limited in capacity (up to 1.2 mb at the time of writing) and have longer read–write access times than fixed disks. Magnetic tape cartridges can have very large capacity, but by their very nature are unsuitable for the rapid retrieval of individual data items. If the primary data are held on magnetic tape, such as might occur in a large database, the tapes must be searched by the computer to pick out the relevant information (e.g. the references on a particular topic in a library retrieval system) and this may

take several minutes, even in a very large system. Tape cartidges are commonly used as data back-up devices, to provide protection against catastrophic failure as may occur if a hard disk 'crashes' during use.

Some peripheral devices (such as a hard magnetic disk) may be connected directly to the data bus. However, many peripherals (such as tape decks and printers) are not fully compatible with the data bus, and so must be connected to it via an interface circuit. This is simply a circuit which converts data bus signals into a form intelligible to the peripheral, and vice versa. It also has to synchronize the two devices, since the peripheral will often operate at a slower rate than the CPU. This was particularly important with early systems, which often relied upon perforated paper tape or even cards as a storage medium.

Today, peripherals such as printers are equipped with large data stores (called buffers). These buffers allow data to be transferred in large blocks at high speed, so that the computer itself need spend very little time communicating with the printer and therefore can continue with other tasks.

The input to the computer may be typed in from a keyboard. A modern keyboard is equipped with a dedicated microprocessor which communicates directly with the main processor. Similarly, the most common output device is the screen unit, which also operates under the control of its own microprocessor.

So far, it has been assumed that the computer is linked directly to the data source. This is said to be on-line operation. This is not always possible, because computers often have several users. In the very simple example of pressure waveform analysis we could, instead, have tape-recorded the voltage waveform and replayed the data into the computer at a more convenient time. This is called off-line, real-time processing, because the computer does not receive the data as it is generated, but does receive it at the original rate. A great deal of computer time can, however, be saved by using time-contraction techniques. The tape recorder is replayed at exactly 4, 8 or 16 times the speed at which it was recorded so that processing takes proportionately less time. This poses few technical problems, since ADC can be performed many thousands of times per second if required, each computation literally taking micro-seconds. It is, of course, necessary to tell the program how fast the tape is going, or dP/dt_{max} will be interpreted as being in the 'bionic' range!

LARGE COMPUTERS

Large computers, such as those to be found in university computing departments, are almost invariably unsuitable for the kind of task we have so far considered, since it is uneconomic for a single user to have uninterrupted access to the CPU. These large machines generally operate on a time-sharing basis, so that a large number of operators, using simple terminals or networked microcomputers, can be served almost at once, the amount of central processor time actually used by each operator being very small.

The time-sharing computer can be likened to a chess grandmaster playing numerous exhibition matches simultaneously. He shares his time between opponents, giving each his undivided attention for a brief period, making a move and then going on to the next opponent who is ready for him. Because he analyses problems so quickly and has a large memory, he can effectively oppose each player almost as if the others were not present.

The time-sharing computer, with its extensive program library and vast storage capability, is of great use to a worker who needs to handle very large quantities of data (such as population statistics), but is of relatively little value to the physiologist who requires on-line data computation. In this application, the microprocessor is likely to reign supreme for many years to come.

EEG Signal processing: an of example progress

Electroencephalogram signals are recorded from a number of electrodes placed in designated positions on the scalp, each channel recording the difference in potential between one pair of electrodes. The EEG waveform represents the integrated activity of a large number of neurones so that the resultant signal is complex and relatively non-specific. Although the signals can be displayed on an oscilloscope it is difficult to analyse such a complex signal during a brief display. On the other hand, recording at normal paper speeds generates so much paper that it is quite unsuitable for clinical monitoring. Many attempts have been made to process the output so that the maximum amount of useful data is compressed into a small space on the record.

A low cost instrument which has been shown to be of practical value is the Cerebral Function Monitor (CFM; see Prior, 1980 for a descriptive review). This instrument utilizes two recording electrodes (one on each parietal region) and a third guard electrode which is situated in the midline anterior to the vertex. The EEG signal is passed through a band-pass filter which restricts the amplification of signals to those within the 2–15 Hz frequency range, thus eliminating many of the problems due to interference from other physiological signals or sources of 50 Hz noise. The signal is further compressed by logarithmic transformation, and then rectified and smoothed to yield a continuous line indicating signal amplitude. A slow-speed, hot-stylus chart recorder displays two traces (Fig. 5.5).

The upper trace shows the signal amplitude signal, with the thickness of the trace indicating the variability in amplitude. Thus increases or decreases in EEG amplitude are shown by upward or downward movement of the trace whilst alterations in trace width indicate changing signal amplitude variability.

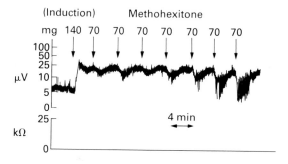

Fig. 5.5. Cortical depression increasing after each increment of methohexitone given at regular time intervals. kΩ: impedance between electrodes in kilo-ohms. (From Dubois *et al.* 1978b.)

The lower trace indicates the electrode impedance and provides a continuous indication of signal validity. Thus artefacts caused by electrode movement are easily distinguished from major physiological events. The recording can be run at speeds as low as $2.5 \, cm \cdot hr^{-1}$ for trend analysis in the Intensive Therapy environment or at $36 \, cm \cdot hr^{-1}$ for monitoring more acute changes in the operating theatre. The instrument is not designed to detect focal activity but has proved useful in monitoring cerebral function in situations in which cerebral perfusion may be impaired (Prior *et al.* 1971; Prior & Maynard, 1986). It has also proved useful in monitoring the response to anaesthetic drugs (Dubois *et al.* 1978a & b).

A more complex approach allowed the frequency content of the signal to be displayed. Here, an analogue frequency analyser used a number of narrow band-pass filters (often known as a comb filter) each of which permitted amplification of signals within a very narrow range of frequencies. The output amplitudes of all the filter channels could then be displayed as a histogram with frequency and intensity on *x*- and *y*-axes respectively.

This approach has been incorporated in a development of the CFM concept; the Cerebral Function Analysing Monitor (CFAM). This presents a similar output to the original CFM but with the addition of a power analyser which displays the output amplitude from four narrow-band filters corresponding to the classical EEG frequency groups ($\delta, \theta, \alpha, \beta$). It thus combines the functions of the original device and those of a simple power spectrum analyser (Sebel *et al.* 1983).

From this crude technique evolved the compressed spectral array (CSA). Using a computer program, Fourier analysis of a recorded epoch yields a power density function (Bickford *et al.* 1971). This can be plotted as a power spectrum, with frequency on the *x*-axis and power on the *y*-axis. A large number of such spectra are shown on the same plot, with successive determinations blanking out the previous ones. The resulting image looks rather like a range of mountains (Fig. 5.6), with the spectra for the previous epochs shown above and behind the more recent ones.

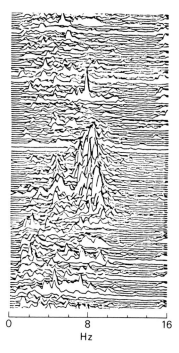

Fig. 5.6. Computer print out of sequential analysis of the EEG. The most recent data is at the bottom of the display.

Using the CSA technique it is possible to display patterns of change in the frequency components of the EEG over any desired period of time. Since the display contains much more information it is more likely to detect ischaemic changes than the CFM (Smith & Rampil, 1983).

Originally, these techniques demanded the use of large computers and were therefore limited to the research laboratory (Smith, 1978). However, the recent development of a single integrated circuit capable of very fast Fourier analysis has made the technique commercially feasible, and a number of instruments are available.

Further development of fast Fourier analysis has enabled complex arrays of EEG channels to be analysed simultaneously (i.e. in parallel), and the information presented as a spatial map on a computer screen using different colours to denote spectral densities.

Many investigators have pursued the idea that the EEG signal must contain information regarding the 'depth of anaesthesia'. The tendency for the frequency power spectrum to shift leftwards with deepening unconsciousness has attracted a good deal of attention, and several indices of this shift have been developed. Of these, the best established are the median frequency and the spectral edge. Both measures are statistical descriptors of the power spectrum: median frequency is that at which equal power density lies above and below that frequency, while spectral edge is that frequency at which some small fraction (usually 5%) of the spectral power density lies above that frequency. The use of processed EEG signals in the assessment of depth of anaesthesia is discussed in greater detail in Chapter 24.

A glossary of computer terms

Algorithm A fixed step-by-step procedure for accomplishing a given task. It is often defined in algebraic terms.

Alphanumeric Alphabetical and numerical symbols.

Analogue signal A continuously varying signal whose magnitude is proportional to that of some stated variable.

Assembly language Program instructions in the form of symbols or mnemonics which are then (very rapidly) converted into machine code by the computer. This is very useful for writing routines which must be executed both often and very rapidly.

Baud One byte per second.

Bit A contraction of 'binary digit'. It always has the value 1 or 0.

Byte A sequence of bits processed as a unit. This will contain a binary number, to which is added a number of further bits for error checking and correction. Some small computers use 8-bit bytes, but 16 bits have become commonplace and some 32-bit machines are now available. Since all the bits are processed simultaneously, 32-bit machines can usually handle data much more rapidly than 8-bit devices.

Character A digit, letter or symbol.

Compiler A program which converts high level language statements into machine code. These can be executed very much more rapidly than the same program written in the same language but executed by an interpreter.

Central Processing Unit (CPU) The section of the computer which controls the operations of the other parts.

Disk storage A data storage medium on which data are stored on a number of concentric circular tracks on magnetic disks. These rotate at high speed and give direct access. 'Floppy' disks are cheaper, slower and less capacious than 'fixed' disks, but can be removed for storage.

Hardware The physical components of a computer system such as the CPU, keyboard, memory and peripheral devices.

Hybrid computer A computer which solves problems using both analogue and digital hardware.

High level language A programming language orientated to the natural language of the programmer. Each instruction generates a number of machine code instructions.

Interface The part of a device which 'communicates' with other devices. Interface circuits are needed to ensure that connections between the devices conform to some common standard. The commonest interface used by monitoring instruments is the RS232 type, which transmits data from one device to another in serial form, thus requiring only very few wires. Parallel interfaces (such as IEEE) are much faster but require more wiring and can operate over short distances only.

Interpreter A method by which each instruction of a high level programming language (such as BASIC) is converted to machine code immediately prior to execution of that instruction. This is very convenient during program development but causes the program to run very slowly. When large computations are required it is more conventional to convert the entire program to machine code before execution (see compiler).

Local Area Network (LAN) A system by which a number of computers are inter-linked so that programs and data can be freely exchanged. It also enables messages ('electronic mail') to be passed between users.

Machine language The lowest-level computer language, each instruction using a numerical code to describe the operation or the location of data.

Memory The part of the computer which stores information for use by the central processing unit. The memory consists of a large number of semiconductor binary cells, mounted in integrated circuits. Some types of memory lose data when the power is switched off, and are known as volatile memory.

Off-line Not directly connected to the computer; not operating simultaneously with the computer.

On-line Equipment or function in the system connected directly to the computer.

Operating system A program which controls the movement of information to and from the disk drive(s). In most small computers, this must be loaded before any other programs can be read from disk. Most small computers use DOS or CPM, while larger machines use UNIX.

Printers Hard copy of computer outputs can be achieved using a variety of technologies. A *'Daisy wheel'* printer has a print head which travels across the page, one line at a time, carrying a plastic print-wheel which has a number of characters embossed around its circumference. As the head moves across the page a 'hammer' strikes the print-wheel such that the embossed characters impact through a conventional typewriter ribbon to create corresponding character images on the paper. Such printers are slow, noisy, restricted in capability and nowadays restricted to very low-cost systems.

The print head of a *dot matrix impact* printer scans across the page carrying an array of steel pins which strike the paper through a conventional typewriter ribbon. As the head moves to each horizontal position an encoded signal activates some or all of the pins to create an image on the paper. A number of such images, set very close together, are necessary to create each complete alphanumeric character.

The *ink-jet* printer uses a similar scanning concept, but here the print head carries an array of *very* fine nozzles through which ink can be projected directly onto the paper. These are generally faster and less noisy than dot matrix impact printers, and create a superior image. The cost-per-page is, however, considerably greater. The *laser* printer provides, without doubt, the best technology available at the time of writing. An electrostatic 'image' is placed on a drum by a scanning laser. Carbon powder adheres (or not) according to the distribution of electrical charge, and is then rolled directly onto the paper. This is simply a development of the familiar xerographic process used by most photocopiers. This method has the advantages of silence, speed and very fine resolution over all other technologies.

Program A set of instructions which tells the computer how to execute a specific task. These may be direct instructions in machine code or higher level mnemonic instructions which themselves control a series of machine-code instructions. High level instructions from a programming language (such as BASIC, PASCAL or FORTRAN) may execute a very large number of processor operations.

Random Access Memory (RAM) Areas of computer memory available for data to be written or read at high speed. Memory areas are directly addressed, so that the time taken to access information does not depend on the location of that information.

Read Only Memory (ROM) Areas of computer memory from which data can be read, but unavailable for data storage. Every computer contains large areas of ROM, which contain essential information for the basic running of the machine. Some computers carry complete operating systems and high level languages in ROM, so that they are instantly available at switch-on.

Real-time Processing of data by a computer sufficiently rapidly for events to be detected or influenced as they occur.

Routine Part of a program, often compiled as an individual section of code, which can be 'called' by the main program when required. In languages such as FORTRAN and PASCAL many such routines lie in highly structured libraries within the programming environment.

Software The programs associated with a computer system. Some of these are provided by the manufacturer, and may be integrated into the computer design but others are written to deal with specific problems.

WORM drive Acronym signifying Write Once, Read Many times. A large-volume non-volatile data storage device based on laser-disk technology (see p. 90).

References

Bickford, R.G., Fleming, N. & Billinger, T.H. (1971) Compression of EEG data. *Transactions of the American Neurological Association* **96**, 118–122.

Dubois, M., Scott, D.F. & Savege, T.M. (1978a) Assessment of recovery from short anaesthesia using the cerebral function monitor. *British Journal of Anaesthesia* **50**, 825–832.

Dubois, M., Savege, T.M., O'Caroll, T.M. & Frank, M. (1978b) General anaesthesia and changes in the cerebral function monitor. *Anaesthesia* **33**, 157–64.

Fukui, Y. & Smith, N.T. (1981a) Interactions among ventilation, the circulation, and the uptake and distribution of halothane — use of a hybrid computer multiple model: I. the basic model. *Anesthesiology* **54**, 107–118.

Fukui, Y. & Smith, N.T. (1981b) Interactions among ventilation, the circulation, and the uptake and distribution of halothane — use of a hybrid computer multiple model: II. Spontaneous vs. controlled ventilation and the effect of CO_2. *Anesthesiology* **54**, 119–124.

Hull, C.J. & McLeod, K. (1976). Pharmacokinetic analysis using an electrical analogue. *British Journal of Anaesthesia* **48**, 677–686.

Prior, P. (1980) Noninvasive monitoring of cerebral function. *British Journal of Clinical Equipment* **5**(2), 54–63.

Prior, P.F. & Maynard, D.E. (1986) *Monitoring cerebral function. Long term monitoring of EEG and evoked potentials*, 2nd edn. Elsevier Biomedical, Amsterdam.

Prior, P.F., Maynard, D.E., Sheaff, P.C., Simpson, B.R., Strunin, L., Weaver, E.J.M. & Scott, D.E. (1971) Monitoring cerebral function: clinical experience with a new device for continuous recording of electrical activity of brain. *British Medical Journal* **ii**, 736–738.

Sebel, P.S., Maynard, D.E., Mayor, E. & Frank, M. (1983) The cerebral function analysing monitor (CFAM). *British Journal of Anaesthesia* **55**, 1265–1270.

Simons, A.J.R. and Pronk, R.A.F. (1983) Automatic EEG monitoring during anesthesia. In Prakash, O. (ed.) *Computing in anesthesia and intensive care*, pp. 227–257. Martinus Nijhoff, Boston.

Smith, N.T. (1978) Computers in anesthesia. In Saidman, L.J. and Smith, N.T. (eds) *Monitoring in anesthesia*, Chapter 13. New York, John Wiley & Sons, New York.

Smith, N.T. and Rampil, I.S. (1983) The use of computer generated numbers in interpreting the EEG. pp. 214–226. In Prakash, O. (ed.), *Computing in anesthesia and intensive care*. Martinus Nijhoff, Boston.

Wesseling, K.H., Smith, N.T., Nicholas, W.W., Weber, H., de Wit, B. & Benekin, J.E.W. (1974) Beat to beat cardiac output from the arterial pressure contour. In: Feldman, S.A., Leigh, J.M. & Spierdijk, J. (eds), *Measurement in anaesthesia*, pp. 150–164. University Press, Leiden.

6: Displaying the Signal

Types of display

In the early years of clinical measurement most biological signals were processed by analogue methods and displayed by a mechanical pointer on a scale or a moving 'spot' on a cathode-ray tube (CRT). However, the micro-processor has revolutionized signal management such that systems based upon analogue technology are disappearing rapidly. Microprocessors with their associated storage elements require much less maintenance, retain their accuracy longer and have much greater inherent flexibility than analogue devices.

However, the human brain is accustomed to receiving analogue information. We are accustomed to judging the height, width, weight, heat or brightness of objects in our physical world in terms of comparative scales rather than numeric values. For instance we look at a tree and instantly assess its height by comparison with other trees or buildings: gauging its height in feet or metres requires a conscious effort.

Thus it is with physiological measuring instruments. A measured variable, such as temperature, has two distinct attributes; a *numeric value* (such as 36.8 °C) and a *comparison* with some intuitive scale of acceptability. Thus a digital presentation would express the value but nothing more, but an analogue display might show the temperature as a point on a vertical scale, on which the average normal value (say 37.4 °C) appears with an indication of some preset range of acceptable values (Fig. 6.1).

Clearly, the analogue display contains more information and also conveys a sense of physiological significance.

The true significance of a measurement can often be assessed only by comparison with previous values. Trend graphs are a popular method of presenting historical information, and form another type of analogue display. However, some information is best conveyed in digital form; the output of a blood gas analyser is a good example. The array of numeric values *could* be presented in analogue form, but the clinician considers such information in numeric terms and therefore prefers to see digits rather than graphs.

In a number of cases a single display medium can be used to present information in a variety of ways. In order to avoid repetition, this chapter considers first a range of display types, with emphasis upon communication rather than technology. In a following section the physical techniques are described in more detail.

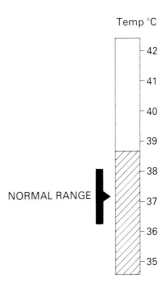

Fig. 6.1. Temperature scale showing normal value and physiological limits.

ANALOGUE DISPLAYS

In scientific terms, an analogue signal is one in which a variable (such as pressure) is represented by some physical quantity whose amplitude (such the deflection of a pointer) represents that of the input variable. Alternatively, the variable could be represented by the number of lights in an illuminated array. Such a *scalar* display is of particular use when it is desirable to indicate whether the signal is within or outside the normal range. By choosing an appropriate scale length for each variable and colour coding the scale in segments for the high, normal and low ranges, an observer is able to monitor many displays simultaneously and quickly identify an aberrant reading. Screen displays (such as a cathode-ray oscilloscope) can provide a continuous indication of the variable, and are easily visible from a distance or in poor lighting conditions. They are of particular value for dynamic signals (such as electrocardiographic or arterial pressure) where the waveform itself is of diagnostic value. Modern screen displays often contain several types of information; thus a dynamic pressure waveform may be accompanied by current *numeric* values of systolic and diastolic pressure and a trend display of mean arterial pressure over the past hour.

Scalar display

The scale may be linear or curvilinear, and the signal may be displayed directly or by electronic means. The simplest example of a direct linear display is that produced by the mercury column in a mercury-in-glass thermometer or sphygmomanometer, or by a rotameter bobbin. Electronic forms of display became essential if the signal is to be processed before presentation to the clinician.

The simplest electrical device is the moving-coil or moving-iron meter, whose pointer takes up a position on a physical scale in proportion to the applied current. This type of display is useful when the signal does not fluctuate too rapidly, and the user wishes to be able to extract such information as peak value with minimal complexity; such variables as heart rate and airway CO_2 concentration can be shown in this way. However, the meter has a number of disadvantages, such as fragility,

non-linearity, limited viewing angle and the need for an analogue input signal.

The electronic bargraph

New techniques have displaced the electrical meter except in a few very specialized applications. In its simplest form, a row of light bulbs can be arranged to form a bargraph. If one end is regarded as zero, a column of illuminated bulbs indicates the magnitude of some variable. For example, an ECG signal can be used to determine the heart rate and the value displayed by showing an illuminated column beside a linear scale. In a more complex application a dynamic blood pressure signal may be analysed to yield systolic and diastolic pressures, and an illuminated bar used to indicate the pulse pressure against a 0–300 mmHg scale. This type of presentation is familiar to doctors and nurses and high/low limit indicators can be added very easily.

Since the bargraph display is composed of discrete elements, it is necessary for the variable to be represented by a linear array of transistors, each responsible for switching a single display element on and off. The on/off signal to each transistor is easily decoded from a digital byte (see Chapter 5). As a display element the simple light bulb has obvious disadvantages, such as high power consumption and a short lifetime. However, new technologies have overcome this limitation and the electronic bargraph is now widely used as a means of presenting scalar information. The first satisfactory device was composed of light-emitting diodes (LEDs) arranged as a linear array. Later developments have made use of liquid crystal, gas discharge and electrofluorescent techniques, and examples are now commonplace in clinical monitoring.

Screen displays of analogue information

Many signals, such as the ECG, require dynamic waveform display. This is most efficiently done using a screen-based device such as the cathode-ray oscilloscope, where the horizontal axis represents time and the vertical axis signal magnitude. Other techniques can also be used; small screens using liquid crystal and electrofluorescent technologies are becoming available.

To an increasing extent the oscilloscope screen is used to display the contents of digital memory stores. In this application the information may be presented in an analogue form, but the technology is entirely digital.

Screen displays can also be used to present trend information. Here, digital signal processing and storage is used to construct an on-screen graph representing the changing value of some variable over a specified period.

DIGITAL DISPLAYS

In many situations, such as the simple electronic thermometer, digital displays are required. Numeric digits may be generated by gas-filled tubes, LEDs, liquid crystal or electrofluorescent devices, displayed on a screen or printed on paper. Obviously, the number of digits available must cover the range and accuracy required. Digital displays can convey more information in a given area than many other forms of display but are often difficult to read when viewing conditions are poor and are not suitable for rapidly changing signals. This type of display eliminates errors due to faulty scale reading, but may introduce others, by, for example, incorrectly identifying the position of a decimal point.

Physical principles of display devices

THE ELECTRICAL METER

The magnitude of a signal can be displayed on an electrical meter. Most meters operate on the principle of the moving-coil galvanometer, which consists of a coil of wire suspended in a magnetic field (Fig. 6.2).

When current is passed through the coil a force is generated which tends to rotate the coil to a different position in the field. This force is opposed by a spring, so that the degree of rotation of the coil is proportional to the applied current. The pivot upon which the coil is mounted is coupled to a pointer, such that it moves against a scale. Since meters are usually used for the display of slowly changing signals, the mass of the moving parts is not critical and a large coil can be used to increase sensitivity.

The movement of a coil may also be displayed

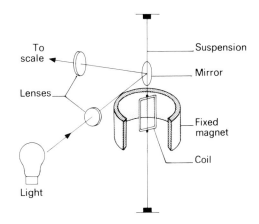

Fig. 6.2. Moving-coil galvonometer using a light source and a mirror to display the signal on a translucent scale.

by shining a narrow beam of light onto a small mirror attached to the coil. The reflected beam is then directed onto a translucent scale. The use of a mirror allows the mass of the moving parts of the instrument to be greatly reduced and so increases the frequency response (p. 87). Furthermore by increasing the length of the light path, usually by reflecting the light back and forth between a system of fixed mirrors, it is possible to increase greatly the sensitivity of the system. Mirror galvanometers are commonly used when it is desired to obtain maximum sensitivity and speed of response. The movement of the light beam can also be recorded by directing it onto a moving photographic film or onto special paper which is sensitive to ultraviolet light (see Chapter 7).

THE CRT (OSCILLOSCOPE)

This form of display is very widely used, since it can convey information in analogue or digital form and can present both rapidly and slowly changing signals with equal facility. It is almost the only type of display capable of presenting very high frequency signals.

Usually, the variable is displayed on the y-axis with time on the x-axis but for some purposes (for example, pressure–volume loops or vectorcardiography) a second variable is applied to the x-axis so that a two-dimensional shape is described on the screen.

There are two types of CRT, electrostatic and electro-magnetic. The electrostatic type is the standard laboratory instrument used to display high frequency analogue signals on a relatively small screen, whilst the electromagnetic tube is employed when a high velocity electron beam is required to produce a bright display over a large area, for example in television and radar receivers. Both types of tube consist of a glass cylinder with a conical or tetrahedral expansion at one end. The narrow part of the glass tube contains an electron 'gun'. This consists of a heated cathode which generates a stream of electrons, a cylindrical grid which controls the intensity of the electron beam (and hence the brightness of the display), and a series of positively-charged anodes which accelerate the beam and focus it onto a fluorescent coating which lines the flat surface at the expanded end of the tube. The electron stream makes the coating fluoresce and a bright 'spot' is seen from outside the tube (Fig. 6.3a). Between the anodes and the screen there is mounted some means of deflecting the electron beam in the x- and y-axes.

Electrostatic deflection

In the *electrostatic* tube the deflection is produced by applying potentials to two pairs of deflection plates situated within the tube. One pair of plates is mounted horizontally and deflects the beam in a vertical direction (y-plates) whilst the other pair is mounted vertically and deflects the spot horizontally (x-plates). Normally a potential from a special time-base circuit is applied to the x-plates. This potential resembles a saw-tooth waveform, since it increases linearly until some preset voltage is reached, then falls abruptly to zero. When this waveform is applied to the x-plates the spot is drawn at a constant rate from left to right across the screen and then suddenly returned to the left side again before commencing another sweep. If an input voltage is now applied to the y-plates, an image representing signal amplitude versus time will be produced, thus re-creating the original analogue input signal. When desired the time-base can be switched off and a second input signal applied to the x-plates; an x–y graphical plot then appears.

Electromagnetic deflection

Electromagnetic tubes are designed to produce much larger images which require correspondingly greater beam deflection angles. In an electrostatic tube such deflections would require impossibly large deflection plate voltages, so some alternative deflection system is required. This is accomplished by electromagnetic deflector coils situated *outside* the tube and mounted between the focus coils and the second anode (Fig. 6.3b).

Multiple trace CRT displays

Both types of display can be used to display more than one input signal on the y-axis.

Multiple y-inputs to an electrostatic system can be displayed by utilizing several separate beams of electrons (each from its own gun) and deflecting each beam independently. However, this makes the equipment bulky and expensive. More commonly a single electron gun is used in association with a beam-switching technique which causes each input

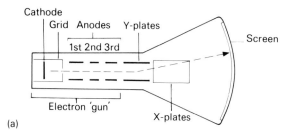

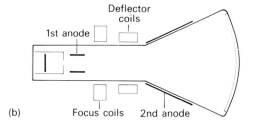

Fig. 6.3. (a) Electrostatic CRT. (b) Electromagnetic CRT.

to be sampled in turn. Each input channel is associated with a certain value of 'y-shift' so that the time-base deflection corresponding to it is located at a certain height on the tube face, the rate of switching between channels being designed to maintain an adequate quality of signal on each trace. Thus a switching rate of at least 10 kHz would be adequate to display concurrently four signals each having a frequency of 1 kHz. (This beam switching can often be identified on the trace when the writing speed is high, for the trace then appears as a series of dots.) At the end of each horizontal traverse of the screen the spot must return to its starting position. Since this would produce an interfering image on the screen, the electron beam is normally switched off temporarily. The same technique is used to suppress unwanted images while the beam is switching between channels. This change in intensity (properly called *z-modulation*) is synchronized with both beam switching and the resetting of the time-base and is known as *fly-back blanking*.

The speed of deflection in an electromagnetic tube is slower than in an electrostatic tube, and this limits the degree to which beams can be 'split' to display more than one input signal. Instead, a 'raster' type of display is used. Here the electron beam is repeatedly moved in a very fine zig-zag pattern over the whole screen, the actual display being generated by altering the brightness of the spot as it moves vertically or horizontally across the screen. This technique permits complex displays (including alphanumeric characters) to be generated, and the frequency of signal that can be handled is a function of the number of times that the spot can cover the screen each second.

In the simplest application (for example, the display of an electrocardiogram (ECG) signal) a vertical raster can be moved across the screen at such a speed that the horizontal movement is equivalent to the paper speed of a direct recorder. As the beam moves up the screen on each raster line the intensity is kept switched off until the raster voltage equals that of the signal. It is then briefly turned on and off so that the screen glows at that point. Successive raster sweeps thus gradually build up a waveform, which can have any number

of traces so long as they all move at the same speed. In this type of display a long-persistence phosphor is essential: this is usually chosen so that the beginning of the trace has disappeared by the time the raster returns to the left-hand side of the screen.

In more advanced systems, such as the visual display unit (VDU) of a computer, the whole raster pattern fills the screen many times a second, the spot modulation being controlled by the computer. This type of display will be considered in more detail in a following section.

Colour CRT displays

In many modern display units there are three guns, as in a colour television tube. Three electron beams traverse the tube in close proximity, so that the magnetic deflection coils affect them all equally. The phosphor is no longer homogeneous, but consists of innumerable groups of three different phosphor materials which fluoresce red, blue or green. Each beam is gated electronically as it traverses the screen, such that it falls only upon one phosphor type and thereby produces a spot of only one primary colour. Because each group of three phosphor dots is so minute, the viewer's eye integrates their emitted light into a single colour: that which represents the 'colour by addition' of the three primary colour spots. Obviously, any desired colour can be produced by suitable adjustment of three beam intensities. Colour displays require sophisticated signal processing, so that they are limited to applications where a computer is responsible for data management; in many cases this is a dedicated processor within an instrument or system.

The storage oscilloscope

Several different principles are employed to permit retention of the image. One type is known as a direct-view bistable storage tube. This is illustrated in Fig. 6.4.

This tube contains two electron guns. In the narrow part of the tube there is a writing gun which can be focused and deflected as in a conventional electrostatic or electromagnetic CRT. The second

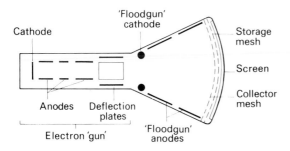

Fig. 6.4. Bistable storage CRT.

cathode, generating electrons for a 'flood' function, is usually annular in shape and situated at the narrow end of the conical part of the tube. Electrons emanating from this gun are collimated by an electrode in the conical part of the tube (often a carbon coating on the inside of the tube itself) so that they form a wide parallel beam of equal density which floods the screen with electrons. Parallel to the screen and close to it are two fine wire meshes, the storage mesh and the collector mesh. The side of the storage mesh remote from the screen is coated with an insulating material which has good secondary emission characteristics. When this material is bombarded with fast-moving electrons it emits more electrons than it receives and so becomes positively charged.

The image on the 'screen' is created by the stream of fast-moving electrons from the writing gun. These electrons impinge on the storage mesh and displace electrons so that the written area is positively charged with respect to the rest of the mesh. Meanwhile the flood gun showers the whole area of the screen with low velocity electrons which have inadequate energy to cause secondary emission. These areas therefore become negatively charged and cease to attract further electrons from the flood gun, the electrons being accelerated instead to the positively charged, 'written' areas. Their velocity is high enough for them to penetrate the storage mesh and so to cause persistence of the image on the screen. This image tends to fade if storage periods are more than about 10 min because the rest of the screen tends to brighten gradually with time. This brightening is caused by leakage of electrons across the insulator surface and

by bombardment with positively charged ions formed within the tube. However, this can be prevented by switching off the flood gun when continued viewing is not required. The image can be erased completely by applying a single positive pulse to the storage mesh. It is also possible to carry out a continuous erase by applying a succession of smaller pulses so that the image fades at a controlled rate (so-called *variable persistence*). This type of display is much used in the radar field, since moving objects appear as a trail with a bright head and fading tail, whilst stationary objects remain uniformly bright as their image is up-dated by each sweep of the writing gun. In the medical field storage tubes are often used for the display of images built up from the output of a gamma camera or ultrasonic imaging device.

Permanent records from an oscilloscope screen

The display on an oscilloscope screen can be photographed with a Polaroid or standard camera or the time-base can be switched off and the vertical deflection of the spot recorded on a photographic film moving in the horizontal plane. Cathode-ray tubes with a fibre-optic face plate produce an image which is bright enough to record directly onto ordinary photographic paper (see p. 112). However, it is often more convenient to photograph the image on a storage oscilloscope.

The 'digital' oscilloscope

If an ECG signal is fed into an ADC, and the resulting stream of numbers then stored in a digital memory large enough to contain all the data arriving during a period of several (say 10) seconds, that digital memory can be 'replayed' very rapidly through a DAC and thence to the y-axis amplifier of an oscilloscope. If this 'replay' is synchronized with the equally rapid movement of a raster across the screen, an image representing all the data in the store (i.e. 10 s of ECG signal) appears on the screen. However, because of short phosphor persistence this fades almost immediately. If the raster 'refreshes' the screen by repeating the process 10 times per second a static, relatively flicker-free display of the ECG record will be displayed. At higher refresh rates (well above the flicker–fusion frequency of the observer), flicker can be eliminated altogether. If, now, the process of reading from the store is slightly desynchronized with respect to the raster movement, the information at any specific storage location is displayed very slightly earlier in the progress of the raster across the screen with each pass and therefore appears to move to the left. Consequently, the stored ECG complexes appear to move smoothly across the screen. If *new* ECG data is written over the oldest data in the store at the same rate as the trace 'moves', the appearance takes on that of an endless strip of paper passing across the screen. An alternative approach is to keep the ECG complexes static, in which case a vertical 'cursor' passes repeatedly across the screen from left to right, erasing old data and leaving new data to its left. Surprisingly, there are those who prefer this curious arrangement.

The display can be 'frozen' at any desired moment to facilitate recognition of individual ECG complexes, and the DAC can be connected to a conventional direct writing recorder to produce a record of the current screen display. The digital information can also be passed to a computer for further processing or storage.

Mapped graphic displays

Many newer devices — especially computer screens — have 'bit-mapped graphic screens'. The CRT viewing area is organized into a very large number of minute areas, called *pixels*. Each lies in a specific place on the screen and corresponds to a specific location in the computer memory. Some 25 times a second, the computer scans the entire 'screen map' as the raster spot scans the physical screen itself. As the raster spot reaches each pixel location the computer map determines whether the spot shall 'bright-up' or not. As a result, a flicker-free display of uniform brightness can be generated. Since the entire display is refreshed many times a second a very short-persistence phosphor is used. Clearly, the complexity of the display is limited only by the resolution of the screen map and the

speed at which the computer can alter it in response to incoming data. Not only can multiple traces be shown, but they may 'move' at individual rates and can be combined with alphanumeric data on the same screen area.

A colour screen requires more memory for its 'map', since colour information must be added to the existing attributes of position and brightness.

NEW DISPLAY TECHNOLOGIES

The oscilloscope screen is large, expensive, clumsy, fragile, dangerous and power-hungry. It continues to survive for one reason only; no-one has (yet) invented anything better for the presentation of complex information. However, there are new technologies struggling to compete, especially since a powerful computer can be put in a case the size of a cigarette packet and run from a small battery. Such computers demand display systems which are cheap, economical, rugged and, above all, portable.

Many small instruments do not require large, complex displays; they need only some means of showing one or two alphanumeric messages which indicate the current value of some measured quantity and perhaps a single, slowly changing dynamic variable. A capnograph is a good example of this type of requirement.

A variety of devices have been developed, each of which has advantages and disadvantages.

Gas-filled indicator tubes

The first digital displays were provided by a gas-filled filament indicator. Inside a glass envelope (similar in appearance to an old-fashioned radio valve) was mounted a complex array of filaments, each in the shape of a numeric character. When a current was passed through an individual filament the surrounding gas glowed (more or less) brightly and the character became visible. A number of such tubes could be mounted in a row to present a multi-digit number. An irritating feature of such tubes was that the displayed characters did not all appear in the same plane, since physical separation of the filaments was essential. A further disadvantage was that high voltages were necessary. The gas-filled tube has evolved into the modern 'plasma' display (see below).

Segmented display units

An important development was the concept of a *segmented character* (Fig. 6.5).

Any numeric digit can be created by illuminating some elements of a seven-segment array. For instance, the digit 1 requires two segments to be visible while the digit 8 requires all seven. If a full range of English characters are to be displayed, larger arrays (often with 14 segments) are required. Several different techniques have been used to illuminate the segments.

Fig. 6.5. Seven-segment numeric display.

Light-emitting diodes (LEDs)

The simplest makes use of the light-emitting properties of some semiconductor materials. Most devices are based upon gallium arsenide technology and are often referred to as GAs diodes. Light-emitting diodes are cheap, easily fabricated into segmental arrays and operate from the same low voltages as microprocessors, etc. They can be made to emit light at a variety of wavelengths. They are most useful where physically small digits are acceptable, since power consumption can be high if bright, 1 inch high characters are required.

Gas discharge displays

The segmented display can be implemented using gas-discharge devices. These are cold-cathode, gas-filled tubes, whose elements can be excited by anode voltages of some 180 V. They have great advantages over LED displays by virtue of much greater size and brightness. However, the need for 180 V power supplies makes them uneconomic unless an instrument requires a number of digit-only displays.

The gas discharge principle has recently been developed further to produce the so-called 'plasma' display tube. By mounting rows of wire electrodes immediately behind a flat screen face, with those in the '*X*' plane separated from those in the '*Y*' plane, an exciting voltage between one wire in the '*X*' plane and one in the '*Y*' plane will produce a bright spot at their intersection. By scanning the electrode arrays many times a second using an electronic decoder, a non-flickering display can be produced, with characters made up from patterns of 'spots' or, more correctly, pixels. Since this type of display panel is bright and clear with a wide viewing angle, it is increasingly used in the manufacture of portable computers.

Liquid crystal (LC) displays

The LC cell is cheap, safe and requires very little motive power. Not surprisingly, it has revolutionized the small instrument market. The cell consists of a thin layer of LC sandwiched between glass plates and connected to two electrodes. Normally transparent, the crystal changes its physical structure when subjected to a minute electrical current such that it appears black when viewed at 90°. Such cells can be very small, and early examples were usually seven-segment digital arrays which could be driven by suitable electronics to create numeric digits. A number of such devices could be placed side-by-side to display large numbers. As the technology improved it became possible to construct an LC screen display, consisting of many hundreds of LC cells in an array which could be addressed by a microprocessor. Since each cell is addressed individually it can be treated by the computer as a pixel and driven, in a similar manner to the plasma display, by suitable scanning electronics.

For good visibility the display panel must be well illuminated and viewed from the correct angle.

In its simplest form, an LC display panel is silvered on its rear surface so that reflected light, passing forward through the cells, creates the image. The back-lit LC display has a low intensity electroluminescent panel mounted immediately behind the liquid crystal sandwich. This device is much more tolerant of wide viewing angles than the front-lit panel, with greatly improved visibility. Very recently, devices known as *super-twisted nematic* LC displays have appeared; these offer even better contrast and greatly increased viewing angle. The main limitations of the LC display are that it is *very* slow by comparison with an oscilloscope, relatively intolerant of viewing angle and is (as yet) only available in monochrome. However, it *does* require very little power and can be built into small portable instruments without difficulty. These advantages have made it an attractive option to the designers of pulse oximeters and capnographs where the (relatively) slow signal can be accommodated without difficulty.

The electro-fluorescent indicator

This very recent development is based upon the same physical principle as the cathode-ray oscilloscope.

A directly heated, oxide-coated tungsten cathode is mounted in an evacuated glass envelope. As in the CRT, electrons are accelerated towards a positively-charged, phosphor-coated anode. However, because the distances are very small, only 12–40 V are required as compared with several hundred volts in a CRT. The anode phosphor is shaped such that when excited by the electron stream it becomes visible as a character segment or pixel dot. A thin metal mesh is placed between cathode and anode, and biased with a low negative voltage. This allows accelerating electrons to pass through but traps any low-velocity stray electrons. This prevents stray electrons from the cathode from causing a 'background glow' on the anode phosphor. A number of anodes can be mounted very close together to create coherent images. These fluorescent devices are available as segmented alphanumeric displays, bargraphs and even matrix screen arrays.

Hard copy displays

For slow analogue signals it is possible to use any of the recorder systems outlined in Chapter 7 as display systems. Some flat-bed recorders have an additional facility which permits separate signals to be recorded on the *x*- and *y*-axes, the paper being kept stationary. These are useful for recording shapes like pressure-flow or pressure–volume loops. By an extension of this principle it is possible to display results in graphical form, each point being printed at the appropriate intersection of the *x*- and *y*-axis.

CHOICE AND POSITION OF DISPLAY DEVICES

It is crucially important that in any application the most effective form of information display is chosen. Choosing the wrong type may lead to inadequate data presentation, an increased likelihood of errors due to data misinterpretation and increased strain on the observer. Although instrument manufacturers have greatly improved the quality of display systems, it is still possible to find examples of bad design where otherwise excellent instruments do not convey information to the user in the most effective way.

Portable instruments are limited to display systems which do not rapidly drain batteries, so that despite their limitations liquid crystal devices are often used. Instruments which always operate from mains power supplies may use a variety of systems. Those which have very simple outputs, such as one or two digital numbers, will usually depend upon LC, LED, plasma or electroluminescent displays, but instruments with more complex outputs are likely to have oscilloscope screens which can convey information of all types, given suitable control electronics.

Display units should be placed in situations where they are easily visible to the appropriate observer, but not to the patient, and lighting conditions should be adjusted so that the display stands out clearly from the background. It is often difficult to achieve such conditions in the hospital environment but strenuous efforts should be made to do so, for the patient's life may depend on the presentation of accurate information to the observer in a form which he or she can most readily assimilate.

7: Recorders and Data Storage Devices

A recorder may be defined as a device which stores information in a durable form. This may be a hard copy image (i.e. on paper) or a non-volatile record on some storage medium from which the information can be retrieved when required (Cashman 1980).

Recorders

There are four main types of recorders:

1 Signal recorders and plotters which make a direct imprint onto paper by means of an ink pen or jet (Figs. 7.1 and 7.2).

2 Photographic or ultraviolet recorders, in which an impression is made by a beam of white or ultraviolet light onto photosensitive paper (Fig. 7.3).

3 Digitally controlled printers and plotters which create permanent images under the control of a computer. These devices require the data to be digitized and then encoded into a form which is suitable for the output device concerned.

4 Tape recorders, using direct analogue or frequency modulation (FM) techniques. Unlike direct analogue tape recorders, FM devices can accept very low frequency or even direct current (d.c.) signals; this is particularly useful when recording signals from pressure transducers, etc. Frequency modulation recorders can replay data directly into pen or ultraviolet recorders when a hard copy is required. When the recorded signals contain a wide range of frequencies, the tape may be replayed at a much lower speed than that used for recording. This reduces the frequencies by the ratio of tape speeds and therefore allows the use of a pen recorder with restricted frequency response.

Digital data storage devices

It is becoming commonplace to store digital data, especially when generated by computers, on bulk-storage devices from which they may be retrieved at some later time. Such devices have similar functions to recorders, and may be described as such. The technologies involved include magnetic

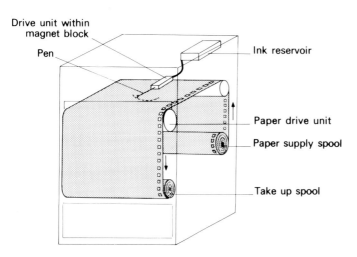

Fig. 7.1. A simple pen recorder.

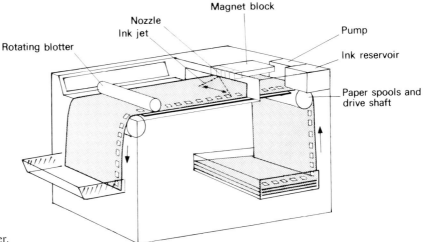

Fig. 7.2. An ink-jet recorder.

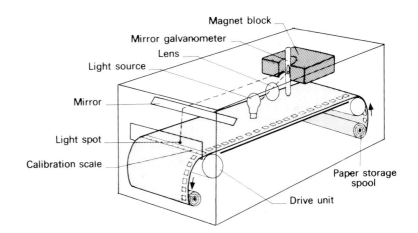

Fig. 7.3. An ultraviolet galvanometer recorder.

disk, magnetic tape, WORM drives (Write Once, Read Many times optical disk storage) or Bernouilli effect (magnetic bubble) devices.

Suitability of recorders for specific applications

The choice of recorder is determined mainly by the range of frequencies which comprise the signal which is to be recorded. The frequency components of some typical biological signals are shown in Table 7.1.

It may be seen that they vary from a steady current or voltage (d.c.) to a frequency of 5000 Hz. Potentiometric recorders can only deal with d.c. or low frequency signals. Few recorders with a me-chanical writing arm are capable of accurately recording frequencies above 75–100 Hz. Ink-jet recorders can handle frequencies up to 500 Hz whilst photographic and ultraviolet recorders may be capable of reproducing frequencies up to 8000 Hz. Even higher frequencies can be recorded by photographing the movements of an electron beam on the fluorescent screen of a cathode ray tube (CRT). To an increasing extent, signals are digitized and then held in a computer-based store of some kind. They can be further processed and finally converted to hard copy at any convenient time, using a graphics (laser or ink-jet) printer. The great advantage of this off-line approach is that printing speed is no longer important and the

Table 7.1. Frequency and magnitude of some typical biological signals

Signal	Approximate frequency range (Hz)	Approximate magnitude
ECG	0.1–100	1 mV
EEG	0.5–70	50 μV
EMG	10–70	100 μV (skin electrode)
	3–5000	1 mV (needle electrode)
EOG	d.c.–120	0.5 mV
Arterial pressure	d.c.–20	
Left ventricular dP/dt_{max}	d.c.–100	
Phonocardiogram	20–2000	
Respiratory airflow	d.c.–30	

errors inherent in pen recorders (see below) are eliminated altogether.

The second factor to be considered is the accuracy and resolution required from the recording. For example, when recording arterial blood pressure it may be adequate to display the trace on a 50-mm wide paper strip. With the recording system gain adjusted to produce a full-scale deflection of 250 mmHg, each millimetre on the record then represents 5 mmHg. This is quite satisfactory for most clinical purposes. On the other hand, a dye-dilution curve should be recorded with an amplitude of at least 10 cm so that the logarithmic replotting of the exponential part of the curve can be accomplished with sufficient accuracy (p. 216). Since the dye curve has only low frequency components and since most galvanometric pen recorders become non-linear when the deflection is large, it is better to choose a potentiometric recorder for this application. Modern instruments for cardiac output determination fit exponential functions to dye-dilution curves and compute final values automatically.

The third factor determining the choice of recorder is the environment in which it is to be used. For example, heated stylus recorders are usually more robust and reliable than ink-pen recorders and are ideal for the clinical situation. Photographic or ultraviolet recorders do not produce an immediate image and are more difficult to adjust, but may be essential if high frequency recordings are required or if more than four to six channels are to be recorded simultaneously. Tape recorders

are clean, compact and can incorporate a voice channel, thus obviating the need to write down details or events. However, it is often neccessary to display the data (on a chart recorder or oscilloscope) as it is acquired, so that the user can monitor the signal quality. Computer-based recording systems allow many different types of data to be recorded simultaneously (physiological signals, events, numeric data from other measuring systems, information typed onto a keyboard, etc.), and have the added advantage that the data can be displayed on a suitable screen at the same time.

The fourth important factor is cost. Pen recorders are relatively cheap to buy and to operate. Heated stylus recorders are more expensive and require special recording paper, as do ultraviolet and photographic recorders. Paper costs must be considered in relation to likely consumption. For example, electroencephalograph (EEG) recordings are usually made with pen recorders on plain paper because the cost of photographic or heated stylus papers would be prohibitive when continuous recordings may extend to 30 min or more. Magnetic tape and computerized storage systems are relatively expensive, but are able to record many data channels for extended periods on reusable storage media.

Recorder performance

When analysing the performance of a recorder it is necessary to consider the frequency response, linearity and the possibility of timing errors.

FREQUENCY RESPONSE: AMPLITUDE AND PHASE DISTORTION

If a writing arm is driven at progressively greater frequencies by a sine wave signal of constant amplitude it responds in a characteristic fashion (Fig. 7.4a).

At low frequencies it faithfully follows the sine wave input but as the frequency rises the excursion of the pen arm begins to increase. At a particular frequency the excursion of the arm reaches a peak but then at higher frequencies declines progressively until it is scarcely discernible. This increase in amplitude is due to resonance, which is a property of any oscillating mechanical system having both mass and compliance (elasticity). The frequency at which the greatest over-emphasis occurs represents the resonant frequency (f_0) of the vibrating system. At high frequencies the movement of the pen fails to follow the applied waveform and simply indicates the mean value.

The response illustrated in Fig. 7.4a is that of a freely oscillating system with a natural frequency determined by the effective mass of the writing arm and the tension of the spring tending to return the writing arm to its zero position. The resonant frequency can be increased by reducing the effective mass of the arm (by decreasing its weight or its length) or by increasing the stiffness of the spring. This will permit higher frequencies to be recorded without approaching the resonant frequency but will still leave much of the potential of the system untapped.

As well as needing an adequate frequency response, an efficient and accurate system needs to be

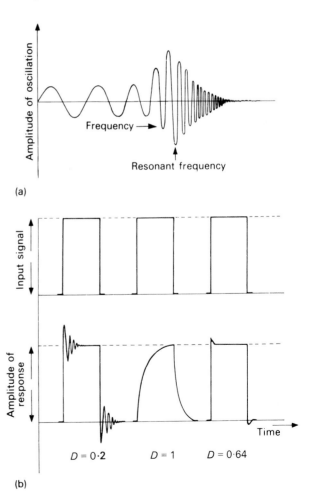

(a)

(b)

Fig. 7.4. (a) Effect of increasing frequency on amplitude of recorded signal with constant amplitude sine wave input. (b) Response to square wave input. Left: minimal damping showing overshoot and oscillation. Centre: critically damped (overshoot just abolished). Right: damping 64% of critical showing maximum speed of response with minimal overshoot, D = damping factor.

appropriately damped if all frequencies within the working range are to be drawn with equal amplitude. This may be done hydraulically (for example, by suspending the driving galvanometer in a viscous fluid) or electronically (by incorporating an inductance in the system). A system is said to be critically damped when it follows a step change at the input with maximum velocity but does not overshoot (Fig. 7.4b). However, this degree of damping markedly slows the response to a square wave input signal. The optimal rate of response with minimal overshoot (approximately 6–7%) occurs when the damping is adjusted to be about 64–66% of critical. The degree of damping is expressed as a damping factor D, such that for a critically damped system $D = 1$. Over-damped systems have damping factors greater than 1 and under-damped systems have values less than 1.

An optimally damped system has a 'flat' response (i.e. the amplitude distortion is less than $\pm 2\%$) up to 66% of the undamped natural frequency. Thus to record the higher harmonics of an arterial pressure waveform (usually considered to be about 20 Hz) it is necessary to use a recorder with an undamped natural frequency of 30 Hz and then adjust the damping factor to 0.64. Optimal damping minimizes amplitude distortion and enables a large proportion of the frequency range below f_0 to be used (Fig. 7.5).

When considering frequency response it is important to take note of phase delay as well as amplitude distortion, because both of these factors will distort the output signal (see p. 167 *et seq.*). Phase delay occurs because the inertia of the vibrating system causes it to lag behind the applied waveform. The phase lag varies with both the frequency and with the degree of damping (Fig. 7.6).

Phase lag is small at low frequencies but increases to 90° at the resonant frequency of the system. To secure an accurate registration of all the harmonics of a complex wave it is essential that the time delay imparted to all harmonics should be the same so that their phase relationships with each other are undisturbed. Now a 1 Hz sine wave with a phase lag of 90° is subject to a delay of 0.25 s, whereas a 2 Hz signal with 90° lag would be delayed by only 0.125 s. To secure the same time

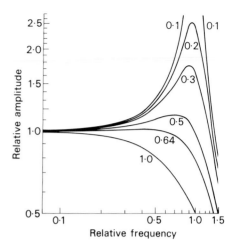

Fig. 7.5. Amplitude distortion with increasing frequency. The number by each curve is the damping factor (D). $D = 1.0$ represents critical damping, $D = 0$ is undamped. When $D = 0.64$ the recorded amplitude is accurate to within $\pm 2\%$ up to about two thirds of the undamped natural frequency. (Relative frequency = fraction of undamped natural frequency.)

delay it is therefore essential that the phase lag should increase in proportion to the frequency. As shown in Fig. 7.6 this condition is satisfied when the damping factor is 0.64. Thus optimal damping

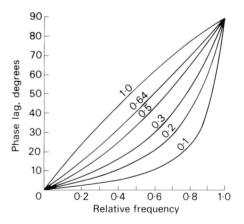

Fig. 7.6. Phase lag with increasing frequency, $D = 1.0$ represents critical damping, $D = 0.1$ is underdamped. Phase lag is proportional to frequency when $D = 0.64$. (Relative frequency = fraction of undamped natural frequency.)

Fig. 7.7. Sources of distortion in a pen recorder. The pen (of length r) describes an arc whose length is $r\theta$ radians. The vertical displacement of the pen tip is $r \sin \theta$ and the timing error is $t = r - r \cos \theta$. The sine error causes the vertical displacement to be less than it should be at large angular displacements.

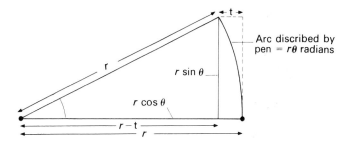

secures the optimal frequency response and also minimizes both amplitude and phase distortion.

LINEARITY AND TIMING ERRORS

An ideal recorder would respond to a square wave input signal by producing an identical square wave on the recording paper. Such an ideal response is very difficult to achieve.

Consider a step increase in applied signal to a pen recorder in which the angular displacement of the pen is proportional to the amplitude of the applied signal. The pen will not draw a vertical step, but describes an arc across the paper. While the length of the arc is a true representation of the signal amplitude, the height of the drawn line is not. Since we are concerned with both the amplitude of the signal (i.e. vertical displacement) and the timing of the signal (horizontal displacement) we must assess the magnitude of the errors introduced by this method of recording. Since the length of the arc is directly related to the length of the

writing arm (r) and the angular displacement (θ radians) the length of the arc must be directly related to the input signal (Fig. 7.7).

However, the vertical displacement of the writing point from the zero position is given by $r \sin \theta$. Each successive increment of angular displacement will therefore produce a smaller vertical displacement than the previous one, so that the recorded

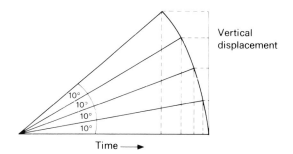

Fig. 7.8. Angular displacements of writing arm of 10°, 20°, 30° and 40° to show relative magnitudes of sine error and timing error with 10 cm long arm.

Table 7.2. Effect of angular displacement of writing arm on sine, timing and tangent errors

Angular displacement (degrees)	Length of arc (cm)	Linear displacement (cm)		
		Vertical	horizontal	vertical
	($= R\theta$ radians)	($= R \sin \theta$)	($= t$)	($= R \tan \theta$)
0	0.00	0.00	0.00	0.00
10	1.75	1.74	0.15	1.76
20	3.49	3.42	0.60	3.64
30	5.23	5.00	1.34	5.77
40	6.98	6.43	2.34	8.39

Displacement along the arc, vertical and horizontal axes calculated for a writing arm 10 cm long. Since a tangent error arises from an effective lengthening of the writing arm it is assumed that the arm is 10 cm long at zero displacement (see Figs 7.7, 7.8 and 7.12).

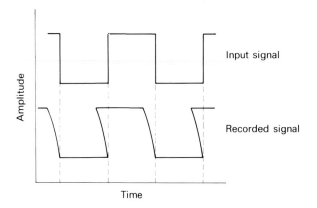

Fig. 7.9. Use of curvilinear co-ordinates to eliminate pen distortion. Although the time and amplitude of the event are now correctly recorded the shape of the waveform is distorted.

amplitude is not linearly related to the input signal. This sine error is minimized by limiting the pen movement to small angular displacements and is not significant with a 10-cm pen arm moving though an angular displacement of $\pm 20°$.

A larger error is produced on the time axis (Fig. 7.7). This timing error (t) can be calculated from the expression $t = r - r\cos\theta$.

As may be seen from Table 7.2 and Fig. 7.8 this error can create major inaccuracies in timing even with relatively small angular displacements of the pen.

The simplest method of overcoming these problems is to mark the recording paper with curvilinear co-ordinates which parallel the arc inscribed by the pen (Fig 7.9).

This eliminates both sources of error but yields a trace whose shape does not reflect that of the applied waveform. This limitation can be overcome by forcing the paper to lie in a curved trough, such that the sweep of the pen now draws an exactly vertical line on the paper (Fig. 7.10).

This is a simple solution in single-channel recorders but creates insuperable problems when a number of signals must be recorded on the same roll of paper.

A more satisfactory alternative is to draw the paper over a knife-edge and to use a heated stylus to mark heat-sensitive paper. (This type of paper has a coloured base and is covered with a thin layer of white cellulose; when the cellulose is melted by a hot stylus the coloured base shows through.) The heated stylus is usually about 1–2 cm long, and mounted at the tip of the writing arm in its long

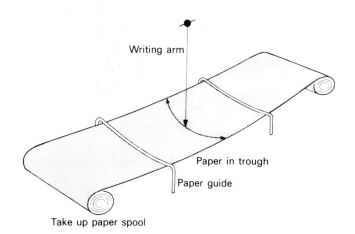

Fig. 7.10. Use of curved trough and vertical writing arm to overcome sine distortion.

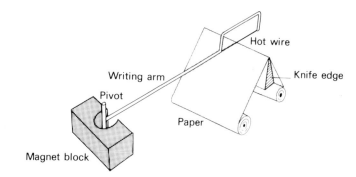

Fig. 7.11. Use of knife-edge and heated stylus to overcome the timing error.

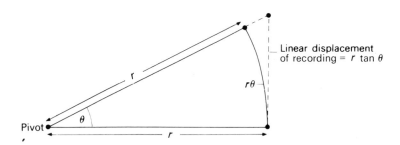

Fig. 7.12. Tangent error which must be corrected in recorders using knife-edge and heated stylus, ink-jet or mirror galvanometers. The error in vertical displacement gets larger as the angular displacement increases.

axis. The knife-edge is mounted at right angles to the direction of travel of the paper (Fig. 7.11).

When the writing arm is deflected the point of contact between the heated stylus and the knife-edge approaches the tip of the writing arm. This has the effect of lengthening the arm as it moves laterally and so ensures that the time co-ordinate is unaffected by lateral displacement of the writing arm. A similar effect is achieved in the ink-jet recorder where the jet is mounted above the paper and the angular displacement of the jet results in a vertical displacement of the trace (Fig. 7.2). As the deflection increases, the length of the 'ink' writing arm increases with the distance from jet to paper.

Unfortunately both these methods introduce yet another problem, that of tangent distortion (Fig. 7.12).

In this case the deflection along the vertical axis is $r \tan \theta$. Again, the error is not significant at small angles of deflection (Table 7.2) but if larger deflections are used (as in the ink-jet and galvanometer recorders) the error must be corrected electronically.

In a few recorders sine distortion is overcome by lengthening the arm mechanically. To accomplish this without compromising the frequency response demands high precision engineering; such recorders are always very expensive (Fig. 7.13).

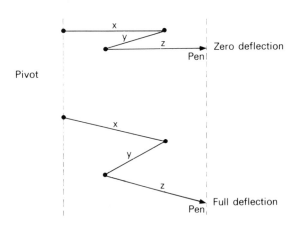

Fig. 7.13. Use of mechanical linkage to lengthen the writing arm and so obviate time distortion.

Direct-writing recorders

The disadvantages of pen recorders have already been outlined. Nevertheless their relative simplicity, the immediacy of the image and the cheapness of the recording paper make them a popular choice for many types of recording where linearity and time distortion are not of paramount importance (e.g. EEG, ECG). Indeed, by suitable modification many of the disadvantages can be minimized. Although heat-sensitive paper is much more expensive than plain recording paper, the hot stylus/knife-edge technique is easily implemented and forms the basis of many currently available recorders. Other methods of producing an image are a cold stylus writing on pressure-sensitive paper or a pen acting as an electrode which creates an image when contacting specially coated, electro-sensitive paper. In the latter case, both writing-arm mass and pen/paper friction can be minimized, thus enabling high frequency responses to be achieved. Several high-quality recorders are based on this technique.

Any mechanical writing arm will display hysteresis, i.e. the pen does not return exactly to zero after it has been deflected. However, suitable design of the zero-return spring can limit hysteresis to no more than 2% of the maximum deflection.

The flat frequency response of most pen recorders is limited to 70–100 Hz. Some recorders contain very simple amplifiers, which may require an input signal of 0–1 V to achieve a full-scale deflection (f.s.d.), but many have sophisticated pre-amplifiers which will accept signals in the microvolt range with input impedances of more than 1 MΩ, together with adjustable damping characteristics.

Ultraviolet optical recorders with mirror galvanometers

Photographic recorders utilizing the mirror galvanometer (Fig. 7.3) have been used for many years, but they have suffered from the disadvantage that the trace had to be developed and fixed before the image could be inspected. However, the introduction of ultraviolet sensitive paper, on which an image appears after a short delay, brought the mirror galvanometer recorder back into popularity, though the image does lack the contrast which is obtainable with most other kinds of recording. The image is semi-permanent, but the paper blackens if it is exposed to bright light for prolonged periods. The image can be preserved by chemical treatment, by spraying the paper with a protective yellow varnish or by photography. In some cases the image will survive xerographic reproduction. Whatever method of image preservation is used, it is essential that exhaustive tests be carried out before risking paper containing data. Once faded, the image is not recoverable.

The mirror galvanometer has a number of advantages. Many channels (sometimes up to 50 or even 100) can be recorded on the same strip of paper with the traces overlapped so that each can sweep the full width of the paper. Identification marks can be superimposed on each trace and a time scale and calibration grid can be printed onto the paper as it passes through the recorder. The light spots can also be projected onto a ground-glass screen so that the zero and calibration points can be adjusted and the recording monitored visually. Perhaps the greatest advantage is the wide choice of galvanometers which permits each channel to be matched exactly to the frequency requirements of the input signal. Since each galvanometer is carried as a complete unit in a compact, 5–6 cm long cylinder it is a simple matter to change types when required.

MIRROR GALVANOMETERS

The sensitivity of a mirror galvanometer depends on the length of the optical writing arm (mirror to paper distance) and on the deflection of the mirror produced by a given current or voltage. In many ultraviolet recorders the optical writing arm is greatly extended by the use of mirrors, so that the light beam travels several times back and forth within the enclosure before reaching the paper. The deflection can be enhanced by increasing the density of the magnetic field or by increasing the size of the coil. There is a limit to the density of the magnetic field which can be achieved and the larger the coil the greater is the mass and therefore the lower is the undamped natural frequency. Although the sensitivity is also affected by the internal resistance of the galvanometer, sensitivity is approximately inversely proportional to the square of the natural frequency. There is therefore no advantage to be gained from using a galvanometer with a higher frequency response than that required for the purpose in hand. For this reason the first step in choosing a galvanometer is to decide on the maximum frequency which it will be called upon to handle. The undamped natural frequency is then calculated by multiplying this by a factor of 1.6 since, if it is correctly damped, the frequency response should be flat to 66% of its natural frequency.

In addition to undamped natural frequency and sensitivity it is necessary to ensure that damping is optimal. In galvanometers with undamped natural frequencies up to 300–400 Hz damping is applied electromagnetically, but with galvanometers with undamped natural frequencies above about 1 kHz fluid damping is used.

Electromagnetic damping is achieved by inserting a known resistance into the galvanometer circuit such that the reverse current induced in the coil by its own deflection produces the required degree of damping. The magnitude of this resistance can be calculated if the resistance of the current source is known, for optimal conditions exist when the resistance of the source equals the resistance of the damping resistance. When these resistances are not equal, a series or parallel resistance may need to be incorporated in the circuit. Details are given in the manufacturers' literature. Ideally, each galvanometer is driven by a matching pre-amplifier, and high-quality instruments have pre-amplifiers which can be configured to drive a wide variety of galvanometers.

Some typical values for galvanometer characteristics are given in Table 7.3. This illustrates how sensitivity decreases as frequency response increases.

Oscilloscope recorders

An oscilloscope may be used to make a hard copy record as well as to display the dynamic waveform. The simplest method is to photograph the screen of a storage oscilloscope on which the signal is temporarily captured. Special oscilloscope cameras make this a simple procedure, and may even illuminate the screen with ultraviolet light in order to induce background screen luminescence such that the graticule appears on the processed image. The use of a polaroid camera overcomes the problem of incorrect exposure time, since a poor image is immediately apparent.

When prolonged periods of recording are required the time base on the oscilloscope may be switched off and the film moved continuously through the camera. The oscillations of the light spots on the y-axis then produce continuous traces on the film. This form of recording greatly enhances the versatility of the instrument but some care is necessary to ensure correct exposure. Although some experience with the technique is necessary to produce good records, there is little alternative to the oscilloscope when one wishes to record components of a waveform having a frequency greater than 8 kHz.

Recent developments in design have widened the application of oscilloscopes in the recording field, since those equipped with fibre-optic face plates produce such bright images that traces can be recorded directly onto photographic or ultraviolet-sensitive paper.

Table 7.3. Typical values for galvanometer characteristics

Natural frequency (Hz)	Frequency response (±5%) (Hz)	Galvanometer sensitivity	
		(mA cm)	(mV cm)
35	20	0.0008	0.038
450	300	0.05	6.0
1000	600	0.34	25
5000	3000	25	1050

Potentiometric recorders

This type of recorder is used when a slowly changing signal is to be recorded onto a wide (10–30 cm) strip chart with high accuracy. Sensitivity can be made very high (e.g. 1 mV f.s.d.) by the use of suitable, usually built-in, pre-amplifiers. However, the frequency response is very low by comparison with galvanometric recorders. In low-cost instruments the pen may take 2 s to traverse the full width of the paper although it is possible to obtain slewing speeds of 75 cm·s^{-1} in sophisticated models.

This type of recorder is based on the potentiometer circuit (Fig. 7.14). A battery or power supply supplies a constant current to a slide wire A, B. The slide wire has a uniform cross-section throughout its length so that the resistance per unit length is constant. The input voltage is applied between one end of the slide wire and the moving contact, C. When the position of the contact is such that the voltage drop between B and C is the same as the input voltage there will be no current flow through the galvanometer. In the potentiometric recorder the galvanometer is replaced by a servo-amplifier which drives a motor which, in turn, moves the

sliding contact along the potentiometer wire. Thus if the input voltage to the recorder exceeds that across B–C the bridge will be out of balance and the servo-motor will move the sliding contact in the direction which tends to minimize the difference in potential between the input and B–C. If the input voltage is less than B–C it will move the contact in the opposite direction. Thus the position of the contact is continually adjusted to match the input voltage. Since the pen is directly linked to the contact a continuous record of the input voltage is obtained.

Potentiometric recorders are used in many monitoring applications for very low frequency signals such as indicator dilution curves or chromatograph detector outputs. Sampling recorders, printing out distinctively marked traces for a number of different variables in rotation, are used for such applications as the monitoring of temperature from a number of different probes. Another variation is the *x–y* recorder, in which two potentiometric mechanisms drive the pen along two axes at right angles to each other. This may be used for plotting two simultaneously changing variables, such as pressure and volume in lung mechanics measurements. They may also be used as curve plotters at the output of analogue computers. The best modern recorders can follow signals up to about 10 Hz.

Magnetic recorders

Magnetic recording is used for both analogue and digital data. Analogue data are stored on magnetic tape but digital data can be stored either on magnetic tape or disk.

TAPE RECORDERS FOR ANALOGUE DATA

There are basically two types of analogue tape recorder. The first utilizes a direct recording system in which the magnitude of the signal is recorded by altering the magnetic flux on the tape. This is the method used in audio recorders. The highest frequency which can be recorded depends on how small an area of the tape may be independently

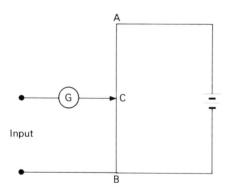

Fig. 7.14. Principle of a potentiometric recorder. A constant current is passed along the slide wire A–B. A sliding contact, C, is moved along the wire by a servo-amplifier and servo-motor which is activated when a potential difference is detected at G. The motor thus moves the sliding contact in such a way that the potential difference across B–C always matches the input voltage. Since the pen is linked to the sliding contact it produces a record of the input voltage.

magnetized and on the tape speed. In general, direct recording systems provide a relatively wide frequency bandwidth even with low tape speeds. However, they have several disadvantages: the handling of signals below 100 Hz is poor, the amplitude response varies markedly with frequency and the signal-to-noise ratio is relatively low.

The second type of recorder uses FM. Here the input voltage is represented on the tape by an audio tone whose frequency is directly proportional to the input voltage (p. 43). For example, the modulator might produce a 1000 Hz signal when the input voltage is zero. This is known as the carrier or centre frequency. Input voltages of $+10$ or -10 V might then be represented by frequencies of 1300 and 700 Hz, respectively, so that the full range of input voltages would be covered by a bandwidth of 600 Hz. On playback, the modulated signal is retrieved from the tape and the original input waveform reconstructed by a demodulator which transforms frequency back to voltage.

Frequency modulation systems have the advantage that the amplitude response is relatively flat from d.c. to the upper frequency limit of the recorder and that the signal-to-noise ratio is relatively high. Indeed, so long as the modulated signal is clearly recovered from the tape, the demodulator is almost entirely unresponsive to tape hiss, capstan rumble, etc. However, their upper frequency limit is generally less than that obtained in direct recording systems. The multichannel FM recorders used for physiological work are generally known as instrumentation tape recorders.

One of the main problems in FM tape recording is the maintenance of a precisely constant tape speed, since any such variation causes corresponding changes in signal frequency on playback. As with audio recording, low frequency variations are known as 'wow' and high frequency variations as 'flutter'. Whereas they lead to frequency aberrations in audio recorders, the FM playback demodulator converts them to errors in signal amplitude. There are two methods of reducing the FM recorder's sensitivity to variations in tape speed, both methods requiring the sacrifice of a tape channel. In one method a reference voltage is recorded on one channel as a constant frequency signal. Then, on playback, variations in the demodulated reference signal are used to correct any synchronous variations on the other channels. In the second method a stable, high repetition rate pulse train is recorded on one channel and then on replay, used to control the servo-motor driving the tape transport capstan.

Analogue recorders can be used for temporary data storage or for prolonged monitoring. Recorders using 0.6 cm (0.25 in) tape can provide up to four parallel data channels whilst 1.25 cm (0.5 in) tape can carry up to eight channels. It is often useful to use one channel to record a spoken commentary and the remainder for recording the physiological signals.

One example of the use of magnetic tape for temporary storage of data is the tape loop. This consists of a complete loop of tape which can be varied in length to provide a period of recording which suits the chosen application. As the tape passes through the recording head the previous signal is erased and the new signal is recorded. This system can be used for monitoring patients who are likely to develop a cardiac arrhythmia or arrest. If the nurse stops the tape when such an arrest occurs, the ECG for the previous 5–10 min will be retained and can be played back to reveal the pattern of events leading up to the arrest. Magnetic tape may also be employed when it is desired to select small periods of a long recording for detailed analysis, for example when analysing the incidence of arrhythmias over a period of 24 hours. The tape can be replayed at high speed and relevant portions of the record played back into a direct-writing recorder to obtain a permanent visual record. The tape can then be re-used. Compact cassette tape recorders running at slow speed have also proved useful in monitoring the response to drugs used in the treatment of hypertension (Stott, 1977).

MAGNETIC TAPE RECORDERS FOR DIGITAL DATA

Just as complex audio signals can be recorded on tape, so can simple binary data. While a simple audio recorder could be used, it is now usual to use a specially designed machine. Many digital tape decks use 1.25 cm (0.5 in) tape with seven or nine tracks. Digital tape is specially inspected for defects before use and one track is usually used for error-detecting or error-correcting procedures. The remaining six or eight tracks are used to store the binary information in parallel, i.e. each byte is stored as a column running cross the tape.

Digital tape recorders are used to record data for subsequent computer processing, and for 'backing up' other storage media such as magnetic disks. While many modern instruments have digital data output ports (usually conforming to RS 232), analogue data must be digitized and suitably formatted before digital recording is possible. This is most easily achieved by a small computer with analogue input channels.

'HARD' AND 'SOFT' MAGNETIC DISK STORAGE

Magnetic disk devices are very similar in principle to the simple tape recorder. The disk operates as a series of concentric tracks, with read/write heads very close to the surface. The flexible or, more popularly named, 'floppy' disk can be removed from the drive so that large libraries of data can be held in this form. However, the technical difficulties inherent in aligning the disk in the drive to *exactly* the position it occupied on a previous occasion limits the density of the recorded data. At present, the highest density available allows 1.2 Mb to be placed on a 3.5 or 5.25 in flexible disk.

The 'hard' disk is a different matter. This is a fixed, high precision disk in constant rotation with the read/write heads mounted *very* close to the surface. While considerably less rugged than flexible disks, hard disks permit much higher recording density so that 100 Mb can be achieved easily at modest cost. Even low-cost personal computers are commonly fitted with 20 or 40 Mb disk drives.

Other data storage media

There are several types of storage media for digital data. Very early computers used 'magnetic storage', and a few such devices survive as museum pieces. The store consisted of an array of ferrite rings, each

of which could be magnetized in a specific direction to record a binary '0' or '1'. Since ferrite rings are permanent magnets the information was non-volatile: in other words it could be retained by the store when the power supply was cut off.

Modern computer memory consists of microscopic semiconductor devices which place tiny electrical charges on even more microscopic capacitors. The size of each device is such that many thousands can be mounted on a small silicon wafer and encapsulated within a 'microchip'.

These devices are generally used for short-term storage and have become widely used in small items of equipment such as oscilloscopes, monitoring systems and analytical apparatus. For example, the modern ECG monitor contains an analogue-to-digital (ADC) converter which continuously samples the ECG waveform and updates a digital memory. This is continuously scanned and the resulting analogue signal displayed on the screen. By using digital techniques it is possible to make the trace move across the screen so that the image appears to have been written by an invisible pen behind one edge of the screen. Alternatively the trace can be 'frozen' at any time for closer inspection. Digital storage also forms the basis of one type of storage oscilloscope (p. 74).

Several entirely new technologies have emerged very recently, in response to demand for very large, low-cost data storage media. The most important is the so-called WORM drive.

In Write mode, a laser beam writes very high density binary data onto a disk rather similar to the compact audio disk. In Read mode, the laser 'reads' the data and sends it to the controlling computer. The advantage of this method lies in the data density, since many megabytes can be held on a single small disk. However, each area of disk can only be 'written' upon once so that once full no new material can be added. However, it is strongly rumoured that high-capacity optical disks from which data can be erased and re-used are just around the corner.

In the Bernouilli storage system the binary data are converted into a stream of magnetic 'bubbles' which pass around a minute, convoluted semiconductor 'race-track' before being re-read. They are not, of course, bubbles in the conventional physical sense. This remains a fairly expensive device, but has the advantage of great capacity, rapid retrieval and no limitations upon the number of read/write cycles.

References

Stott, F.D. (1977) Ambulatory monitoring. *British Journal of Clinical Equipment* **2**, 61.

Cashman, P.M.M. (1980) Foundations of medical technology. Recording methods. *British Journal of Clinical Equipment* **5**(5) 172–175.

8: Electromagnetic Radiation and Optical Measurements

The various forms of electromagnetic radiation are usually given distinct titles such as *ultraviolet*, *infrared*, *radiowaves*, etc., although it should be remembered that they all form part of a continuous spectrum and are qualitatively identical. The spectrum of electromagnetic radiations which is shown in Fig. 8.1 stretches from the very short wavelength and highly energetic cosmic and gamma rays through to the relatively low energy radiowaves. Out of the whole range of these electromagnetic radiations only a small segment of wavelengths is capable of stimulating the eye. This is the visible region. The limits of this band are ill-defined but

may be regarded as terminating at a wavelength of about 390 nm at the ultraviolet end and at 750 nm towards the infrared zone.

These radiations are all examples of energy being transmitted in a waveform in accordance with the laws:

$$\lambda f = c$$

and

$$E = hf$$

where λ is the wavelength (m), f is the frequency (Hz), c is the velocity of light (3×10^8 m·s^{-1} in a vacuum), h is the Planck's constant (Joules·s) and E is the energy (Joules).

These relationships apply when radiation is propagated as if it were a wave motion. However, it should be appreciated that when electromagnetic radiation interacts with matter, it exhibits both wave and particle properties. Some of the interactions can best be described by considering the wave-like properties while other phenomena suggest particle behaviour.

For the purpose of this chapter a detailed understanding of electromagnetic radiation is not required and no further distinction between the two characteristics will be drawn. As can be seen from the expression above, frequency and wavelength are inversely related, while energy is proportional to frequency. Thus the radiowaves with their long wavelengths have low frequencies with little energy whilst the gamma-rays at the opposite end of the spectrum have short wavelengths, high frequencies and considerable energy. Although it is possible to define any particular point within the spectrum by referring to its wavelength, frequency or energy, the wavelength is the usual term (except in scientific circles where frequency or wave num-

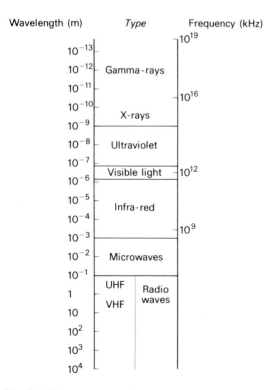

Fig. 8.1. The electromagnetic spectrum.

ber — the reciprocal of wavelength in centimetres — is often used). The units of wavelength in use nowadays are the nano-, micro- and centimetre, but the terms millimicron (mμ) and Angström (Å), now becoming obsolete, are still encountered.*

The tremendous importance of electromagnetic radiations to the scientist resides in their interactions with matter. From the standpoint of the biological and medical sciences, most of the interest concerns the narrow part of the spectrum with wavelengths from 200 nm to 10 μm — the near ultraviolet to the far infrared. Within this range many organic molecules absorb radiation, a process which can be exploited in two ways. Firstly, when dealing with an unknown compound, it can be used for identification or the interpretation of particular structural features. Secondly, the concentration of the absorbing component can be calculated by measuring the amount of energy that is absorbed. Thus the techniques that have grown up based on these interactions have several attractions; analyses can be performed more rapidly and specifically than with chemical procedures, information is gained about molecular structure that is inaccessible by other means and the radiation rarely destroys the material under investigation.

All molecules have natural vibration frequencies which correspond to the molecule oscillating between two states. Most have many such natural vibration frequencies. These states may be electronic transitions where an orbital electron passes from a low energy (ground) state to a higher energy (excited) state or positional movements of atoms with respect to each other, for example, the stretching, flexing or rotation of bonds. Atoms or molecules can only absorb or emit energy in discrete quantities, in fact integral multiples of hf. These packets of energy are referred to as quanta. If the molecule receives electromagnetic radiation of a frequency corresponding to one of its natural vibrations, the radiation will be absorbed. Generally speaking more energy is required for an electronic transition than a vibrational oscillation, which, in turn, is at a higher level than rotational

movement. The electronic transitions are found in the ultraviolet and visible regions, vibrational in the infrared and rotational in the microwave. It is perhaps easier to consider the process involved by concentrating the discussion on the absorption of visible light.

Within a molecule, certain groupings, termed chromophores, absorb light of particular wavelengths. These chromophores have structural features such that energy of the light quanta at that wavelength coincides with the energy required for a particular energy transition. The molecule absorbs the energy and passes into an excited state. Having moved to the higher energy state the excess energy is dissipated via one of several routes:

1 To neighbouring molecules as heat.

2 The energy may be sufficient to rupture a bond so causing the molecule to dissociate.

3 After certain internal rearrangements the molecule may re-emit the excess energy as electromagnetic radiation — a process termed fluorescence.

Different molecules exhibit these three modes of energy dissipation to varying degrees although in the vast majority of cases loss of energy as heat predominates. Light of other wavelengths possesses incorrect energy to cause the transition to the excited state; it is not absorbed and passes unhindered through the sample. Thus, within a molecule each grouping absorbs selectively certain components of the spectrum. When the substance is viewed in white light only the remaining parts of the spectrum are transmitted or reflected so that the substance appears to be coloured. When the substance is placed between a source of white light and the prism system of a spectroscope, the spectrum obtained is not continuous but has dark bands corresponding to those wavelengths which are removed. If the sample absorbs all the incident light, it will appear black. By measuring the extent of the light absorption as a function of wavelength, an absorption spectrum is obtained which, because of its dependence on chemical structure, is a diagnostic characteristic of the compound.

By considering the absorption process that takes place when a quantum of light interacts with a chromophore, certain laws may be derived. If a beam of monochromatic light (light of a single

* 1 mμ = 1 nm = 10^{-9} m or 10^{-7} cm
  1 Å = 0.1 nm = 10^{-10} m or 10^{-8} cm.

wavelength) passes through a solution of a chromophore, the extent of the absorption depends upon three factors: (a) the thickness of the absorbing material through which the radiation passes, (b) the concentration of the chromophore and (c) the efficiency of the chromophore at absorbing light at that wavelength.

As the quanta pass through a thin layer of the solution, the interactions between quanta and absorbing chromophores can be expressed in terms of probabilities of collision. Thus the probability that within a given time interval a particular chromophore will absorb a quantum of light is proportional to the number of quanta passing through the solution, i.e. the quantum flux, which is itself proportional to light intensity. Therefore, the thin layer of solution will absorb a certain proportion of the light which falls on it regardless of the intensity of that incident light. For example, if the incident light intensity is 10 arbitrary units and 10% is absorbed by the layer of solution, the emergent light intensity will be 9 arbitrary units, while an increase in incident intensity to 100 units will result in an emergent intensity of 90 units, namely still 10% absorption. The total absorption

of the cell containing the solution can be considered to comprise a large number of these very thin layers of chromophore and each of these layers absorbs the same proportion of the light which falls upon it (Fig. 8.2a). If the light intensity is 100 arbitrary units and each section removes 10%, then 90 units emerge from the first layer and enter the second. Thus, $90 \times 90\%$ emerge from the second; $(90 \times 90\%) \times 90\%$ emerge from the third, etc. This type of decrease in light intensity across the cell is termed an exponential decay (Fig. 8.2b), which mathematically can be expressed:

$$I = I_0 e^{-kl} \qquad \text{(i)}$$

where k is a constant, l is the length of lightpath through the solution, I_0 is the incident light intensity and I is the emergent light intensity. Taking logarithms and rearranging:

$$\log_{10} \frac{I_0}{I} = \frac{k}{2.303} l. \qquad \text{(ii)}$$

The entity $\log_{10} I_0/I$, which is the logarithm of the ratio of incident to emergent light intensities, is referred to variously as the absorbance, extinction or optical density. The first term, absorbance, is

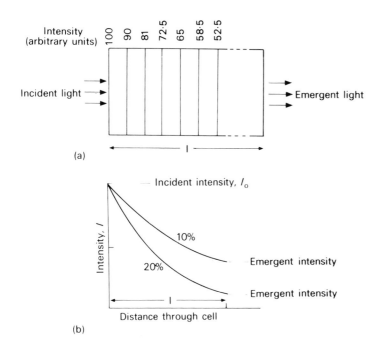

Fig. 8.2. Absorption of light passing through a solution.

preferred. Thus the expression (ii) states that the absorbance is proportional to the thickness of the absorbing layer. This is Lambert's Law.

The probability that a particular quantum will interact rather than travel unimpeded through the solution is dependent upon the density of the chromophores, i.e. the concentration. By doubling the chromophore concentration, the probability of a quantum being absorbed is doubled. Taking the example quoted above, the thin layer of chromophore absorbed 10% of the incident light. If the concentration is doubled, then 20% of the light is absorbed. This is repeated through the series of layers of which the total thickness of solution is composed. The variation in the light intensity across the solution for the two situations is shown in Fig. 8.2b. Note that doubling the concentration does not halve the emergent intensity.

Mathematically, it is found that the concentration term is present in the constant, k, of equation (i) thus

$$I = I_0 e^{-k'cl}$$

where k' is a constant and c is the concentration of chromophore. Taking logarithms:

$$\log_{10} \frac{I_0}{I} = \varepsilon cl$$

where ε is the absorption coefficient. However, since $\log_{10} I_0/I$ is the absorbance (A) this equation can be written:

$$A = \varepsilon cl. \qquad \text{(iii)}$$

In words, expression (iii) states that the absorbance is proportional to the chromophore concentration. This is Beer's Law.

If concentration (c) is measured in moles$\cdot$L^{-1} and length (l) in cm, ε has units of L$\cdot$moles$^{-1}\cdot$cm^{-1} and is referred to as the *molar absorption coefficient*. It is the absorption which would be recorded at that wavelength of a 1 M solution in a 1 cm lightpath cell. The magnitude of the molar absorption coefficient reflects the probability that radiation at that wavelength will cause an electron to be excited. If the probability is high that the structure of a molecule will result in absorption, then the absorption coefficient is large.

If the coefficient is small, it signifies that the efficiency of absorbing radiation is poor. Thus the positions of the absorption maxima and their intensities provide information on the structure of the molecule in question and constitute a fingerprint for identifying it. Because the efficiency of light absorption varies with wavelength, the molar absorption coefficient will likewise be dependent upon the wavelength.

Although these laws have been discussed from the standpoint of the absorption of visible light, the concepts are just as valid for the non-visible parts of the electromagnetic spectrum. The absorption of ultraviolet, infrared and other forms of radiation obeys exactly the same principles. It is in spectrophotometry, the application of these concepts, that the relationships between absorbance, concentration and wavelength are exploited as an analytical technique. The importance of spectrophotometry in the analytical laboratory resides in its reliability in terms of accuracy and reproducibility, and also because it is possible to detect and measure many materials at low concentrations. Usually these measurements are unaffected by the presence of other compounds. The technique may be extended to chemicals which do not themselves absorb. Often such compounds which are transparent to visible light can be easily converted into a coloured, and therefore absorbing species, through a simple chemical procedure.

To take advantage of the potential of spectrophotometry it is essential to be able to measure light intensities accurately at defined regions of the spectrum. The photometric instruments which achieve this all contain the same four basic units, namely, (a) an energy source generating radiation in the appropriate region of the spectrum, (b) a system for selecting particular limited parts of this spectral region, (c) a sample chamber and (d) a means of detecting the intensity of the radiation in use. On the second part of the instrument, wavelength selection, it should be remembered that the Beer and Lambert Laws are based on the assumption that the incident radiation is all of one wavelength. This is difficult to achieve without incurring a high cost penalty, for example, by using lasers. In practice, the instruments have either monochromators which will produce light that has a very narrow bandwidth of wavelengths or filters which transmit a broader spread of radiation. The former type of instrument is termed a spectrophotometer while the latter is a colorimeter. Since the filters in colorimeters transmit light of non-absorptive as well as absorptive wavelengths through the sample, deviations from the Beer and Lambert Laws are more likely with this type of instrument.

Colorimeters

The original analytical technique of colorimetry was performed by eye. In the early instruments colours were matched visually in white light against either a selection of permanent coloured-glass standards or a series of solutions prepared from known concentrations of the substance under assay. The analyst used his own judgement in estimating which of the standards most closely matched the unknown. This subjective approach has disappeared and has been replaced with a photoelectric device that converts the residual or unabsorbed radiation emerging from the sample into an electric current. The magnitude of the signal is related in a defined way to the intensity of the light. Two further advantages were gained by the use of such photoelectric devices: determinations could be performed in the presence of interfering colours and the technique could be applied to the analysis of pale colours or absorptions outside the visible range.

The present-day colorimeter is a fairly simple instrument in which the light detector is either a selenium photocell which generates a current proportional to the light intensity or a cadmium suphide resistor whose resistance varies with light intensity, so changing the current flowing in the circuit. The current is measured by a galvanometer which is calibrated logarithmically in absorbance units. The light source is an incandescent tungsten filament lamp and the required region of the spectrum is selected by filters. A diagrammatic representation is given in Fig. 8.3.

As mentioned above, it is the filter system of wavelength selection which creates the primary limitation and source of inaccuracy in using a colorimeter. Some wavelengths transmitted by the filter (those close to the wavelength of maximum absorption) are absorbed by the chromophore, while the remainder are less efficiently removed. Thus even when the concentration of the chromophore is very high and absorbing all the light at the wavelength of maximum absorption, light of other wavelengths will be unabsorbed and be converted into an electric current by the photocell, so giving a false reading.

Spectrophotometers

In a spectrophotometer a monochromator placed between the light source and the sample replaces the filter system of the colorimeter. The light entering the monochromator is dispersed by either a prism or a combination of a prism with a diffraction grating into a continuous spectrum. Since a very narrow part of this spectrum is selected the sample is illuminated by light that is almost monochromatic and the Beer–Lambert Laws are more closely obeyed.

For operation in the visible region the radiation source is a tungsten filament lamp, although recently quartz-halogen bulbs have been used by some manufacturers. The voltage applied to the lamp is stabilized to prevent variation in filament

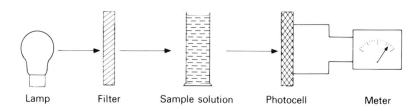

Lamp   Filter   Sample solution   Photocell   Meter

Fig. 8.3. Diagram of a colorimeter.

temperature which would create fluctuations in the intensity of the emitted light. The light detection system of a spectrophotometer is likewise more elaborate than that of a colorimeter, the two devices in most common usage being the phototube and photomultiplier. A phototube is a vacuum tube whose cathode emits electrons in proportion to the light intensity. These electrons are collected by the anode and the resultant small signal amplified before display. Instruments designed for operation at low light intensities usually have photomultipliers as their detectors. These devices are effectively photocells which have several stages of internal amplification but they have the disadvantage of requiring a stabilized high voltage supply. The resultant signal is displayed either in analogue form, for example as a deflection of a meter needle, or in a digital form. Most spectrophotometers have provision for the external recording of the readings on a chart recorder or an automatic printout unit. The layout of a spectrophotometer in diagrammatic form is given in Fig. 8.4. The collimated beam of white light is dispersed by the prism (or diffraction grating) so generating a spectrum which falls on the slit plate. The sample is illuminated only by the portion of the spectrum which passes through the narrow slit aperture. By rotating the prism the spectrum is caused to move along the slit plate, past the aperture, so changing the wavelength of the light emerging from the slit. The wavelength of the selected narrow band may be read off a graduated scale that is related through a suitable gearing system to the angular position of the prism.

Most laboratory spectrophotometers are also capable of operating in the ultraviolet region although certain design modifications are required. A second radiation source is needed, and this is a deuterium arc lamp. The glass prisms and lenses are replaced with quartz equivalents because glass is an efficient absorber at wavelengths shorter than 330 nm.

A feature often encountered in spectrophotometers is a double beam capability. With this type of instrument the light from the monochromator is split into two beams — one of which passes through the test sample and the other through a reference sample. The detection system, usually a photomultiplier in this type of instrument, generates two signals corresponding to the sample and reference light intensities by sampling each in turn. The

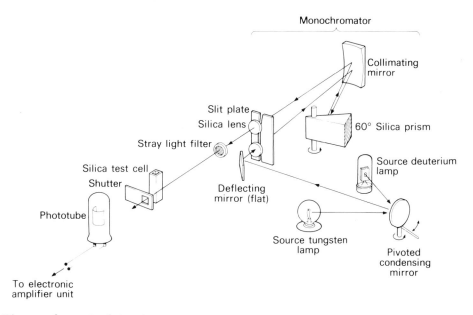

Fig. 8.4. Diagram of a spectrophotometer.

electronic system compares the two signals and generates an output proportional to the difference. This gives greater stability because fluctuations due to the instrument will affect both reference and sample beams equally and thus the difference remains constant. Furthermore, when scanning the absorption spectrum with the double-beam spectrophotometer it is unnecessary to 'zero' the instrument each time the wavelength is changed: the reference beam automatically compensates for the source emitting different intensities of radiation at different wavelengths and the detector having a sensitivity that is wavelength dependent. In view of the greater complexity of spectrophotometers they are larger and considerably more expensive than colorimeters.

When making a measurement the first criterion is selection of the appropriate wavelength. Normally this should be the wavelength that gives maximum absorption, for at this wavelength the sensitivity is the greatest and thus the error on the reading will be the least. Sometimes this rule does not hold. For example, many biological oxidation–reduction processes involve the redox pair NAD^+ and NADH. These two compounds have different and characteristic absorption spectra (Fig. 8.5). The best wavelength to employ in monitoring the interconversion is not at the absorption maxima but at 340 nm, the point of maximum difference

between the two forms. At 340 nm NADH has a molar absorption coefficient of 6.2×10^3 while NAD^+ is transparent. This change in absorption as NAD^+ is reduced or NADH oxidized is the basis of many biochemical assays. Similar considerations apply if two or more components are present and their absorption spectra overlap. Usually by judicious wavelength selection a point can be chosen where the interfering components contribute little absorption compared with the substance of interest. Quite gross variations in the concentration of interfering components will then have little effect on the total absorption, although small changes in concentration of the test substance are easily detected.

The same basic principles are employed in oximetry. Here we may regard the two mutually interfering substances as the oxygenated and unoxygenated forms of haemoglobin. Their relative spectra are illustrated in Fig. 8.6 and it can be seen that the maximum difference in the absorption of the two forms of haemoglobin occurs at a wavelength around 650 nm, while at 800 nm the *absorption coefficient* is the same in both forms. In any mixture of two components, a point at which the absorption coefficients are identical is referred to as an *isobestic* point. Applying Beer's Law the concentration of oxyhaemoglobin is proportional to the absorption difference of the two forms at 650 nm. Unfortunately by making a measurement at a single wavelength of 650 nm the oxyhaemoglobin content cannot be calculated because both forms are contributing to the absorption and the total amount of haemoglobin present in the sample is unknown. However, a measurement of the light absorbed at the isobestic point is independent of the degree of oxygenation and standardizes the system in terms of the quantity of haemoglobin. It also serves as a reference point for the adjustment of the oximeter to compensate for variations in sample size and fluctuations in light intensity. Having created a reference point, the difference between the absorption value at 800 nm and that at 650 nm is proportional to the degree of oxygenation. A full discussion of the design and operation of various types of oximeters has been given by Reichert (1966).

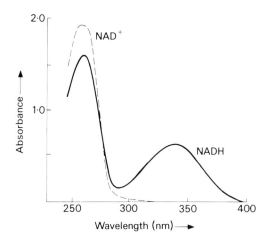

Fig. 8.5. Absorption spectra of NAD^+ and NADH, both solutions in 0.1 mM.

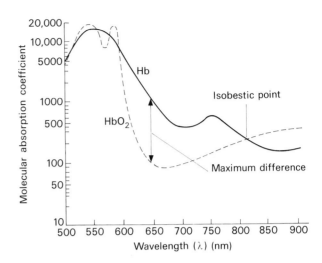

Fig. 8.6. Absorption spectra of reduced (Hb) and oxygenated haemoglobin (HbO$_2$).

In a colorimeter or spectrophotometer the length of the lightpath is fixed usually by the availability of cuvettes with defined dimensions. Commonly these range from 0.2 to 4 cm with the 1 cm light path cuvette being by far the most widely used. In the case of liquids, having decided on the wavelength and light path, the absorbance is proportional to concentration. However, where gases are concerned, changes in pressure affect the quantity of substance in the light path and thus the determination is performed at a defined pressure.

The concentration of a chromophore may be calculated by comparing its absorbance with that given by a solution of known concentration. However, rather than rely on the accuracy of one standard, it is better to plot a calibration curve using a series of standards of known concentrations. This also serves to verify that the Beer–Lambert relationship holds for the particular system being studied. If the Beer–Lambert laws are known to be valid for the system and if the molar absorption coefficient is known for the particular wavelength, an alternative procedure is to apply equation (iii) on page 95, directly.

The term absorbance as defined in equation (iii), is a ratio — the logarithm of incident light intensity to emergent intensity. Thus effectively two readings are required. Firstly the instrument is set for zero absorbance by placing a cuvette containing water or other suitable reference solu-

tion in the light beam. This value is taken as equivalent to the incident light intensity. In addition this reference solution provides a correction for the small absorbance of the cuvette windows and a stable absorbance to refer to in case the energy emitted by the light source changes. Having obtained a 'zero' reference, the second reading, the unabsorbed light emerging from the sample, is taken and displayed as an absorbance value. Some assays depend on the generation of a coloured derivative via a sequence of chemical reactions in which the reagents themselves may contribute to the light absorption. By processing blanks through the entire procedure this error is minimized.

The optical clarity of solutions is essential. Light is scattered by particulate matter so creating the illusion that the solution is absorbing more light than is actually the case. Although normally such particles are removed before taking an absorbance reading, in certain specialized situations advantage is taken of the scattering effect. For example, a standard procedure for estimating the density of a bacterial suspension is to measure the amount of light able to penetrate the culture. As the bacterial density increases during growth the turbidity increases and less light reaches the photocell.

If the solution contains semi-absorbent particles, such as red blood corpuscles, some light is reflected back, and some is absorbed in passing through the corpuscles. Both components may then be reflected off other corpuscles and scattered in all directions, including the forward direction. The high degree of transmission through blood is due to the fact that a proportion of the light is subject to multiple reflection and is thus transmitted through the liquid without passing through the solid elements. A simple instrument which utilizes this property is the pulse detector, in which a light source and a photosensitive detector are positioned so that either reflected or transmitted light impinges on the detector. By using a detector which is only sensitive to red light, outside daylight interference is minimized. The rhythmic electrical output can be displayed either by a moving pointer, via a rate-meter or used to actuate an intermittent light or audible device.

The use of time versus concentration curves of dye dilution, sensed by an oximeter type of cuvette, has been a common method for measuring cardiac output. The dye, indocyanine green, was chosen because its peak absorption occurred at 800 nm, the isobestic point on the oxygenated and un-oxygenated haemoglobin spectra (Fig. 8.6). Consequently, the sensing device was unaffected by any changes in the state of oxygenation of the haemoglobin in the sample during the course of sampling the dye curve. The determination of cardiac output is discussed in detail in Chapter 16.

Infrared spectroscopy

Many molecules of biological interest absorb in the infrared region. The absorptions occurring at infra-red wavelengths originate from the natural vibrations of the bonds between atomic nuclei. The bond linking two atoms behaves rather like an elastic force and thus will vibrate in much the same way as a spring with a weight at each end. For a diatomic molecule in which the masses and electric charges of the two atoms are different, for example CO or NO, the oscillation of the atoms creates a similar regular fluctuation in the magnetic dipole moment. This arises because as the atoms move apart the lighter atom moves further than the heavier one in order to keep the centre of the mass for the molecule stationary (Fig. 8.7). An analogy can be drawn to balancing two dissimilar weights on a beam across a fulcrum: to achieve equilibrium the heavier weight is the closer of the two to the fulcrum. Should the heavier weight be displaced away from the fulcrum, the lighter one must be moved a much greater distance in the opposite direction to restore the balance. To return to the oscillating diatomic molecule, the distance apart of the two charges carried by the atoms is varying and because the charges are dissimilar a fluctuating magnetic field or dipole moment is created. Such a system absorbs energy from an oscillating electromagnetic field, provided the field frequency and the vibration frequency of the dipole are identical. Radiation of this resonant frequency will be absorbed and removed from the spectrum. The frequency at which the absorption occurs is dependent on the bond strength and the masses of the atoms linked by the bond. The stronger the bond and the lighter the atoms, the faster is the vibration

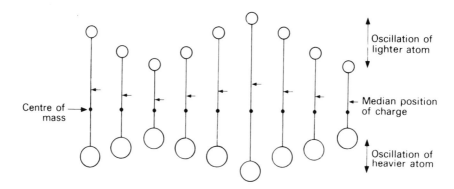

Fig. 8.7. Stretching vibration of an asymmetric diatomic molecule.

and the higher the absorption frequency. (For symmetrical diatomic molecules such as O_2 and N_2, in which the atoms have equal masses, the atoms move equal distances and since the charges are identical, no change in dipole moment occurs and hence there is no absorption.)

There are other influences which can lead to a fluctuation in the dipole moment of an asymmetric diatomic molecule, for instance, the rotation of the molecule around its axis. All such oscillations in the dipole moment lead to absorption of electromagnetic radiation in the infrared region, each absorption being characteristic of the type of bond.

In the polyatomic molecule the situation is considerably more complex and is beyond the scope of this chapter. Basically all absorptions originate from factors which cause dipole moments to oscillate, such as stretching and bending of bonds, but these frequencies may be modified by the environment in which the particular bond occurs. At first sight it would seem that with so many oscillations the absorption spectrum of a complex molecule would have too many absorption bands to be useful. In practice, compounds possessing particular functional groups do have absorption bands at characteristic wavelengths. Examples of such groups are OH (stretching) at $2.8 \, \mu m$, C=O (stretching) at $5.7 \, \mu m$ and C—O—H (bending) at $8 \, \mu m$. Thus with relatively simple molecules the infrared spectrum is characteristic of the molecule itself while for more complex compounds it aids the detection of specific features within the molecule.

The principles underlying the design of an infrared spectrophotometer are essentially the same as described above for ultraviolet and visible light instruments. The differences are necessary to cope with the longer wavelengths being studied. Two common sources of infrared radiation are a heated nichrome wire and the Nernst filament (zirconium oxide together with other rare earth oxides). In the instruments that use prisms rather than diffraction gratings to disperse the radiation, the prism material is NaCl, KBr or a similar salt, glass not being transparent to infrared radiation. KBr, which exhibits very little absorption throughout the infrared region, is used also as a supporting medium for

studying solid samples. The material under investigation is ground into a fine powder with KBr and compressed to form a translucent disk. This form of sample presentation overcomes the problem of finding suitable solvents that do not absorb in the infrared region. Materials that are liquid or gaseous are analysed directly. The unabsorbed radiation is focussed on a thermal detector, the change in temperature of which is measured with a thermopile* or Golay cell. The Golay thermal detector is a pneumatic device which, although responding to a wide range of wavelengths from ultraviolet to microwave, is normally only encountered in infrared instruments. It is similar in principle to the Luft analyser (see p. 235). The radiation enters the detector through a window that forms one end of a closed, gas-filled chamber. In the middle of the chamber a membrane of very low thermal capacity absorbs the radiation, so warming up the gas, usually xenon. The other end of the chamber is sealed with a membrane that incorporates a mirror. When the gas expands, this mirror moves in sympathy. An optical system monitors the small movements of the mirror.

Fluorescence

The spectroscopic techniques described so far have centred on the absorption of energy while the fate of this energy within the excited molecule has been ignored. As mentioned earlier in this chapter most molecules, on absorbing energy, dissipate it as heat. On the other hand, after excitation, the electrons in certain molecules instead of returning directly to the ground state pass to a metastable state intermediate in energy between the ground and excited states. The electrons return from this metastable state to the ground state with the emission of energy in the form of electromagnetic radiation. The process is termed fluorescence. Since the energy gap between metastable and ground states is less than the energy absorbed during excitation, the

---

* A thermopile consists essentially of a number of thermocouples connected in series, one set of junctions being exposed to the heat source and the other set being shielded from the radiation.

wavelength of the emitted radiation will be longer than that of the absorbed light. (If no loss in energy occurred during the process, the emitted and absorption wavelengths would be identical.) A characteristic of fluorescence is that the compound absorbs radiation, so exhibiting an excitation spectrum, and re-emits at longer wavelengths in the form of an emission spectrum (Fig. 8.8). Furthermore, the fluorescent radiation is emitted in all directions, not just following the path of the original beam.

Fluorescence is studied by modifying the arrangement of the sample chamber and detector of a spectrophotometer. The sample is illuminated with monochromatic light of a wavelength at which the molecule absorbs energy. Since the fluorescent emission has lost the directionality of the excitatory beam, it is measured usually at right angles to the incident light. This confers on fluorescence as a technique several advantages over absorption spectroscopy. The main benefit is much increased sensitivity for although the emitted light intensities are low, they are measured with reference to no light. This contrasts with absorption spectroscopy where the measurements depend on the difference in the intensities of the light entering and leaving the sample or comparing the light beams emerging

from the sample and reference cells. An analogy might be loosely drawn: the contrast is between comparing two light bulbs, one of 100 W and the other of 99 W, and viewing a 1 W light bulb in an otherwise completely dark room. It is far easier to measure accurately the emission from a 1 W bulb than to detect a 1% change in a 100 W bulb.

Unfortunately, fluorometric measurements are susceptible to interference from a variety of factors. These originate partly from the sensitive nature of the technique. For example, trace impurities in reagents that would not have affected an assay based on absorption, can pose significant problems with fluorescence. Another technical difficulty concerns particulate matter such as dust which scatters the incident light into the detector. Interference from this effect is minimized by using two monochromators; one to select the excitatory radiation and another to analyse the emitted radiation — the scattered light being of the same wavelength as the incident beam is ignored by the emission monochromator. This arrangement involving two monochromators increases the cost of the instrument considerably. A compromise is to eliminate the scattered light with a filter. A further variable that must be controlled is temperature. In fluorescence, an excited molecule loses its energy via two routes — to other molecules by collision or release as light. As the temperature increases, the kinetic energy of the molecule is raised, so making intermolecular collision more probable. With a greater proportion of the absorbed energy being dissipated in collisions less is emitted as fluorescence. Thus for accurate quantitative measurements, temperature control is vital.

Atomic absorption spectrophotometry and flame photometry

The technique of flame photometry was developed many decades ago and has become a standard procedure in clinical laboratories for it constitutes a rapid and accurate method for the determination of many inorganic ions. Many flame photometers are fully automated to dilute the sample into the

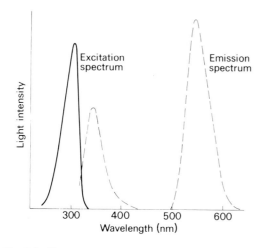

Fig. 8.8. Flourescence spectrum of 5-hydroxytryptophan in acid solution: solid line, excitation spectrum; dashed line, emission spectrum.

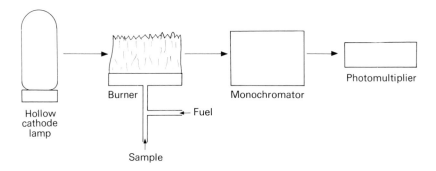

Fig. 8.9. Schematic representation of an atomic absorption spectrophotometer.

correct concentration range, inject it into the flame and, by reference to the response given by standards, calculate and print out the concentration in the original sample.

With flame photometry the sample is dispersed into a flame from which the metal ions draw sufficient energy to become excited. On returning to the ground state, energy is emitted as electromagnetic radiation in the visible part of the spectrum, usually as a very narrow wavelength band. These coloured emissions — sodium (orange), potassium (lilac), calcium (red) — have long been recognized as characteristic of many metals. The radiation is filtered to remove unwanted wavelengths and the resultant intensity measured.

The related technique of atomic absorption is more recent, but it has already developed into an extremely sensitive and specific technique, in routine use in most laboratories, for the analysis of metals and semi-metals.

In atomic absorption the sample is injected likewise into a flame which imparts sufficient energy to dissociate it into the constituent atoms but not enough to move the individual atoms out of their ground state. These atoms can absorb energy from a light beam passing through the flame if the wavelength of the radiation is correct for the promotion of an electronic transition. The Beer–Lambert Laws also apply to this system so the absorbance is proportional to the concentration of atoms in the flame. The absorption wavelengths are characteristic of the element in question and unlike the spectrophoto-

metric absorptions described previously, have very narrow bandwidths. As an analytical technique atomic absorption is far more sensitive than flame photometry. The detection limits for most metals using atomic absorption are in the nanogram per millilitre range. The reason for this difference in sensitivity is that in flame photometry only a small proportion of the atoms are excited and hence emitting radiation while with atomic absorption all the atoms present can contribute potentially to the absorption, thus giving a much greater response. In addition to sensitivity, atomic absorption has the further advantages of simplicity and speed. Because interference from other materials in the sample very rarely causes a problem, sample processing prior to analysis is usually very straightforward.

The organization of the components of an atomic absorption spectrophotometer is shown in Fig. 8.9. The instrument itself closely resembles a spectrophotometer. In place of the sample chamber there is a burner in which sample, fuel and oxidant are mixed. Typical fuel mixtures are air/acetylene and N_2O/acetylene. The burner is designed to generate a long flat flame aligned so that the light beam passes along the length of the flame. This arrangement ensures that the maximum number of atoms are in the beam.

The sample is illuminated with radiation created by a special type of source, termed a hollow cathode lamp, which emits radiation only of the wavelengths characteristic of the element under analysis. Thus the sample is illuminated only by the wavelengths that it is capable of absorbing. A different hollow cathode lamp is required for each element to be analysed.

Magnetic resonance

Electron spin resonance (ESR) and nuclear magnetic resonance (NMR) are a pair of related techniques which, although still concerned with the absorption of electromagnetic radiation, differ considerably from other spectroscopic procedures. Both phenomena arise from the magnetic property possessed by certain atoms; this property enables them to absorb electromagnetic radiation. The difference between ESR and NMR lies in the origin of these magnetic properties: in ESR the electrons are responsible while with NMR the composition of the subatomic particles in the nucleus creates the magnetic field.

NUCLEAR MAGNETIC RESONANCE

Each of the protons within the nucleus carries a single positive charge. The protons usually form pairs; one proton having opposite spin characteristics to the other so that from a magnetic point of view they cancel each other out. For an atom having an odd number of protons one of the protons remains unpaired and, because it has both spin and charge, the nucleus will behave like a small magnet. Normally, the nuclei have no directional organization but point randomly in all directions. However, when they are placed in the field of another magnet the two fields interact, leading the nucleus to adopt one of two orientations; the first being alignment with the external field and the second against this field. These orientations possess different energy levels, the lower energy state being where the alignment is with the field. Imparting energy in the form of electromagnetic radiation causes the nuclear magnets to jump from the low to the high energy states, and the absorption of this energy can be measured. This is the basis of the technique of NMR. The energy required to effect this transition is quite

small and therefore the radiations absorbed are at the comparatively long wavelengths in the radiowave part of the spectrum.

The great advantage of NMR as a technique is in the ability to study a single type of atom within a molecule to the exclusion of all other nuclei. Only those atoms with magnetic properties are accessible so within organic molecules the isotopes ^1H, ^3H, ^{13}C, ^{17}O and ^{31}P, are potentially open to study. Most investigations have centred on ^1H because it has a high natural abundance and does not require the chemical synthesis of the compound from suitably labelled precursors. When studying a hydrogen atom in a particular molecule the other atoms, while not participating in the magnetic resonance phenomenon themselves, are not without influence for they create local environments that slightly disturb the natural resonance of the hydrogen atom. For example the hydrogen atom within a methyl group has a different resonance to the same atom in an hydroxyl group. In consequence, the oscillation of the magnetic nucleus in the external magnetic field yields considerable information on the structure of the parent molecule.

One such hydrogen containing molecule which is amenable to study is water. The ability to investigate the state of hydration within the soft tissues has recently been the subject of interest since the freedom of movement of water molecules in tumour cells and normal tissue appears to differ.

ELECTRON SPIN RESONANCE

With ESR the magnetic properties arise from the spin and charge possessed by unpaired electrons. In much the same way as described for NMR, if the molecule containing such an atom is placed in a magnetic field, it can adopt one of two possible attitudes, each possessing different energy levels. Absorption of electromagnetic radiation will promote the transition to the higher energy state although the frequencies required to observe this resonance are in the microwave region rather than the radiowave range employed in NMR. ESR has proved particularly useful for studying transition metal ions and so has been employed in investigating natural metalloproteins.

Reference

Reichert, W.J. (1966) The theory and construction of oximeters. In Payne, J.P. & Hill, D.W. (eds) *Oxygen measurement in blood and tissues and their significance* Churchill, London.

Further reading

Knowles, P.F., Marsh, D. & Rattles, H.W.E. (1976) *Magnetic resonance in biomolecules.* John Wiley, New York.

Metzler, D.E. (1977) *Biochemistry*, chapter 13. Academic Press, New York.

Stern, E.S. & Timmons, C.J. (1970) *Electronic absorption spectroscopy in organic chemistry.* Edward Arnold, London.

Van der Maas, J.H. (1969) *Basic infrared spectroscopy.* Hayden Book Co., New York.

9: Ultrasound

Ultrasound techniques permit tissue interfaces to be detected and their shape and size described: they are of most use in situations where X-rays yield poor images, such as the definition of soft tissues, or are contra-indicated, as in pregnancy. They have the additional advantage that the movement of surfaces within the body can be detected and measured with a useful degree of accuracy, whilst information about the composition of a tissue can often be obtained. The introduction of Doppler techniques has also provided a useful means of deriving qualitative information about blood flow. Since the energies used in diagnostic ultrasound techniques appear to be harmless, the measurement can be used repeatedly on the same patient and there is no risk to the operator.

However, there are a number of problems. It is often difficult to locate the structures of interest and the interpretation of ultrasonic images can be difficult. Image detail is somewhat limited in many machines and instruments have a large number of controls. Successful ultrasonic diagnosis therefore depends on the appropriate choice of instrument and on the correct use of its facilities by a skilled operator.

Before dealing specifically with the generation and special properties of ultrasound it is necessary to consider some of the general properties of wave motion.

Wave motion

The simplest way to visualize wave motion is to consider the action of a plunger which is moved up and down in a regular manner on the surface of water (Fig. 9.1). The plunger interacts with the

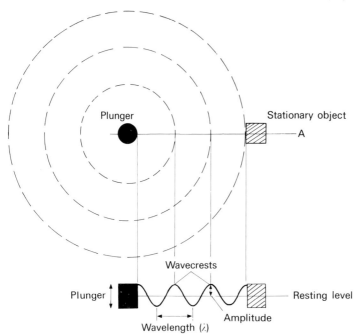

Fig. 9.1. Above: surface view of plunger creating ripples on surface of water. Below: section through water surface from plunger to A showing movement of water molecules at right angles to direction of propagation of wave.

water particles immediately surrounding it and causes them to oscillate in a similar manner. This oscillatory motion is transmitted in an outward direction from one group of particles to the next and so forms a series of ripples. The maximum displacement of the water surface from its resting level represents the *amplitude* of the wave, the distance between the crests of the waves defines the *wavelength* (λ) whilst the number of ripples impinging on a stationary object in their path each second indicates the *frequency* of the oscillation (f). All wave motions can be simply defined by just these three terms. The speed with which the wave front moves (c) is then given by the equation:

$$c = \lambda f.$$

When waves are formed on the surface of water the particles move at *right angles* to the direction of wave propagation, the transmission of the wave thus being similar to the transmission of an oscillation imparted to one end of a piece of rope.

Sound waves

Sound waves, however, are usually transmitted by the oscillation of particles in the *same direction* as wave transmission. The motion is thus similar to the oscillation seen in a row of railway trucks when a shunted truck hits the end of the row. This is illustrated in Fig. 9.2. In this type of wave motion the distance between the successive peaks of high pressure defines the *wavelength*, and the amplitude (the difference in pressure between ambient and the peaks of the waveform) governs the loudness or *intensity* of the sound. The *pitch* of the sound is determined by the frequency, which is again defined by the number of high (or low) pressure pulses which can be detected per unit time by a

pressure transducer placed in the path of the oncoming wave.

The human ear can detect frequencies within the range 20–20 000 Hz although in the elderly the upper limit of audibility is commonly reduced to 15 000 Hz or less. Sound waves generated at a frequency above that which can be detected by the human ear (i.e. >20 000 Hz) are therefore termed ultrasound. Nowadays it is possible to generate sound waves with frequencies up to 10 000 000 000 Hz, i.e. 10 000 MHz, and more. In diagnostic ultrasonics the most commonly-used frequencies are in the range 1–10 MHz. Since the speed of wave propagation (c) in tissues is about 1500 m·s^{-1}, the resulting wavelengths can be calculated from the equation given above, and show that for a frequency of 1 MHz the wavelength will be 1.5 mm whilst for a frequency of 10 MHz the wavelength will be 0.15 mm (150 μm). Since the ability to resolve small distances increases as wavelength is reduced, the best resolution is achieved with the highest frequencies. However, at higher frequencies penetration is reduced.

In practice the oscillating source does not energize a single line of particles but imparts its energy to particles in contact with the whole of its oscillating surface, producing planes of high and low pressure which move at right angles from the oscillating surface of the generator, and so creating a beam of ultrasound (Fig. 9.3a). This beam normally tends to diverge but by making the shape of the oscillating surface concave it is possible to focus the beam so that the diameter of the beam becomes narrower before diverging again (Fig. 9.3b). Acoustic lenses and mirrors can also be used to control the width and direction of the beam. However, in ultrasound apparatus the lenses are of opposite curvature to their optical equivalents (Fig. 9.3c)

Fig. 9.2. Above: longitudinal propagation of sound wave. The position of the oscillating source is shown on the left, the dense areas showing how the zone of high pressure is transmitted along the line of particles. The intermediate low pressure zones travel in the same direction. Below: the pressures recorded in the transmitting medium.

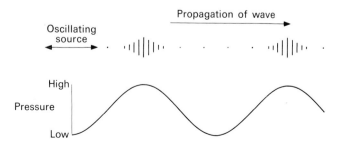

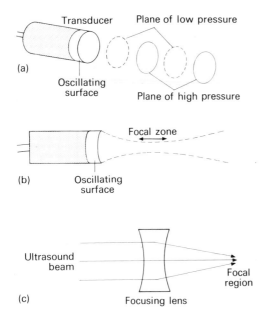

Fig. 9.3. (a) Generation of a plane wave by a flat oscillating source. (b) Generation of a focused beam using a concave oscillating source. (c) Focusing by lens.

because ultrasound travels faster in the solid lens material than in the surrounding medium, whereas light travels slower in glass than in air.

Natural sources of ultrasound are few. Bats and porpoises transmit and receive information at frequencies up to 100 kHz whilst grasshoppers can generate similar frequencies. The paucity of naturally occurring sources of ultrasound has hampered investigations into the long-term effects of ultrasound on man. However, the evidence is that the short-term diagnostic use of ultrasound is free from hazard.

Generation and detection of ultrasound

Most diagnostic apparatus produces a narrow beam of ultrasound which is highly directional and can thus be aimed at the target. Some instruments transmit ultrasound continuously but in others the ultrasound is emitted in a series of short bursts. The resulting pulse travels through the medium at a speed which is determined by the medium; but because the pulse duration is characteristically only

two or three cycles in length the pulse only affects a limited region of tissue 2–3 mm thick at any particular instant. Very short pulses of ultrasound contain oscillations of varying frequencies and amplitudes and this complicates the way in which they are affected by tissues. Pulsed ultrasound has proved invaluable in many clinical applications for it forms the basis of the pulse-echo techniques to identify tissue interfaces.

The generation and sensing of ultrasound is performed with transducers which are manufactured from materials displaying the piezo-electric effect. When such materials are subjected to pressure an electrical charge appears on the surfaces. The charges are positive on one side and negative on the other and are generated because the structure of the material is disturbed when pressure is applied. Such materials are used both to sense the pressure waves produced by ultrasound and also to generate the ultrasound beam. Ultrasound is generated by applying a high frequency alternating potential difference to the two sides of the transducer which changes its thickness and so produces ultrasonic radiation of the same frequency as the applied voltage.

Most ultrasonic transducers are now made from ceramic materials containing lead zirconate and lead titanate. These substances are cheap, easily shaped and very efficient in transforming mechanical to electrical energy and vice versa. The thickness determines the operating frequency of the transducer and must be matched to the alternating voltage which excites it. The front and back surfaces of the crystal are coated with metal and connected by wires to the electronic circuits which generate or detect the alternating voltage. The whole transducer is surrounded with an accoustic insulator (Fig. 9.4). Pulsed ultrasound is produced by applying a step change of voltage which shocks the crystal into a brief burst of vibration, much like tapping a bell.

Ultrasound can be produced by other types of transducers such as the magnetorestrictive transducers used in ultrasonic cleaning baths. However, they are much less efficient at the frequencies used for diagnosis.

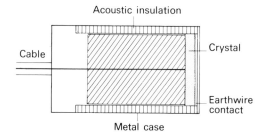

Fig. 9.4. Ultrasound transducer.

Properties of ultrasound

The characteristics of a continuous ultrasound beam are described by its frequency, wavelength and its amplitude. It has already been pointed out that wavelength determines the limits of resolution of an image. Amplitude determines the intensity of the ultrasound beam. The intensity, which would correspond to loudness in the audible range, is defined as the rate of flow of energy crossing a unit area held at right-angles to the beam at that point, the units being watts per square metre ($W \cdot m^{-2}$). The intensity of the beam determines the sensitivity of the instrument and thus governs the number and size of echoes recorded. It may also be relevant to the safety of the method. The total power of the instrument is the product of the intensity and the cross-sectional area of the beam. Its dimensions are:

$$\frac{watts}{m^2} \times m^2 = watts.$$

Ultrasound is absorbed by tissues and reflected and refracted at tissue interfaces. The intensity of the beam decreases exponentially as it passes through any tissue so it is convenient to express the intensity at any point with respect to an arbitrary reference level. For example, when the attenuation of ultrasound by a given medium is being measured the reference intensity and amplitude levels are normally taken to be those on the surface of the medium nearest the generator. The intensity and amplitude levels within the medium are then said to be a given number of decibels 'down' with respect to the initial levels, i.e.

relative level (dB)

$$= 10\log_{10} \frac{\text{power of observed wave}}{\text{power of reference wave}}.$$

Attenuation is expressed in terms of decibel loss per centimetre or sometimes in terms of the $d_{1/2}$ — the distance at which the intensity is reduced to half (approximately 3 dB down) at a frequency of 1 MHz (Table 9.1). Attenuation is affected not only by the character and temperature of the tissue but, most importantly, by the frequency of the ultrasound, attenuation increasing linearly with frequency in soft tissues. Thus the greatest penetration of the beam is generally achieved with the lowest frequency. However, at low frequencies resolution is poor because the wavelength is long. It is therefore common practice to utilize the highest frequency which will ensure adequate penetration of the tissues being investigated. For example, frequencies of 3–5 MHz are used for abdominal scanning whereas frequencies in the 10 MHz range may be used in ophthalmic investigations.

The absorption of ultrasound by the tissues results in the generation of heat and this is probably the basis for its use in physiotherapy. However, it is the reflection of the ultrasound beam from the junction between two tissues or from tissue–fluid or tissue–air interfaces which forms the basis of the majority of diagnostic techniques. An echo is generated if the characteristic impedances of the two tissues are different, the magnitude of the echo depending on the difference between the two impedances. The characteristic impedance is the product of the density of the tissue and the speed of sound in that tissue. The difference between the characteristic impedances of most tissues is quite small whilst there is a large difference between most soft tissues and the values for

Table 9.1. Attenuation of ultrasound by tissues at 1 MHz

	Attenuation coefficient	$d_{1/2}$(cm)
Strong (bone, lung)	>10	>0.1
Intermediate (fat, muscle)	>1	~3
Weak (blood)	0.2	~15
Very weak (water)	0.002	~1500

Table 9.2. Speed and characteristic impedance of ultrasound in some materials

	Speed of sound ($m \cdot s^{-1}$)	Characteristic impedance ($kg \cdot m^{-2} \cdot s^{-1}$)
Air (STP)	330	0.0004×10^6
Blood	1570	1.61×10^6
Bone	4080	7.80×10^6
Fat	1450	1.38×10^6
Kidney	1560	1.62×10^6
Liver	1550	1.65×10^6
Muscle	1580	1.70×10^6
Water (20 °C)	1480	1.48×10^6

air (very low) and for bone (very high) (Table 9.2). Reflections at most soft tissue interfaces are therefore very weak (less than 1% of the energy being reflected) whilst a bone–fat interface may reflect 50% and a soft tissue–air interface 99% of the incident energy. This renders detailed examination of structures through the lung and the skull and other bones almost impossible.

The angle of reflection from a tissue interface equals the angle of incidence (in just the same way as light is reflected from a mirror) but some degree of scattering also occurs. The intensity of the reflection is very much affected by the angle of the incident beam, the detected reflection being strongest when the beam is at right angles to the tissue plane. When such a beam strikes an interface at anything other than a right angle the non-reflected ultrasound is refracted in a manner analogous to light passing through a lens or prism. Although the deviation of the beam produced by this mechanism is usually relatively small it can lead to errors of location in some applications (Fig. 9.5).

Display of ultrasound information

Since the signals developed by most ultrasound apparatus have a short duration and high repetition rate the only practicable form of display for many applications is the cathode-ray oscilloscope (p. 71). However, the choice of instrument is governed by the scanning technique and the type of information being sought.

SCANNING TECHNIQUES

A-scan (amplitude scan or A-mode)

This is the simplest technique. The crystal, acting as the transmitter and receiver of pulsed ultrasound, is coupled to the skin by a liquid coupling medium, such as oil or water, and pointed at the area of interest. The echoes which are reflected back to the crystal are delayed by time intervals which are determined by the distance of the interface from the transducer and the speed of sound in the intervening tissues. In soft tissues a time delay of 1 μs corresponds to a tissue distance of about 1.5 mm (i.e. a tissue *thickness* of 0.75 mm). The scan is displayed by initiating the sweep of the time base on the oscilloscope at the moment that the pulse is transmitted. When an echo is received the spot is deflected vertically for the duration of the echo. It then returns to the baseline and continues its horizontal traverse until another echo is received or another sweep of the time base is initiated by another pulse of ultrasound. If the tissue planes are stationary the echo pattern will be repeated in exactly the same place at each sweep of the time base. Because of the persistence of vision the display will appear to

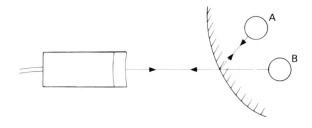

Fig. 9.5. Effect of refraction of ultrasound beam on apparent position of interface. Object A is interpreted as being at position B, if there is a difference in the speeds of ultrasound in the media on each side of the boundary. This effect is usually negligible in soft tissues.

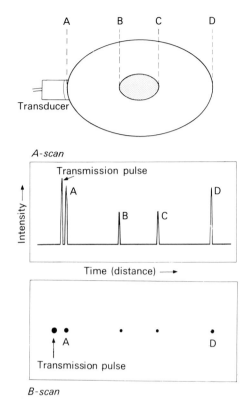

A-scan

B-scan

Fig. 9.6. A-scan and brightness modulation displays showing reflections from surfaces A, B, C and D. The brightness modulation (B-scan) quantifies the amplitude of the deflections in the A-scan in terms of brightness on the screen.

remain static provided that the pulse repetition frequency is at least 20 Hz. The size of the vertical deflection represents the amplitude of the echo whilst the position of the deflection along the time base is a measure of the time taken for the echo to return to the receiver and hence is related to the distance of the tissue interface from the crystal (Fig. 9.6). In fact, it is rare to receive a single echo from biological tissues for there are usually many interfaces and scatterers and, sometimes, multiple reflection artefacts.

Since echo signals from deep structures are attenuated more than those from superficial structures most machines incorporate a swept gain function generator which progressively increases the amplification of the echo signal as the time base

moves the spot from left to right. This provides a substantial improvement in the usefulness of the information provided.

The A-scan is most useful where the anatomical structures are not complex and where accurate measurement of dimensions is required. Examples are the measurement of fetal dimensions and the measurement of the depth of the chambers of the eye. It is also useful for differentiating solid from cystic lesions (e.g. in the kidney).

Brightness modulation of the display (B-scan)

It often proves difficult to identify the source of all the echoes received during A-scanning and identification may become impossible if the structures are moving. The use of brightness modulation obviates some of the difficulties by modifying the form of the display. The depth of the echo is still recorded by the sweep on one axis of the oscilloscope but the site of the echo is now recorded by a bright spot on the sweep line, the brightness of the spot being proportional to the intensity of the echo. The principle is illustrated in the lower part of Fig. 9.6.

Time-position (M-Mode) recording

In its simplest form time-position recording can be achieved as shown in Fig. 9.7a. The vertical axis displays the depth of the reflecting surfaces from the transducer with varying degrees of brightness. If any of the echoes are moving this will be shown by movement of the bright spots up and down along the vertical axis. Since this scan is produced by rapid repetition of the ultrasonic pulses a graphical display of the movement can now be obtained by adding a time base on the horizontal axis and moving the display across the screen to yield an M-mode scan (Fig. 9.7b). The horizontal time base is relatively slow in comparison with the vertical time base. For example, in studies of the movement of cardiac valves the traverse may take 3 s so that one or two cardiac cycles are displayed. The screen can then be photographed by a time exposure (Fig. 9.7b) or the image can be displayed on a long-persistence screen or on a storage oscillo-

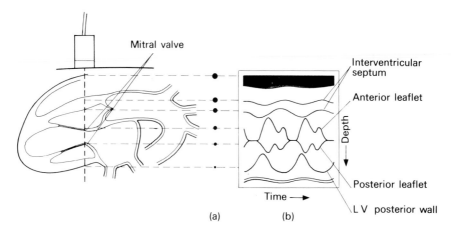

Fig. 9.7. Time–position recording on oscilloscope, (a) static brightness modulation, (b) with addition of slow horizontal time base (M-scan).

scope (p. 73). If more prolonged periods of recording are required the B-scan is displayed on a cathode-ray oscilloscope with a fibre-optic face plate. This produces an extremely bright image of the B-mode scan depth axis which can then be converted to a continuous record by driving ultraviolet recording paper across the face plate at right angles to the direction of the depth scan (Fig. 9.8). Such scans are also called time–motion scans (T–M scans) or time-position scans (T–P scans). They are of most use in assessing the movement of heart valves or ventricular wall.

Two-dimensional scanning

Another application of the brightness-modulated display is illustrated in Fig. 9.9. In this type of scan the transducer is typically moved linearly across the object and the movement of the transducer is linked mechanically and electronically to the horizontal sweep of the cathode-ray oscilloscope. The depths of the reflecting surfaces are marked in the vertical direction by spots of varying brightness, and the shape of the underlying structure is then built up as the transducer is moved across the object. The scan can be displayed on a storage oscilloscope and then photographed.

The accurate registration of the movement of the transducer and its synchronization with the oscilloscope trace naturally add greatly to the complexity and cost of such apparatus. There are also problems associated with the coupling of the transducer to the skin. However, the tremendous improvement in the images obtained has greatly extended the scope of ultrasound imaging.

Although the principles of two-dimensional B-scanning can perhaps be most easily understood by reference to the simple system just described, in

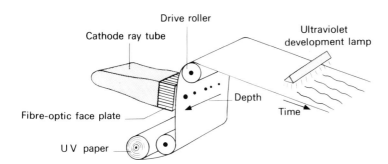

Fig. 9.8. M-scan: time–position recording on ultraviolet paper.

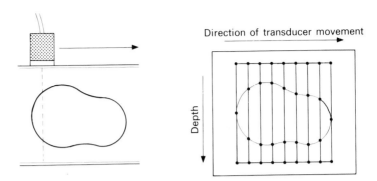

Fig. 9.9. Two-dimensional B-scanning principles.

Direction of transducer movement

Depth

practice the movement of the probe needs to be able to follow the contours of the surface of the body. Instruments of this type — known as 'static B-scanners' — have now largely been abandoned in favour of 'real-time' systems, as described below.

Real-time scanning

In pulsed ultrasound, the maximum pulse repetition rate is limited by the time taken for the echoes and their reverberations to return to the transducer. For a penetration of, say, 15 cm one sweep of the time base takes about $200\,\mu s$. This is followed by a dead period of about $100\,\mu s$ in order to allow the reverberations to die down. The resultant maximal pulse repetition rate is thus about 3000 per second. Since each pulse can contribute a single line to the B-scan, the rapidity with which an object can be completely scanned will depend on the number of scan lines required to build up a satisfactory image. A conventional television has 625 lines but for ultrasound images, 100 scan lines are sufficient. For a pulse repetition rate of 3000 per second an image built up from 100 scan lines can be scanned completely 30 times per second. Because of the persistence of vision, the eye thus sees a series of moving images which are comparable to those recorded by the separate frames on a cine-film. Instruments which produce and display images at more than 20 frames per second are said to operate in 'real-time' and permit moving structures to be studied in great detail.

There are basically three types of real-time scanners. In one, the probe contains a linear array of about 150 separate transducer elements which are operated sequentially in small groups to produce a rectangular image of the anatomy lying underneath the probe. A second type of machine incorporates a high speed mechanical scanner using one or more transducer probes. If this is in contact with the skin its movement is limited to rotation or oscillation around the point of contact. The third type of apparatus uses a phased array of transducer elements. The probe consists of about 50 transducer elements mounted in parallel so that they would normally view a field in their long axis. However, by introducing time delay circuits in the signal paths associated with each transducer element it is possible to steer the beam through a sector and to record the image as the sector is scanned.

Recently, the potential usefulness of scanners which can be inserted into the body has become apparent. Compact versions of the scanning systems used for transcutaneous imaging have been mounted on probes and endoscopes and some ingenious designs have been described. Of particular interest to anaesthetists is the endoscopic approach which allows the heart to be scanned from the oesophagus. A sideways-looking transducer array, mounted on a steerable probe, can produce very clear pictures without interference from structures which may be troublesome when scanning through the chest wall.

Real-time scanners need an operator to observe the display, and when an image which seems to contain useful diagnostic information appears, the operator stores the image for later study. This can be done by means of a digital frame store which retains the image in TV-compatible form, each line of the raster being divided into a number of picture elements called 'pixels'. In the digital store, each pixel can have one of several different grey-scale levels; for example, if the store is capable of retaining four binary bits of information per pixel, there can be $2^4 = 16$ different levels of grey. The operator can 'freeze' the image in the frame store by operating a convenient control, often a foot switch. Images stored in this way can be archived, either photographically or on video tape, or digitally, using a floppy disk.

Clinical application of ultrasonic two-dimensional scanning

Ultrasonic scanning now has a vast range of applications in clinical diagnosis. Real-time scanning is indispensible in obstetrics and gynaecology, cardiology, internal medicine, ophthalmology, and in many less well-defined clinical specialties. Indeed, so large has the subject become that it is now beyond the scope of a single review.

From the point of view of the anaesthetist, probably the most important application of two-dimensional real-time ultrasound scanning is in cardiac investigations. M-mode recording of the motion of the ventricular walls allows cardiac output to be estimated, along with measurements of cardiac function such as the shortening rate of the myocardium. The performance of cardiac

valves can also be assessed. By combining measurements of blood vessel dimensions made by real-time ultrasound imaging with Doppler studies of blood flow, as described later in this chapter, blood flow can be measured in accessible vessels.

Detection of motion by the Doppler effect

When an ultrasound beam is reflected from a stationary object the frequency of the reflected wave equals that of the transmitted wave. However, when the reflector is moved towards the transmitter it encounters more oscillations in a given time than a stationary reflector so that the frequency of the waves impinging on the reflector is apparently increased (Fig. 9.10). This is known as the Doppler effect. For a transmitted frequency of f_0, a wavelength λ and the velocity of sound in the medium c, $f_0 = c/\lambda$. If the ultrasound beam hits a reflecting object moving towards the source at velocity v, the frequency of the waves impinging on the reflector will be:

$$f = \frac{c + v}{\lambda}.$$

Since the reflector then acts as a source which is moving towards the transmitter/receiver the actual frequency sensed by the receiver (f_r) must be:

$$f_r = \frac{c + 2v}{\lambda}.$$

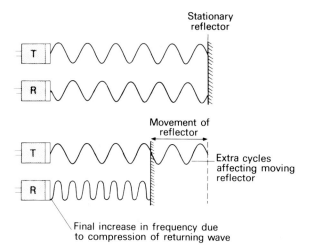

Fig. 9.10. Doppler effect. An object moving towards the transmitter encounters more cycles per second than a stationary object so that the reflected waves have a higher frequency than those from the transmitter. The increase in frequency sensed by the receiver is doubled because the reflected waves are also compressed into a shorter distance, thus decreasing their wavelength and increasing the apparent frequency further. For clarity, the incident and reflected waves are shown as parallel beams though in reality they are superimposed. T = transmitter, R = receiver.

Thus, the apparent *increase* in frequency is given by:

$$f_r - f_0 = \frac{c + 2v}{\lambda} - \frac{c}{\lambda} = \frac{2v}{\lambda}$$

or, since $\lambda = c/f_0$

$$f_r - f_0 = \frac{2vf_0}{c}.$$

This equation assumes that the speed of the reflector is small compared with the speed of sound in the medium, a condition which exists in most clinical situations. Substituting some typical values in the equation, e.g. $c = 1500 \text{ m} \cdot \text{s}^{-1}$, $f = 2 \text{ MHz}$, $v = 0.1 \text{ m} \cdot \text{s}^{-1}$ indicates that:

$$f_r - f_0 = \frac{2 \times 0.1 \times 2\,000\,000}{1500} = 267 \text{ Hz}$$

Since the signal is within the audible range of frequencies the output can be made to drive a loudspeaker or earphones. The resulting sound often proves vividly descriptive. For example, pulsatile flow in a blood vessel sounds like a high-pitched murmur whilst movements of the fetal heart sound very like real fetal heart sounds.

The application of the Doppler principle is not restricted to the detection of movement in the direction of the beam. When the ultrasound beam is at an angle θ to the direction of movement (Fig. 9.11) the resulting frequency shift is given by:

$$f_r - f_0 = \frac{2f_0 v \cos \theta}{c}.$$

When making comparisons between blood flow in different vessels it is therefore necessary to ensure that due account is taken of the angle between the beam and the direction of blood flow. Note that when the beam is at right angles to the motion of the reflecting surface (i.e. aligned with

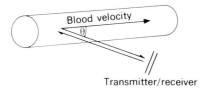

Fig. 9.11. Use of Doppler principle to measure flow in a blood vessel.

the long axis of the vessel) $\cos \theta = \cos 0° = 1$. Furthermore, small deviations from a right angle (e.g. $\cos 10° = 0.98$) cause relatively small errors in $f_r - f_0$.

DOPPLER INSTRUMENTS

In most simple continuous-wave Doppler-shift instruments, separate transmitting and receiving crystals are mounted side by side in a hand-held probe. Although the receiver senses echoes from both static and moving objects the output is related to frequency shift so that static reflections are not detected. Although the direction of movement can be derived from the direction of the frequency shift this requires additional signal processing. In most inexpensive instruments the output is therefore restricted to an indication of the speed of movement, but there is no indication of its direction.

Continuous-wave Doppler systems are sensitive only to motion; they cannot determine the depth along the ultrasonic beam at which movement is taking place, nor can they distinguish between moving targets at different points along the beam. However, by pulsing the ultrasound and assuming that each pulse travels through tissue at $1500 \text{ m} \cdot \text{s}^{-1}$, it is possible to calculate the depth of the tissue at which the reflections are occurring. Gating circuits are then used to select the signals coming from the desired depth. In this way the desired area of investigation can be selected without any interference from other targets along the beam.

The Doppler signals from some structures and blood vessels can be identified with confidence; for example, it is relatively easy to position the ultrasound beam so that it passes through the carotid artery by listening to the Doppler signals. The same applies to the thoracic aorta with the probe positioned in the suprasternal notch. In many situations, however, it is not possible to identify the anatomical location of the origin of the Doppler signals without the additional information available from imaging. Instruments which combine Doppler detection with real-time pulse–echo imaging are known as 'duplex' scanners; they allow the sample volume to be positioned precisely in a region of interest identified on the scan, with the scan and the Doppler information available simultaneously (if the real-time scanner is of the transducer array type) or in rapid sequence (with a mechanical real-time scanner).

An extension of the duplex principle combines two-dimensional real-time grey scale imaging with two-dimensional real-time Doppler mapping, the Doppler information relating to flow and motion being colour coded and superimposed on the anatomical image. This allows blood flow velocity to be estimated and, as explained later, from this it is possible for blood flow rate to be calculated.

An alternative method of measuring blood flow, which has recently been developed, depends on obtaining two Doppler signals from the vessel being studied: one signal corresponds to the blood flow velocity distribution and is obtained with a wide ultrasound beam uniformly irradiating the whole cross-section; the other signal is obtained with a narrow beam with the sample volume entirely within the blood vessel so that the power of this signal is related to the attenuation of ultrasound in the overlying tissues. The instrument, called the 'attenuation compensated blood flow volume rate meter', does not require estimates to be made of the vessel dimensions or of the Doppler angle.

CLINICAL APPLICATIONS

One application of the Doppler method is the detection of fetal heart movements. These are almost always detectable by 12 weeks. Doppler monitoring of fetal heart rate during labour is now widely practised, since it is greatly superior to the simple stethoscope.

Another application is the sensing of flow in blood vessels, for example to determine the patency of a peripheral vessel after suspected thrombo-embolism, or in sensing the onset of systolic flow in indirect blood pressure measurement. In the latter application the small transducer head is placed over a peripheral artery with the ultrasound beam aligned at an angle of about 45° with the long axis of the artery. As the cuff is deflated the systolic point is marked by an audible signal corresponding to the intermittent flow through the vessel.

The Doppler technique has also been used to sense the movement of the arterial wall under a sphygmomanometer cuff so that systolic and diastolic points can be established (p. 178). The output signal from most Doppler units is complex because there are usually many components of flow moving at different speeds and directions within the ultrasonic beam. In simple instruments, such as those designed to detect the presence of air emboli in the blood stream or the presence of flow in an artery, the output is conveniently presented by loudspeaker or earphone, because pulsatile flow produces a sound which aptly mimics the pulsatile flow of blood through an orifice. However, for more complex applications it is necessary to analyse the Doppler signal into its frequency components and also to indicate the direction of flow.

Of special interest to anaesthetists is the capability of the ultrasonic Doppler method to study blood flow. A Doppler signal proportional to the blood flow can be obtained from the ascending aorta using the suprasternal approach; in any given patient, changes in cardiac output and function are reflected by changes in the Doppler signal.

In principle, there are two methods by which the actual value of volume flow rate can be measured using Doppler ultrasound. The first depends on the measurement of the mean velocity of blood flow and the cross-section of the blood vessel. It is associated with several sources of error: the estimation of mean velocity requires either a knowledge of the flow velocity profile or that the entire cross-section of the blood vessel should be uniformly irradiated with ultrasound so that the contribution to the Doppler signal of each element of blood is equal; the angle between the direction of blood flow and the effective direction of the ultrasonic beam needs to be known and the potential error becomes larger as the angle becomes greater; if the cross-sectional area is calculated assuming that the vessel is circular, the diameter needs to be measured by the pulse-echo method. Unfortunately, the ultrasonic beam cannot be favourably positioned for both Doppler and dimensional measurements simultaneously.

The second method of measuring blood flow depends on the attenuation compensated approach described above. It is easy to use and gives results which compare well with dye dilution and other techniques for measuring flow.

Further reading

Chambers, J.B., Monaghan, M.J. & Jackson, G. (1988) Echocardiography. Information on morphology and function. *British Medical Journal* **297**, 1071–1076.

Goldberg, B.B. & Wells, P.N.T. (eds) (1983) *Ultrasonics in clinical diagnosis*, 3rd edn. Churchill Livingstone, Edinburgh.

Lancee, C.T. (ed.) (1981) *Echocardiology*. Martinus Nijhoff, The Hague.

McDicken, W.N. (1981) *Diagnostic ultrasonics: principles and use of instruments*, 2nd edn. John Wiley, New York.

Rifkin, M.D. (ed.) (1987) *Intraoperative and endoscopic ultrasonography*. Churchill Livingstone, New York.

Taylor, K.J.W, Burns, P.N. & Wells, P.N.T. (eds) (1988) *Clinical applications of Doppler ultrasound*. Raven Press, New York.

Wells, P.N.T. (1977) *Biomedical ultrasonics*. Academic Press, London.

Winsberg, F. & Cooperberg, P.L. (eds) (1982) *Real-time ultrasonography*. Churchill Livingstone, New York.

10: Radionuclides and their Use in Clinical Measurement

Use of radionuclides in imaging

Nuclear medicine utilizes the nuclear properties of radioactive and stable nuclides to make a diagnostic evaluation of the anatomical and/or physiological conditions of the body and to provide therapy with unsealed radioactive sources. However, this chapter will be concerned mainly with the investigation of metabolic and physiological functions in various organ systems using tracer kinetics and functional imaging.

ISOTOPES (OR NUCLIDES)

All matter is composed of atoms, each consisting of a small dense nucleus and a surrounding 'cloud' of moving planetary electrons. Atoms can differ from one another in the constitution of their nuclei and the arrangement of their electrons. The nucleus, simplistically at least, can be seen as consisting of two types of particles — protons and neutrons, either particle being referred to as a nucleon. Protons carry a positive charge, equal in size but opposite in sign to that carried by the negative electrons, while neutrons have no charge. The mass number of the atom is the total number of protons and neutrons in the nucleus.

Careful measurements have shown that even the purest elements consist of a mixture of different atomic species, with the *same* extranuclear structure, but *different* nuclear masses i.e. different mass numbers. Atoms composed of nuclei with the same number of protons, but a different number of neutrons, are called isotopes. An isotope may be represented in shorthand notation as the appropriate chemical symbol with the mass number as superscript, e.g. the isotope of iodine with mass number 131 can be written as ^{131}I. Since isotopes have the same number of electrons they have the same chemical properties and so cannot be separated from one another by chemical means. However, since they have different masses, they can be separated by physical means.

Isotopes can be stable or unstable depending on the number of neutrons and protons in the atom. In stable atoms, which are usually small and simple, the numbers of protons and neutrons are essentially equal. However, as atoms become larger and more complex, relatively more neutrons must be present for stability. If this is not the case and the proton/neutron ratio does not lie in the stable range, the change to a more stable ratio takes place by means of the ejection of particles in a random atom-by-atom fashion. The ejection of such a particle is known as a *disintegration*, and the nucleus will continue to eject particles until a stable isotope is obtained. An unstable isotope is termed a radioactive isotope or radionuclide.

In a stable nucleus, no particle ever acquires enough energy to escape, but in a radioactive nucleus it is possible for a particle, by a series of chance encounters, to gain enough energy to escape from the nucleus. The ejection of a nuclear particle is pure chance, and there is no way of deciding when any particular nucleus will disintegrate. However, if there are many nuclei, a certain percentage will disintegrate in a given time so, on the average, one can predict that in a given time, called the half-life, half of the atoms will disintegrate. Similarly, in the next half-life, half of the remaining atoms will decay. This physical half-life (T_p) must be distinguished from the biological half-life (T_b), which is the time taken by the body to reduce by elimination the amount of radioactivity by half. This combines with the physical half-life to give an 'effective half-life (T_e)'. The effective half-life is less than either the physical or the biological half-lives and is given by:

$$\frac{1}{T_e} = \frac{1}{T_p} + \frac{1}{T_b}$$

or

$$T_e = \frac{T_p T_b}{T_p + T_b}.$$

Transformation of a radioactive atom is accompanied by the emission of elementary particles and electromagnetic radiation. There are three kinds of radioactivity: alpha, beta and gamma. Alpha particles are composed of two protons and two neutrons, but they are the least penetrating and associated only with the relatively few heavy naturally-occurring radioactive nuclei, for example uranium-235 and radium-226. For practical purposes in nuclear medicine, therefore, they warrant no further discussion.

Beta particles may be negatively or positively charged. Radioactive atoms that contain too many neutrons decay by emission of negatively-charged beta particles, which are really electrons. They are more penetrating than alpha particles and require a few millimetres of aluminium to stop them. If emitted within the body, they are absorbed locally and not emitted from the body, implying that they can not only cause local tissue damage, but are also not detectable externally. They therefore form the basis of radionuclides used in therapy for killing cells rather than in diagnosis for external imaging. However, beta radiation can be used for measurement when samples can be removed from the body.

Positively-charged beta particles are called positrons and appear in nuclei that have an excess number of protons and sufficient energy to convert a proton into a neutron. They interact with negative electrons to produce so-called annihilation gamma-rays, which are emitted in opposite directions.

Gamma-rays are, like X-rays, electromagnetic radiations which travel with the speed of light and differ from them only in origin. They are propagated as waves of very short wavelength and are emitted as packets of energy called photons. They are very penetrating, so do not cause much local ionization and are detectable outside the body if emitted from within.

The nucleus of any radionuclide, being unstable, approaches a stable state through a process of decay which involves the emission of beta particles which may or may not be accompanied by gamma radiation. The energy of the emitted particles and gamma-rays is usually expressed in mega-electron volts (MeV) or in kilo-electron volts (keV) where 1 MeV = 1000 keV. For example, the energy of the annihilation gamma-ray is 511 keV.

The unit of radioactivity is the becquerel (Bq) and indicates one disintegration per second. As this is a very small and impractical amount of activity, one usually works in megabecquerels (MBq), where 1 MBq = 10^6 disintegrations per second.

DETECTION SYSTEMS

In nuclear medicine imaging (sometimes called nuclear radiology) the imaging device is nowadays usually a gamma camera, a stationary device which appeared in 1958 as a result of the pioneering efforts of Hal Anger. The camera is consequently often referred to as an 'Anger Camera'.

All types of detector depend on the fact that radiation interacts with certain crystals and organic materials to produce tiny flashes of light as a result of the so-called photoelectric effect. The intensity of light so produced is directly proportional to the energy of radiation. Such substances are called scintillators and the most commonly-used crystal scintillator is sodium iodide.

A scintillation detector (Fig. 10.1) consists of a lead collimator, which determines the size of field from which radiation is detected, and a crystal which produces a flash of light whenever radiation is received. The light flash is converted to an electrical signal by means of a photomultiplier, which produces an electrical pulse, the size of which is proportional to the intensity of the light flash and thus to the energy of the initiating gamma-ray. This small electrical pulse is amplified, first by a pre-amplifier in the detector head and then transmitted along a cable to a further pulse amplifier.

The signal then usually goes through a discriminator, followed by a pulse-height analyser. The discriminator will prevent electrical pulses below

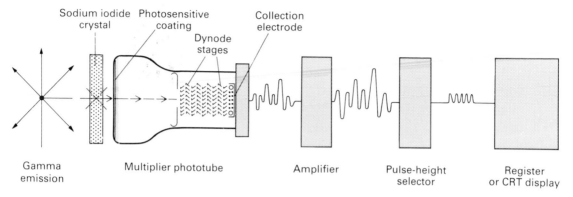

Sodium iodide crystal Photosensitive coating Dynode stages Collection electrode

Gamma emission   Multiplier phototube   Amplifier   Pulse-height selector   Register or CRT display

Fig. 10.1. Essential features of a scintillation detector. Gamma-rays from the patient strike a sensitive sodium iodide crystal, where they are converted into light photons. These, in turn, strike a photosensitive coating and are changed into electrons. The electrons are multiplied by the dynode stages in the photomultiplier until a large number are available to constitute an electrical current. The current is amplified and eventually reaches a television screen. The pulse-height selector filters out pulses produced by the wrong kind of radiation, e.g. cosmic ray activity and unwanted radionuclides administered previously.

any set arbitrary level (for example from spurious electronic sources) from reaching the output system. The pulse-height analyser has a similar action, and can not only reject pulses below an arbitrary level, but also those which are too large. This enables radiation from isotopes with different energies to be counted simultaneously.

The earliest detection devices were true 'scanners' in that the scintillation assembly was automatically moved to and fro in straight lines over the area of interest in raster fashion. They were thus known as rectilinear scanners. The gamma camera, on the other hand, does not scan in this way, but records the activity in all parts of the organ under review at a given instant. The heart of the device is a sodium iodide crystal about 29 cm in diameter and 13 mm thick (Fig. 10.2). This crystal is 'looked at' by a large number of photomultipliers arranged in an hexagonal array. Light flashes from the crystal are transmitted to the photomultipliers by means of a Lucite coupling plate. The crystal is covered by a lead collimating device designed so that only gamma-rays from the organ of interest strike the crystal. While such a collimator may be of the 'pinhole' variety, it is usually a multichannel device consisting of hundreds of holes about 3 mm in diameter which can be parallel, converging or diverging in the manner

of 'lenses'. Generally, the camera is provided with a series of interchangeable collimators of different thicknesses. Thicker ones are necessary when penetrating gamma-ray emitters are used and thinner ones for low-energy emitters.

The crystal photomultiplier assembly is surrounded by lead to exclude extraneous irradiations. In use the unit is held in a fixed position over the organ of interest and the distribution of radioactivity in the organ is presented on the screen of an oscilloscope, where it can be photographed. Alternatively, it may be led to a computer or made to activate a light source which can in turn form an image on X-ray film. The image finally produced, often called a 'scan', is correctly termed a scintigram to distinguish it from scans produced by other modalities, e.g. ultrasound, computed tomography or magnetic resonance imaging. This imaging technique is therefore known as scintigraphy.

The excellence of any imaging device depends upon its resolution and sensitivity. In principle, one would like a very sensitive detector so that recordings occupy a short time, but at the same time have a device which will observe detail and so have high resolution. Unfortunately the two properties are inversely related and a compromise pertinent to the case under investigation must be made.

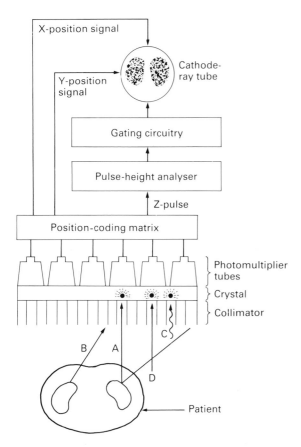

Fig. 10.2. A schematic view of the gamma camera and its circuitry. The lead collimator will only allow parallel rays such as A, C and D to reach the crystal. Rays such as B will be absorbed by the lead. The pulse-height analyser and gating circuitry will later filter off D (cosmic radiation) and C (scattered radiation) because their energies will not be appropriate. The position-coding matrix circuit will assign the pulse to the correct position on the television screen, which will obviously correspond to the coordinates of the photomultipliers which are activated. The Z-pulse provides intensity.

In recent years the use of computer interfacing has added much to the flexibility of the technique in that it is now possible to record, store and play back a number of procedures. During the playback a variety of manipulative techniques can be carried out. One of the chief advantages of such a system is that data can be recorded while the patient is present, but all the subsequent analyses performed

later. Images can be recorded in 'dynamic' or 'static' mode. The former will provide rapid, sequential views of the flow of radioactive material through the body or through a particular organ (Fig. 10.3). Quantification of the image can also be obtained as facilities are available to convert information electronically from any specified 'region of interest' on the image into activity-time curves or absolute counts. This technique is often used in cerebral, cardiac and renal studies.

Images produced with the gamma camera in a fixed position are called *planar* scintigrams, an example of which is shown in Fig. 10.4. However, it is now also possible to produce cross-sectional images using a rotating gamma camera and computing techniques similar to those in computed tomography and magnetic resonance imaging. In fact the method was first worked out by Kuhl and Edwards (1963) some 10 years before the work of Hounsfield (1973).

In laboratory-based nuclear medicine investigations, where extreme sensitivity is required and even beta particles have to be detected (but, of course, not imaged), use is made of the *liquid scintillation* counter. Here the sample is introduced into a glass vial which is then placed between two photomultipliers in a well-shielded lead castle. When a gamma-ray or beta particle is ejected from the sample it produces an ionizing track in the surrounding scintillation fluid and the emitted photons are detected by the photomultipliers. The rest of the technology is similar to that described for the gamma camera, but these devices are designed to count sequentially a large number of samples and record only the activity of each. For high-energy beta particles the device is nearly 100% efficient, but for gamma-rays the efficiency is limited by the fraction of the emitted gamma-rays which interact with the scintillating fluid, the remainder of this penetrating radiation passing through without causing an ionizing event.

One problem in liquid scintillation counters is that certain samples contain compounds that quench, i.e. interfere with the generation or emission of light pulses. This problem can be overcome by counting samples containing known quantities of radionuclide and graded quantities of quenching

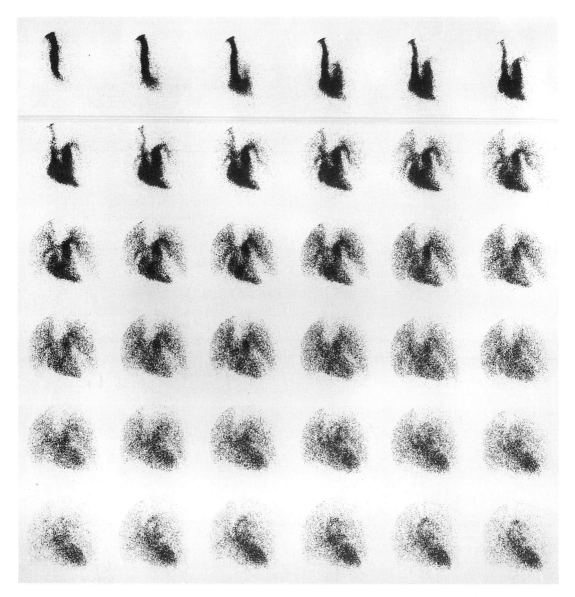

Fig. 10.3. A first-pass cardiac study using technetium-99m-labelled red cells. The tracer enters the heart by way of the superior vena cava and the right atrium and ventricle, thence via the pulmonary outflow tract to the lungs. The left ventricle and the aorta are then seen before mixing takes place (lower line).

agents. These values can subsequently be used to correct count rates for the presence of such agents.

RADIOPHARMACEUTICALS

For most nuclear medicine applications the radio-nuclide must be incorporated in some other sub-stance so that it can be transported to the site of measurement and then act as an indicator of the function being studied.

An ideal radionuclide would be rapidly removed from the blood and taken up by the organ of interest so that activity of the organ could be 'viewed' in low-activity surroundings, i.e. a so-called high

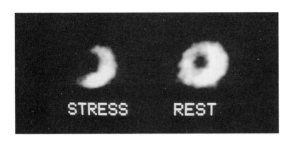

Fig. 10.4. Myocardial scintigram using Thallium-201 chloride, taken in the left-anterior oblique position (looking up the axis of the left ventricle) showing lack of perfusion in the territory of the left-anterior descending coronary artery on stress, but re-perfusing on rest. This demonstrates ischaemia rather than scarring.

target-to-non-target ratio. No radionuclide fully satisfies this ideal. The radiopharmaceutical used must, of course, be sterile and pure both from a radionuclide and a biochemical point of view.

The vast majority of nuclear medicine investigations are performed with a small number of radionuclides (Table 10.1). The recent trend has been to concentrate on the short-lived radionuclides, such as technetium-99m, which for a given activity at the time of scintigraphy produce a lower absorbed dose to the patient than the same activity of longer-lived radionuclides. The 140 keV gamma-ray energy of technetium-99m has satisfac-

Table 10.1. Examples of radiopharmaceuticals used in the investigation of the lungs and the heart

System	Radionuclide	Half-life	Chemical form	Maximum usual activity per test (MBq)*	Effective dose equiv. (mSv)†	Investigation
Heart	Technetium-99m	6 h	Labelled red cells via tin intermediary	800	8	Labels blood within cardiac chambers and allows quantitative measurements of (especially left) ventricular function
	Technetium-99m	6 h	Phosphonate and phosphate compounds	600	4	Detects myocardial infarcts, which take up these agents
	Thallium-201	73 h	Thallium ion	80	7	Detects poor myocardial blood supply and scarring (i.e. an infarct)
	Indium-111	2.8 d	Antimyosin monoclonal antibody	80	1	Detects myocardial necrosis
Lung	Technetium-99m	6 h	Human albumin macroaggregates or microspheres	80	1	Diagnosis of pulmonary emboli
	Xenon-133	5.3 d	In isotonic sodium chloride solution	200	0.2	Lung ventilation imaging by inhalation
	Technetium-99m	6 h	DTPA	40	0.3	Lung ventilation imaging by means of aerosol inhaler.
	Krypton-81m	13 s	Gas	600 (per min)	0.06	Lung ventilation imaging by inhalation
	Xenon-133	5.4 d	Gas	40 (per litre)	0.05	Lung ventilation imaging by rebreathing

* MegaBecquerels.
† mSv = milliSieverts.

tory tissue penetration and yet is readily collimated. The short half-life of about 6 h and the absence of beta activity enables high doses to be used with relative safety, so yielding high counting rates and improved spatial resolution.

Technetium-99m is obtained from a generator or 'cow'. The parent radionuclide, molybdenum-99 (produced in a reactor as a fission product of uranium) is absorbed into an alumina column and daughter technetium-99m is eluted as the pertechnetate ion (TcO_4^-) by passing 0.9% sodium chloride solution over the column. The pertechnetate is then shaken up with the appropriate radiopharmaceutical designed for the organ under investigation and the whole injected intravenously into the patient. Occasionally radionuclides are also inhaled, e.g. krypton-81m and xenon-133.

Technetium-99m is by no means the only radionuclide used in nuclear medicine. Indeed, the first one used was iodine-131, which became available as a fission product from the splitting of uranium-236 by thermal neutrons in a reactor. If the uranium-235 captures a neutron the resulting nucleus uranium-236 is highly unstable and splits into two nuclei of approximately equal mass, plus two or three high-speed neutrons. These neutrons can be slowed down by graphite or heavy water and are then called thermal neutrons. Such neutrons can more easily be captured by other uranium-235 nuclei, so setting up a chain reaction. Today it has been largely replaced clinically by iodine-123 and iodine-125, but it is still used in therapy. Other commonly-used radionuclides include sodium-22 and sodium-24, potassium-42 and potassium-43, chromium-51, cobalt-57 and cobalt-58, gallium-67, selenium-75, bromine-77, krypton-81m, indium-111, xenon-133 and thallium-201.

A radionuclide on its own will, with certain exceptions, not be sufficient for organic localization and must be incorporated as the tracer into a medium that is appropriate to the organ or system under examination. Sometimes this is a simple process. For example technetium-99m may be incorporated into a chelate such as diphenyltriaminepentacetic acid (DTPA), which is simply filtered through the kidneys and can be used to study renal function. However, the process is usually more complicated. For example, to image liver, spleen or bone marrow we make use of the fact that all three of these organ systems contain reticulo-endothelial cells which have the ability to ingest small colloidal-sized particles. Consequently, they can be imaged by injecting sulphur or tin colloids labelled with technetium-99m into the patient (Fig. 10.5). To image the lungs, on the other hand, technetium-99m is attached to small aggregates of human albumin, which, after injection into a vein and passage through the right side of the heart, will impact in the capillary bed of the lungs, the diameter of such capillaries being on average smaller than the small clumps of albumin.

To look at bone, labelled phosphates are employed which, after being carried by the nutrient arteries to bone, are incorporated into the bone by active bone cells or osteoblasts (Fig. 10.6). Similarly, heart muscle is imaged by injecting thallium-201 chloride. This is handled by heart muscle cells as though it were potassium, the actual potassium radionuclides themselves having too short a half-life and being too expensive to use routinely. Thyroid scintigraphy utilizes a similar deception. This organ takes up iodine avidly and so we can use iodine-123 (or less preferably, iodine-131) but an image can also be obtained by injecting technetium-99m in the form of the so-called 'pertechnetate ion', which quite fortuitously has the same ionic radius as iodine! This may also be the mechanism of uptake of gallium-67, which certain cells mistake for the more-commonly available iron. Finally, it is also possible to label blood cells: red cells with technetium-99m using tin compounds as intermediaries and white cells and platelets with indium-111 using oximes or tropolinates (which are also chelates) as intermediaries. Chromaffin tissue can be imaged by using a noradrenaline analogue called metaiodobenzylguanidine (MIBG) labelled with iodine-123 or 131.

Following the success of hybridoma biotechnology and the ability to produce monoclonal antibodies, the exciting possibility now exists of labelling especially the $F(ab')_2$ fragments of the immunoglobulins (IgG_1 and IgG_2) with iodine-123 and indium-111. This enables a number of tumours

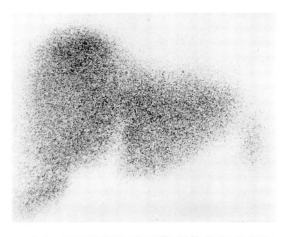

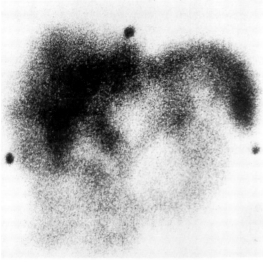

Fig. 10.5. A normal hepatosplenic scintigram obtained using technetium-99m-labelled sulphur colloid which is phagocytosed by the Kupffer cells in the liver and the reticulo-endothelial cells in the spleen. The lower scintigram shows a liver containing multiple metastases, which appear as photon-deficient areas as the tumour displaces normal Kupffer cells.

to be detected. The immunoglobulins may be thought of as Y-shaped molecules with the ends of the two shorter arms known as the variable Fab regions. These constitute the binding sites, the vertical lower portion being known as the constant region (Fc). Papain treatment will separate the molecule into the Fc and two monovalent Fab fragments. Pepsin, in turn, will remove part of the

Fc to produce a bivalent F(ab')$_2$ fragment. The lower molecular weight of the fragments induce rapid elimination and low-background activity, but tumour uptake is also less. For example, malignant melanoma can be detected by an iodine-131 labelled monoclonal antibody against the high molecular-weight epithelial antigen on malignant melanoma cells.

EMISSION TOMOGRAPHY

Much emphasis is now being placed on the radionuclide equivalent of computed X-ray tomography. This is known as 'emission computed tomography', or simply as 'emission tomography'. Two varieties exist: single-photon emission (computed) tomography (SPET or SPECT) and positron-emission tomography (PET). The former mainly utilizes technetium-99m or iodine-123 or 131 and any conventional computerized gamma camera with a rotating detector. Computer technology builds up the cross-sectional images, using a mathematical technique which has been known since 1917 when a French mathematician called Radon worked out how to reconstruct two- or three-dimensional images from the infinite set of all of its projections.

Some of the most spectacular successes of SPECT have been in the elucidation of cerebral pathology not detectable by conventional computed tomography or magnetic resonance imaging. In accordance with the demonstration by Winchell *et al.* (1980) that a large number of amines pass the blood–brain barrier, the search for labelled amines intensified and resulted in the discovery that n-isopropyl-p-iodoamphetamine labelled with iodine-123 is extracted by the brain in proportion to blood flow. More recently, technetium-99m hexamethylpropylene amine oxime (HM-PAO or Hexametazime) has been developed by Amersham International. Figures 10.7 (a) to (c) shows some SPECT cross-sections using this agent in the investigation of neuro-psychiatric disorders. It localizes in normal brain tissue, lesions being identified by photon-deficient areas in the brain image or deviations from the normal distribution patterns.

Perhaps even more exciting is the prospect of imaging so-called 'recognition-site ligands' if appropriate tracers can be found. For example

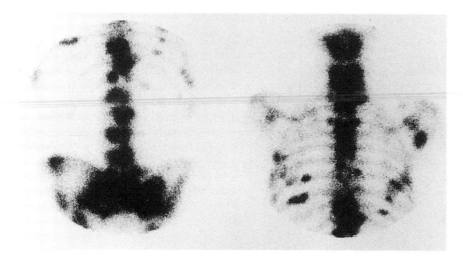

Fig. 10.6. Part of a skeletal scintigram obtained using Technetium-99m methylene diphosphonate. The very black areas are foci of increased uptake due to increased blood flow to and osteoblast stimulation around skeletal metastases from a primary breast cancer.

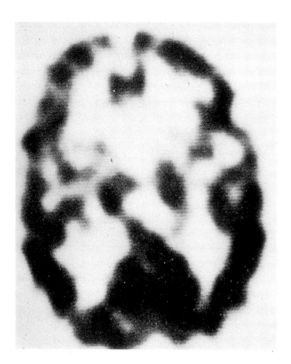

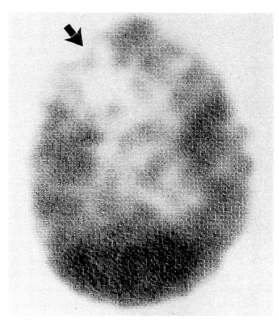

Fig. 10.7(a). SPECT image of the brain using technetium-99m HMPAO showing a normal cross-section at the level of the basal ganglia. Activity is present mainly in the cortex, visual centre and the basal ganglia.

Fig. 10.7(b). SPECT image using technetium-99m HMPAO showing a section through the brain of an 8-year old girl with partial seizure disorder. The image shows a photon deficient area in the right frontal zone (arrow).

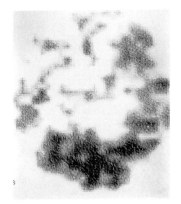
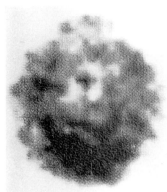

Fig. 10.7(c). SPECT images from a schizophrenic middle-aged woman after an injection of technetium-99m HMPAO. The scintigram at the left was acquired while she was severely disabled by classical schizophrenic symptoms such as auditory and visual hallucinations and shows very poor frontal-zone uptake (the 'hypofrontality' of psychoses). The scintigram on the right shows her in remission, when the equivalent section is indistinguishable from normal. Her medication had not changed.

iodine-123 iodospiroperiodal can already be used to image dopamine receptors.

By contrast positron-emission tomography is high-level technology, involving the expenditure of millions of pounds, as all positron emitters are cyclotron-produced and generally have very short half-lives, e.g. carbon-11 (20 min), oxygen-15 (2 mins), nitrogen-13 (10 min) and fluorine-18 (110 min). Thus the investigations can only be performed close to a cyclotron, which must also have the staff and facilities for sophisticated on-line radiochemistry and a positron camera able to detect the two high-energy gamma-rays resulting from the annihilation of the diametrically-opposite emissions of a positron and electron from a point source within the patient (Fig. 10.8). Such gamma-rays are not easily attenuated in tissue, with consequent superior image retention. The above radionuclides are, of course, also vitally important biologically as they either form part of, or can be incorporated into, many important compounds. For example, the use of glucose labelled with fluorine-18, has revolutionized the non-invasive study of neurophysiology and neuropathology, whilst oxygen-15 has been extensively used for the measurement of cerebral oxygen utilization and blood volume. The uptake of nitrogen-13-labelled ammonia has also been used to estimate blood flow.

The impetus provided by the success of PET views has stimulated research on more practical single-photon-emitting radiopharmaceuticals. Positron emission tomography has been spectac-

ularly successful in the identification of the dopamine and opiate receptors. In the case of the D_2 receptors, whose distribution is abnormal in some psychoses, medication for these patients can be titrated against the number of available receptors.

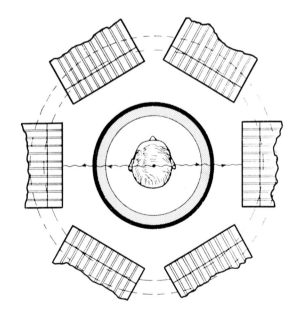

Fig. 10.8. Schematic representation of a positron-emission tomographic device. The annihilation gamma-rays travel in opposite directions from a point source within the brain. Using diametrically opposed detectors, the twin gamma-rays are selected for coincidence and a cross-sectional image is built up from the coincident scintillations.

Carbon-11 and fluorine-18 free fatty acids are also being used for cardiac imaging.

Table 10.1 gives examples of radiopharmaceuticals used in the investigation of the lungs and heart. A comprehensive list of tracers used for other body systems would be out of place in a book devoted to clinical measurement. The interested reader is referred to the bibliography, particularly the manual by Mistry (1988).

As in any form of radiodiagnosis, it is important for the nuclear medicine physician to be totally conversant with the normal appearances and normal variants. Then, by recognizing deviations from these normal patterns pathology can be diagnosed. Some examples of normal and abnormal scintigrams are shown in the figures.

One of the most useful imaging studies which warrants somewhat separate attention is pulmonary perfusion-ventilation scintigraphy in the diagnosis of pulmonary emboli (Fig. 10.9). The perfusion study is performed with macro-aggregates of human serum albumin tagged with technetium-99m which lodge in the capillary bed of the lung in proportion to perfusion. The ventilation distribution is best imaged with the patient breathing krypton-81m gas washed out of its generator with oxygen. An unmatched perfusion defect is indicative of pulmonary embolus. Matched defects may be due to chronic obstructive pulmonary disease or to any condition that causes an opacity on the chest radiograph. In addition to consolidation, neoplasm, oedema, effusion, collapse and fibrosis, this could unfortunately also be due to an established infarction at a stage when it cannot be uniquely diagnosed.

It is important to remember that although nuclear medicine studies are highly sensitive, they are not always as specific as in other branches of imaging. For example, while the slightest lesion can be detected in bone (such as stress effects resulting from a jogging session), it is impossible to distinguish the causes of such a lesion without an appropriate history and/or clinical details. It could just as well be due to a secondary cancer.

The most important thing to keep in mind about nuclear imaging is that it is a *functional* study. If the organ under investigation is not working, no image can be obtained.

Nuclear pathology

Following the isolation of deuterium, an isotope of hydrogen, about 50 years ago by the famous Nobel Laureate chemist, Harold Urey, this isotope was used as a tracer to study the amount of water in the body. Radioactive sodium was also used about this time and the early studies of thyroid physiology were also started.

Thus began the non-imaging branch of nuclear medicine, often referred to as nuclear pathology. Some of the tests under this heading are given in Table 10.2.

RADIOIMMUNOASSAY

Paramount among these tests is the ability to estimate accurately almost infinitesimal amounts of certain hormones, enzymes and drugs in the blood stream using the techniques of competitive binding assays, especially those using so-called radioimmunioassay techniques involving radioactive tracers, particularly iodine-125.

The principle of radioassay is as follows: when a labelled peptide (*A) is mixed with an antiserum raised against the unlabelled peptide (anti-A), it becomes bound to this specific antibody. This binding will be progressively diminished if unlabelled native peptide (A) is progressively added (e.g. as endogenous hormone) and may be measured by counting radioactivity after suitable separation. This equilibrium may be expressed as follows:

(*A) + (anti-A) + A = [*A: anti-A] + [A: anti-A].

The amounts of [*A: anti-A] and [A: anti-A] will be inversely related.

The radioactivity associated with the amount of A in an unknown blood sample can be estimated and, by reversing the process and adding different known amounts of exogenous A, a standard curve can be derived from which the amount of endogenous A can be read off.

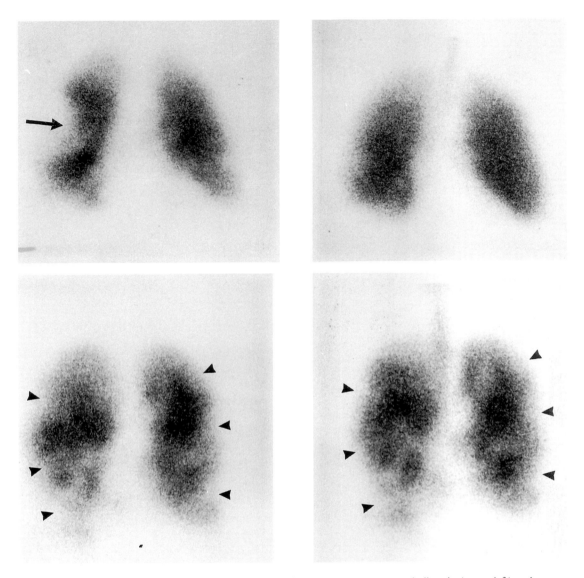

Fig. 10.9. Perfusion-ventilation scintigrams using technetium-99m macroaggregated albumin (upper left) and krypton-81m gas (upper right) respectively. The labelled macroaggregates stick in the pulmonary capillary bed. The upper pair of scintigrams show an unmatched perfusion defect typical of a pulmonary embolus in the right mid-zone. The lower scintigrams show multiple matched defects (arrows) compatible with obstructive airways disease.

Incredibly low levels of a number of hormones (e.g. insulin, thyroxine, triiodothyronine, oestrogen, progestogen, renin), drugs (e.g. digoxin, gentamycin, morphine) and other substances (enzymes, peptides, protein) can be estimated. The method has revolutionized many areas of clinical diagnosis.

Advantages of radioimmunological methods

1 They allow the determination of different compounds in the nanogram (10^{-9} g) or even the picogram (10^{-12} g) ranges.

2 They are generally of higher specificity than colorometric assays.

Table 10.2. Some examples of nuclear medicine investigations not usually resulting in an image

Alimentary tract

Carbon-14-labelled glycocholic acid breath-tests for the detection of increased bile-salt deconjugation

Carbon-14-labelled tripalmitate breath-tests for the investigation of fatty-acid metabolism

Calcium-45 and calcium-47 for the study of gastrointestinal calcium absorption

Chromium-51 for the measurement of gastrointestinal protein loss

Chromium-51-labelled red cells for the investigation of gastrointestinal blood loss

Iron-59 for the study of gastrointestinal iron absorption

Cobalt-57 and cobalt-59 cyanocobalamin (vitamin B_{12}) for the study of gastrointestinal malabsorption, leading to pernicious anaemia.

Selenium-75 tauroselcholic acid (SeHCAT) for the measurement of bile-acid pool loss

Bone

Calcium-47 for the study of bone metabolism

Brain

Xenon-133 gas and technetium-99m HMPAO for the measurement of cerebral blood flow

Cardiovascular system

Sodium-22 for circulation studies

Chromium-51-labelled red cells to measure red-cell volume, red-cell survival, sites of sequestration of effete red cells

Iron-59 for the investigation of iron metabolism

Technetium-99m-labelled normal red cells for the determination of red-cell volume, estimation of ventricular ejection fractions, ventricular volumes, cardiac output

Indium-111-labelled platelets for the study of platelet kinetics

Tritium (hydrogen-3)-labelled folic acid for haematological studies

Iodine-125 iodinated human albumin for the determination of plasma volumes

Xenon-133 gas in saline solution for circulation studies

Electrolyte studies

Tritium (hydrogen-3)-labelled water for the estimation of total body water

Sodium-24 for the estimation of total exchangeable sodium

Potassium-42 and Potassium-43 for the estimation of total-body potassium and total exchangeable potassium

Bromine-77 for the estimation of the chloride space

Kidney

Chromium-51 EDTA for the estimation of glomerular filtration rate

Iodine-125 and iodine-123 orthoiodohippurate for the estimation of effective renal plasma flow.

Pancreas

Carbon-14-labelled para-aminobenzoic acid (PABA) for the study of pancreatic function

Radioimmunoassay

Iodine-125-labelled compounds for the estimation of very small amounts of various drugs (e.g. digoxin, gentamicin) hormones (e.g. insulin, oestrogen, progesterone, thyroxine, renin), tumour markers (alpha fetoprotein, carcinoembryonic antigen, beta-2 microglobulin) physiological substrates (ADP) and many other substances

Thyroid

Iodine-123, iodine-131 and technetium-99m pertechnetate uptake tests in the study of thyroid function

3 Precision is usually higher than with bioassays.

4 They are well suited to automation.

5 Many methods have been simplified as a result of using specific antibodies.

6 In some assays 'direct' measurement in unfractionated extracts of urine or plasma is possible.

7 One technician can analyse 300–500 samples per week.

Disadvantages of radioimmunological methods

1 The necessity of working with radioactive labels.

2 As a result of (1) special equipment, special knowledge and legal controls are needed.

3 The precision is relatively low and certainly less than that reached in chemical techniques.

4 Specificity is not as high as for gas chromatography for certain hormones such as steroids. It can be affected by both cross-reactions and precursor binding.

5 The standard preparations require special storage.

6 The equipment is costly.

7 The more complicated the procedure, the greater is the error.

Quantitative tracer studies

In addition to the imaging studies described earlier, it is also possible to employ radionuclides to assess a number of physiological parameters. This facility has become even more sophisticated recently with the advent of advanced digital data acquisition and analysis.

There are four principal areas in which radionuclides may be used in physiological measurement:

1 Body composition.
2 Circulation and blood flow.
3 Turnover and metabolism.
4 Organ function.

In all these applications it is assumed that the tracer does not affect the system being studied, that it remains attached to the parent compound (or the portion being studied) and that its behaviour in the body is similar to the analogous neutral constituent in the system being investigated. Examples of some of the tracers used are shown in Table 10.2.

BODY COMPOSITION

The general principle underlying the measurement of the distribution of any substance throughout the body is known as the 'dilution principle'. A known quantity of a tracer (in this case a radionuclide, but the technique is also applicable to any other indicator such as a dye) is injected into a body space. After mixing is completed, the volume of the space can be calculated by dividing the quantity injected by the concentration of the diluted sample. This is based on the identity:

Quantity of the tracer injected into space
= Volume of the space
× concentration of tracer in the space.

Thus if a quantity Q injected into a volume V yields a concentration of value C

$$V = Q/C.$$

Q is usually calculated with reference to a known standard.

This technique can be used to measure blood volume and the various fluid and electrolyte spaces in the body. Because they do not correspond with true anatomical spaces, they are called 'dilution volumes'.

Although the principle is simple, the method is actually subject to many errors: mixing may be delayed due to poor circulation; the dilution volume may be reduced by diffusion barriers or reduced local blood flow and the space may be erroneously 'enlarged' by the leakage of tracer during the equilibrium phase. An example of the latter is the loss of serum albumin due to increased capillary permeability during shock. Unfortunately, it is often in such situations that accurate evaluation of body spaces is so important.

Blood volume

Red cells can be labelled with chromium-51 as sodium chromate simply by incubating them together. The tracer will then remain within the erythrocyte as long as the cell is viable. Thus the 27.8-day physical half-life of chromium-51 permits the long-term study of erythrocyte kinetics.

A known volume of the patient's red cells are labelled with chromium-51 and re-injected. After allowing sufficient time for mixing (usually about 10 min) the activity (in counts per ml) in a second volume of blood is determined. Then

$$\text{Blood-volume} = \frac{\text{Activity injected}}{\text{Activity/ml of whole blood}}$$

$$\text{Red-cell volume} = \frac{\text{Activity injected} \times \text{Ht}}{\text{Activity/ml of whole blood}}$$

where Ht = packed cell volume (PCV) of blood sample corrected for trapped plasma.

Determination of red-cell volume is useful, for example, in the differential diagnosis of polycythaemia and in following the response to therapy in this disease. Normal ranges for red-cell volume are: male, 25–35 $\text{ml} \cdot \text{kg}^{-1}$; female 20–30 $\text{ml} \cdot \text{kg}^{-1}$.

Alternatively blood volume may be determined using albumin labelled with iodine-125 or iodine-131. This is usually obtained commercially as radio-iodinated human serum albumin and so avoids incompatibility problems. However, the theoretical fear of HIV contamination makes this compound less attractive nowadays. Radiolabelled albumin is used to measure plasma volume (approx $40 \, ml \cdot kg^{-1}$) and blood volume calculated from the formula:

$$\text{Blood-volume} = \frac{\text{Plasma volume}}{1 - 0.9 \, Ht}$$

where $0.9Ht$ is the whole body haematocrit. Deduction of blood volume from the red-cell volume or the plasma volume is liable to error and so it is better to summate the two volumes.

The measurement of blood volume may be useful to assess a patient for surgery since blood volume is often reduced after prolonged diuretic therapy, in patients with phaeochromocytoma and in cachectic states. It may be totally misinterpreted in situations such as shock and after bypass surgery, when there can be considerable sequestration of part of the circulating blood volume.

Other body spaces

While in theory the distribution volume of any fluid (e.g. water) or electrolyte (sodium, potassium, chloride) can be measured using the dilution principle, the most commonly-used measurements are the determination of body water, the exchangeable sodium space and the extracellular fluid volume.

Whole-body water is estimated using tritiated water (i.e. hydrogen-3); the exchangeable sodium space using sodium-24 as NaCl and the extracellular fluid volume using bromium-85 as NaBr, which is the nearest halogen to chloride available as a radionuclide.

As before, using the sodium space as an example, the radiosodium is injected and the activity of sodium-24 in the plasma determined to give the dilution volume. In this case, as the exchange of sodium throughout the pool is slow, it is usual to delay sampling until 18–24 hours after injection by which time it is assumed that mixing is complete. Corrections must be made for both the radioactive decay of sodium-24 (half-life only 15 h) and for its urinary excretion.

The potassium space can be estimated by a totally different technique entailing the measurement of naturally-occuring potassium-40 in the body, using either a whole-body counter or the technique of neutron activation. In the latter case a shower of neutrons applied to the body results in a number of nuclear reactions leading to new elements which can also be detected by whole-body counting. The technique can also be used to assess whole-body calcium and its relation to loss of bone density in, say, post-menopausal women.

CIRCULATION AND BLOOD FLOW

There are three basic methods available for the determination of cardiac output and the perfusion of other tissue, namely constant injection or bolus indicator dilution and indicator clearance.

Constant injection indicator dilution

This method is applicable only to organs which have single inflow and outflow channels and, furthermore, the outflow channel must be accessible to sampling. The tracer (or other identifiable indicator) is infused at a known rate (F_1) and known concentration (C_1) so that it is completely mixed with the flowing blood. Similarly, a sample is withdrawn from the outflow channel and its concentration (C_2) measured, assuming of course that no indicator is lost between the points of injection and sampling. The unknown is the constant rate of outflow (F_1) of the tracer and it is calculated from the equilibrium identity

$$F_1 C_1 = F_2 C_2$$

or

$$F_2 = \frac{F_1 C_1}{C_2} \, .$$

Bolus indicator dilution

It is always very difficult to achieve the injection of an adequate bolus of any tracer, but it is possible to approximate closely to the ideal under carefully-controlled circumstances. The bolus of tracer must be thoroughly mixed with blood by passing it through a mixing chamber (e.g. the right side of the heart) and a 'dilution curve' is then obtained by withdrawing a blood sample at a constant rate and simultaneously measuring its activity. The outflow activity can be calculated from the dilution curve and a single mixed blood sample. A qualitative assessment of renal perfusion can, for example, be made after a bolus injection of any technetium-99m complex into an antecubital vein and deriving an activity-time curve of its progress through the kidneys. Iodine-123 orthohippurate is structurally similar to p-aminohippurate, which is of course well-known to be cleared by the renal tubules. Excretion of labelled orthohippurate therefore measures the effective renal plasma flow (ERPF). A newer agent, which is handled similarly is technetium-99m mercaptoacetyltriglycine (MAG3); it has all the resolution and safety advantages of a technetium-99m compound.

Clearance methods

A radionuclide is injected into a tissue and its rate of clearance from the tissue is monitored either by sampling or by external counting. When there is no barrier to diffusion between the tissue and the blood, and therefore no delay in transfer, the clearance can be expressed by a simple exponential. Unfortunately, the situation is usually much more complex and sophisticated analyses are necessary. However, it is useful to know that as a *very* rough approximation, blood flow is equal to ln 2, i.e. 0.6931, divided by the half-time, this being the time taken for the activity to fall to half of its initial value. $\ln 2 / T_{1/2}$ is, of course, the rate constant of the presumed first-order process.

Technetium-99m diethylenetriamine penta-acetic acid (DTPA) is cleared by the glomerulus in the same way as inulin and so can be used to measure glomerular filtration rate (GFR). In a well hydrated patient GFR can be measured using technetium-99m DTPA or iodine-125 iothalamate infusion (or even a subcutaneous injection) in order to obtain a constant plasma level during the time that urine is collected for counting. Glomerular filtration rate can also be determined from multiple blood samples following a bolus injection of one of the tracers mentioned above or chromium-51 ethylenediamine tetra-acetic acid (EDTA). In most nuclear medicine departments GFR is estimated from the activity of a single,

timed blood sample and that which accumulates in the kidney 2–3 minutes post-injection as measured by a computerized gamma camera. Effective renal plasma flow can be determined using similar techniques following iodine-123 orthohippurate administration as described previously.

TURNOVER AND METABOLISM

As examples under this heading one can consider certain haematological studies, vitamin B_{12} metabolism, bile-acid resorption and bone densitometry.

While not of as much interest to the anaesthetist as to the haematologist, chromium-51-labelled red cells can be used to measure erythrocyte survival for the evaluation of patients with haemolytic anaemias and it is, of course, also possible to study erythrocyte sequestration in the liver and spleen by external counting. In hypersplenism the spleen destroys cells at a much greater rate than the liver.

Radioisotopes of iron, usually iron-59 or iron-52, can also be used to determine the amount of iron absorbed, transported, stored, utilized and excreted — studies collectively known as ferrokinetics. The studies most commonly employed are plasma-iron clearance, plasma-iron turnover, red-cell iron utilization and iron turnover in the reticulo-endothelial spaces of liver, spleen and bone marrow. Ferrokinetic studies depend on the fact that iron is incorporated into new red cells during their production and so the use of radioiron gives us some idea of the effectiveness of erythro-poiesis and the sites at which it occurs. The anaemias can be studied by investigating the rate of disappearance of radioiron from the plasma as a result of its uptake by the bone marrow during haemoglobin synthesis.

Vitamin B_{12} levels can be measured by means of radioligand assay as outlined above, but the causes of vitamin B_{12} deficiency are not always evident from a measurement of levels alone, and one has to resort to other tests to distinguish between inadequate uptake, malabsorption due to gastric abnormalities, intestinal malabsorption and genetic abnormality in transport proteins. The well-known Shilling test uses cobalt-57-labelled vitamin B_{12} to differentiate pernicious anaemia from the other causes of B_{12} malabsorption and can detect the absence of intrinsic factor when serum B_{12} deficiency or anaemia is not yet present, or when the patient has received folate or Vitamin B_{12} therapy.

Osteoporosis, or decreased bone density per unit volume of skeleton is a very common condition and highly topical in relation to post-menopausal women and its potential therapy with hormone replacement. Quantitative measurement of X- or gamma radiation transmitted through bone provides a unique way of measuring its mineral content. The three most accurate techniques available include X-ray methods; single-photon absorptiometry using a collimated beam of gamma-ray photons from a monoenergetic radionuclide source, and dual-photon absorptiometry, using a radionuclide that emits gamma-ray photons of two different energies. The best instrument to date appears to be one which uses a specially filtered X-ray beam which eliminates all but those X-ray energies appropriate for dual-photon absorptiometry. The spine and the femoral neck are the obvious two sites of interest for this kind of measurement.

The basic principle of measurement is the same in all cases, i.e. the fraction of photons transmitted by the bone is related to the mass, density and attenuation coefficient of that bone for the particular energy being used. The attenuation coefficient is the fractional decrease in the number of photons passing through the tissue and depends on the energy of the photon, its interaction with tissue, the atomic number of the tissue and its so-called electron density. The eventual reading is usually obtained in terms of the mineral content, calculated from all the factors mentioned.

ORGAN FUNCTION

As has been emphasized repeatedly, all imaging studies are dependent on organ function. However, with modern computer technology it is now possible to quantitate virtually all of the studies. In this section, as prime examples of this methodology, analyses related to the heart, brain, kidneys, stomach, and the thyroid will be briefly discussed.

Heart

Although many techniques are now available in nuclear cardiology, one of the most successful has been the evaluation of cardiac function using technetium-99m-labelled autologous red blood cells and the technique of gating the gamma camera to the cardiac cycle via the R-wave of the electrocardiograph. Hence these studies are referred to as multigated acquisition (MUGA) studies. Using this technique estimates may be made of ventricular function (usually the left) and ventricular wall motion.

Images of the heart in systole and diastole are obtained by the summation of counts obtained during end-diastole and end-systole over many cardiac cycles. The cardiac cycle can be subdivided into 16–64 frames and counts for each frame are accumulated from many cycles to form the multiple images of a composite heart beat (Fig. 10.10). Corrections have to be made for arrhythmias. One of the great advantages of this kind of technology, now common in radiology, is that the images from each part of the cycle can be displayed on video as a motion picture of the beating heart. As a result it is easy to spot wall-motion abnormalities.

In the left-oblique position the left ventricle can be seen without overlap from the other chambers. The counts over the ventricle are directly proportional to the ventricular volume and the difference between end-diastolic and end-systolic counts as a fraction of the former, will yield the ejection fraction, i.e.

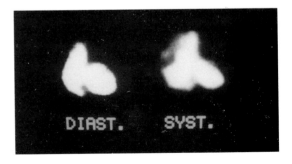

Fig. 10.10. ECG-gated radionuclide ventriculogram using Technetium-99m-labelled autologous red cells showing the left-ventricular blood pool (the area protruding towards the reader's right) at end-diastole (left) and at end-systole (right).

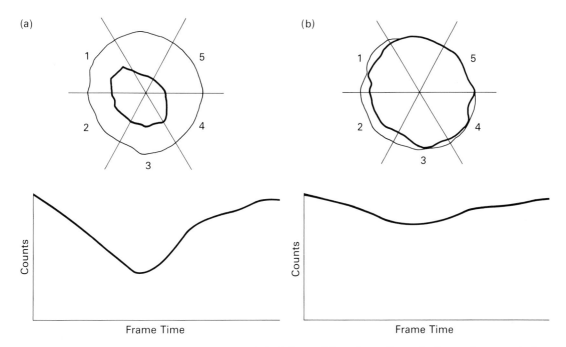

Fig. 10.11. Regions of interest can be drawn around the left ventricle and an adjacent background area producing activity-time curves (volume curves of left-ventricular counts vs. time for a composite cardiac cycle) from which the ejection fraction can be calculated. The curve for a patient with a normal ejection fraction (a) and a poor ejection fraction (b) are shown. The associated circular diagrams show the superimposed end-systolic (inner circle) and end-diastolic (outer circle) outlines (viewed craniad from the apex) in the two instances. Hardly any shift in contour is noted in the patient with low ejection fraction.

Ejection fraction

$$= \frac{\text{End-diastolic counts} - \text{End-systolic counts}}{\text{End-diastolic counts}}$$

The left-ventricular ejection fraction is normally greater than 50% and is a very sensitive indication of its function (Fig. 10.11). It may be reduced following myocardial infarction and is correlated with prognosis. The technique has both a sensitivity and specificity of 87–95% in the detection of stress-induced myocardial ischaemia.* Right ventricular ejection fraction, ventricular volumes and regurgitation fractions in valvular disease can also be estimated. The technique is also of use in evaluating the cardiac response to exercise and chronic pulmonary disease and in the early detection of drug-induced cardiotoxicity.

If the activity over the left ventricle is expressed as a function of time, it produces a complex curve which can be broken down into elementary sine and cosine curves by Fourier analysis (see p. 9). The simple curves are characterized by certain amplitudes (heights of the wave crests above the axis) and phases (angles). Amplitudes and phases can subsequently be calculated over different parts of the ventricle and represented by computer-coloured maps called phase or amplitude diagrams. Any deviations from normal distributions can then easily be detected.

* Sensitivity measures the ability of a test to detect disease when it is present. It is the ratio of true-positive results compared with all of those with the disease (true positive plus false negative). Specificity measures the ability to exclude disease when it is absent. It is the ratio of true-negative results to all those without disease (true negative plus false positive). A graph of sensitivity against the false-positive fraction (1 − specificity) yields what is known as a receiver operating characteristic (ROC) curve.

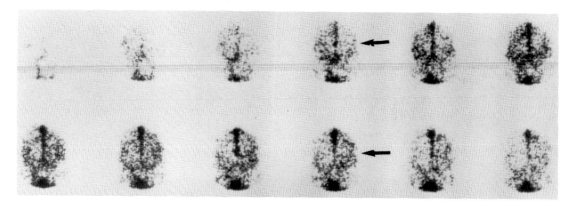

Fig. 10.12. Radionuclide angiogram using technetium-99m as pertechnetate. Delayed appearance of tracer in the left hemisphere (reader's right) due to cerebrovascular disease in the left carotid and/or left middle cerebral artery. During the later venous phase, activity in the right hemisphere decreases to reveal relatively increased flow in the left hemisphere — the so-called 'flip-flop' phenomenon.

Brain

Two tests of function may be mentioned. The first utilizes the ability of the computerized gamma camera to collect counts over time and store these in its memory so that it is possible to obtain sequential images of the radionuclide as it enters the brain. The technique is called radionuclide angiography and provides a simple, virtually non-invasive method of studying the cerebral circulation in health and disease (Fig. 10.12). By defining computer-generated, so-called regions-of-interest[†] in any part of the brain, activity-time curves of the radioactivity can easily be derived.

The second test is used for non-function, i.e. cerebral death. Technetium-99m Hexametazime passes through the blood–brain barrier and so is taken up by normal brain. In brain death there is no perfusion and so no uptake. However the test is not absolute as the brainstem cannot be imaged and so could still be alive. Nevertheless, it is a useful adjunct to the battery of tests used for the establishment of brain death.

[†] A region-of-interest (ROI) is a computer operation whereby a closed border can literally be drawn on the VDU screen around any anatomical region, e.g. a kidney or the left ventricle, in order to produce a graph of the activity within that border as a function of time.

Kidney

Two of the mainstays in the investigation of renal disease are the renogram and the renal scintigram. The former can be carried out with iodine-123 orthohippurate, technetium-99m mercaptoacetyl-triglycine (MAG3) or technetium-99m diphenyltri-amine penta-acetic acid (DTPA). Renal scintigraphy is carried out with technetium-99m dimercaptosuccinic acid (DMSA) which binds to the renal tubules.

The normal renogram is again a computer-generated activity-time curve of the passage of radionuclide through the kidney and is obtained by defining a region-of-interest over the kidney. The normal renogram is shown in Fig. 10.13(a). Analysis of the renogram curve can be very complex, utilizing so-called deconvolutional analysis and deriving transit times, but it seems to be just as useful clinically if it is interpreted simply. The rising part of the curve (Phase I or 'vascular phase') is a function of radionuclide reaching the kidney; the peak (Phase II or 'handling phase') is related to the efficiency of parenchymal function, while the descending part of the curve (Phase III or 'excretory' phase) shows the rate of washout from the renal area. Much of the activity 'seen' by the gamma camera will be background activity and

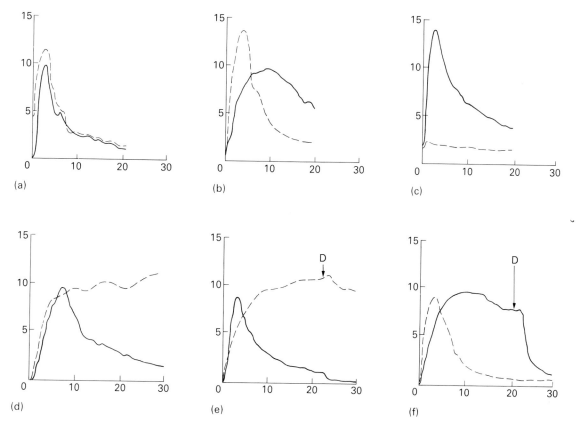

Fig. 10.13. Normal and abnormal renograms. (Solid curve = left kidney; dotted curve = right kidney; Y-axis shows percentage of dose; X-axis shows time in minutes; D = injection of diuretic). (a) Normal gamma-camera renograms each showing rising vascular phase, handling peak and descending excretory phase. (b) Delayed, sub-optimal peak on left side in patient with impaired left renal function. (c) Patient with normal left kidney, but non-functioning right kidney. (d) Renogram showing obstructive pattern on right side. (e) Gamma-camera renogram with diuretic provocation showing normal left renogram, but dilated, obstructed right renal pelvis showing little response to diuretic. (f) Gamma-camera diuresis renogram with normal right kidney and dilated, but non-obstructed left kidney responding to diuretic provocation.

ideally allowances should be made to subtract this from the renal curves. Some obvious deviations from the normal curve and their explanations are shown in Figs 10.13(b) to (f).

One of the most difficult diagnoses to make without invasive angiography is that of renovascular hypertension. However, renography following administration of angiotensin-converting-enzyme (ACE) inhibitors is now reported to increase the sensitivity and specificity of the test in detecting this entity.

Renal scintigraphy using technetium-99m demercaptosuccinic acid not only outlines renal cortical anatomy, but enables the relative distribution of the compound between the two kidneys to be measured — so-called 'divided renal function'. This will be dependent on blood flow and tubular function.

Gastrointestinal tract

Most studies of gastric emptying are either invasive or not quantifiable. By contrast radionuclide methods permit the administration of solid and liquid meals of defined weight and calorie content labelled with appropriate radionuclides to be given to the patient and their progress followed with quantitative imaging. The study can measure the half-time disappearance of the meal from the stomach and deviation from established normal ranges can easily be detected. The test can be used to quantitate abnormal gastric emptying and gastroparesis in diabetes or in those who have undergone surgery or drug therapy. These studies can also be used as an objective tool to monitor therapeutic response.

Thyroid

This is the organ with which nuclear medicine started. Thyroid uptake measurements are based on the fact that the gland requires iodine for incorporation into its hormones. The fraction of radioiodine (usually iodine-123 as sodium iodide) taken up by the thyroid can be determined over selected time intervals and compared to known euthyroid values. The uptake is usually expressed as a percentage of the dose administered and is calculated with reference to a standard (usually counted in a simulated neck known as a 'phantom') that is equivalent to the amount given to the patient.

$$\text{Percentage radioiodide uptake} = \frac{\text{Counts in thyroid} - \text{background}}{\text{Counts in phantom} - \text{background}}$$

Nowadays the procedure is usually combined with thyroid scintigraphy and ultrasound.

These are the most important examples of the use of radionuclides in clinical measurement but the techniques have been applied to many other organ systems. There are even measurements of the degree of testicular torsion and the degree of patency of the fallopian tubes. Radioisotope techniques have been applied to many other disciplines. For example, in microbiology so-called radiomimetric analysis will identify bacteria by means of the labelled carbon dioxide that they produce when grown on substrates containing carbon-14. From the total activity of the radioactive gas an estimate may be made of the number of bacteria present.

Radiotherapy using unsealed sources

Only radionuclides that emit alpha or beta particles are useful for irradiation treatment, for such particles lose all their energy to their surroundings over a very short distance from their origin and this energy is sufficient to kill cells, both benign and malignant, along the path of ionization. Sealed sources such as radium, cobalt-60, iridium-192 and tantalum-182 have been, or are in, common use for radiotherapeutic treatment, but of the unsealed sources — with which this chapter is concerned — only iodine-131, phosphorus-32 and yttrium-90 are important.

As iodine is selectively taken up by the thyroid gland, iodine-131 can be used in the treatment of thyroid tumours, both benign and malignant. It is also being used in iodine-131 metaiodobenzylguanidine (MIBG) treatment of malignant phaeochromocytomas and neuroblastomas. Phosphorus-32 and strontium-89 are used in the treatment of areas of secondary spread of cancer to bone, especially for pain relief. They are also used in the pleural and peritoneal cavities to treat malignant effusions in these spaces. Yttrium-90 is used for joint disorders.

One hopes that in the near future it will be possible to use specific radiolabelled tumour-seeking antibodies for the purpose of treating cancer and its spread.

Safety of nuclear medicine studies

Allergic reactions of the type encountered during the use of conventional contrast media used in radiology (e.g. for intravenous urograms) are virtually unknown in nuclear medicine and most radiopharmaceuticals can be used with impunity, even in highly-sensitive patients.

However, any amount of radiation, no matter how small, has a deleterious biological affect. This assertion is based on the assumption of a linear, non-threshold, dose-effect curve which has been adopted by national and international bodies as the most conservative estimate of risk. Careful consideration has, however, lead to the useful concept of the *lowest practicable* dose. Indeed, the universally adopted policy is to keep radiation exposure at or below this level. It is therefore important that the clinician has a reasonable indication that the potential gain for the patient in using a nuclear medicine procedure will exceed potential risks. Non-essential repetitive examination and the use of radionuclides with large beta-irradiation components must be discouraged. In addition it is essential to use sensitive detection equipment, good handling techniques and highly-trained personnel.

If all of these points are taken into consideration, most nuclear medicine investigations, especially if technetium-99m is the radionuclide used, involve absorbed doses of the same order as those incurred in conventional radiography and often much less. Naturally all diagnostic studies involving ionizing radiation investigations on pregnant women are to be avoided, unless the potential clinically benefit far outweighs the risk.

Future trends

Probably the most exciting of the future possibilities in nuclear medicine is that stated above of using tumour-localizing radiolabelled antibodies, both for diagnosis and therapy. On injection these become fixed to so-called antigenic sites on the primary and secondary tumours. This has become even more likely following the recent discovery of monoclonal antibodies, derived from the fusion of certain cancer cells (myeloma) and the cells which produce antibodies (B-lymphocytes) and which are available in large amounts.

Another enormous area of interest is the development of 'metabolic imaging'. At present this is confined to studies of the distribution of fluorine-18-labelled glucose in the brain and nitrogen-13 ammonia and carbon-11 or fluorine-18-labelled free fatty acids for the heart, but already new vistas of normal cerebral and cardiac physiology are being revealed. For example, it is now quite a simple matter to plot the activity of the visual and auditory centres of the brain non-invasively in response to different stimuli. Its clinical impact will be the greatest in stroke patients, psychiatric illnesses and cardiovascular disease.

References

Hounsfield, G.N. (1973) Computerized transverse axial (tomography) Part 1. Description of systems. *British Journal of Radiology* **46**, 1016–1022.

Kuhl, E.D. & Edwards, E.D. (1963) Image separation isotope scanning. *Radiology* **80**, 653–62.

Mistry, R. (1988) *Manual of nuclear medicine procedures.* Chapman and Hall, London. (A detailed how-to-do-it recipe book.)

Winchell, H.S. Baldwin, R.M. & Lin, T.H. (1980) Development of I-123-labelled amines for brain studies: localization of I-123 iodophenylalkyl amines in rat brain. *Journal of Nuclear Medicine*, **21**, 940–946.

Further reading

Alazraki, N.P. & Mishkin, F.S. (1984) *Fundamentals of nuclear medicine*, 2nd edn. The Society of Nuclear Medicine, Inc, New York. (A simple introductory account.)

Belcher, E.H. & Vetter, H. (eds) (1971) *Radioisotopes in medical diagnosis.* Butterworths, London.

Chilton, H.M. & Witcotshi, R.L. (1986) *Nuclear pharmacy. An introduction to the clinical application of radiopharmaceuticals.* Lea and Febiger, Philadelphia.

Ell, P.J. & Holman, B.L. (eds) (1982) *Computed emission tomography.* Oxford University Press, Oxford.

International Committee for Standardization in Haematology (ICSH): Panel on Diagnostic Applications of isotopes in Haematology. (1973) Standard techniques for the measurement of red-cell and plasma volume. *British Journal of Haematology*, **25**, 801–814.

O'Reilly, P.H., Shields, R.A. & Testa, H.J. (eds) (1986) *Nuclear medicine in urology and nephrology*, 2nd edn. Butterworths, London.

Robinson, P.A. (ed) (1986) *Nuclear gastroenterology.* Churchill Livingstone, Edinburgh.

Rothfield, B. (ed) (1974) *Nuclear medicine in vitro.* J. B. Lippincott Co., Philadelphia.

Royal, H.D. & McNeil, B.J. Qunatitative analysis in nuclear medicine. In Maisey, M.N., Britton, K.E. & Gilday, D.L. (eds), *Clinical nuclear medicine*, pp. 458–479. Publisher, Place. (This is an excellent detailed account of the most important quantitative Nuclear Medicine Studies.)

11: Patient Safety

Electrical power is supplied in the UK at an alternating voltage of 240 V root mean squared (r.m.s.) at a frequency of 50 Hz. This mains supply voltage is extremely dangerous to both patient and clinician unless properly handled. Safety can only be ensured if the hazards are well understood and systematically avoided.

This chapter considers the effect of mains-frequency currents on human tissues, the hazards presented by mains-powered instruments and the techniques used to eliminate electrical accidents.

Effects of mains current

If a gradually increasing 50 Hz current is passed between left and right finger tips, a slight tingling sensation will be felt at the points of contact when it reaches approximately 1 mA (Table 11.1). The exact threshold depends upon the contact area; small contacts require much less current than large ones. When the current reaches 10–15 mA, the sensation becomes very painful, and the muscles of the hands and forearms contract tetanically. Since the flexor muscles are stronger, the hands will close, so that if the electrocuting current enters the body through some grasped object it will be impossible to release it until the current is turned off. This current level is known as the *let-go* threshold.

Table 11.1. The effects of hand-to-hand 50 Hz alternating current

50 Hz current (mA)	Effect
1	Tingling sensation
5	Pain
15	Severe pain, with local muscle spasm
50	Respiratory muscle spasm
80–100	Dysrhythmias with pump failure leading to ventricular fibrillation

As the current is increased further the tetanic spasm spreads to the thorax, so that the respiratory muscles contract with consequent asphyxia. It follows that currents of this magnitude (around 50 mA) cannot be survived for very long. If the current is increased still further the electrical activity of the heart is disturbed by multifocal extrasystoles and an associated reduction in cardiac output. Finally, at 90–100 mA, ventricular fibrillation occurs, with functional cardiac standstill which leads rapidly to fatal hypoxaemia unless the subject is resuscitated quickly.

The effect of a 50 Hz alternating current upon a particular tissue depends upon the current density, which is defined as milliamperes per square centimetre ($mA \cdot cm^{-2}$). Thus the threshold of sensation at the fingertips depends on the current passing through each square millimetre of skin rather than the total current. If the contact area is halved whilst the current is unchanged, the current density will be doubled, with a corresponding increase in the intensity of sensation.

This principle applies to the heart. Much less current is needed to fibrillate the heart when one of the points of contact is within or on the ventricle itself than when the current is diffused across the whole thorax, and point contacts are much more likely to cause fibrillation than large contact areas.

Two other factors determine the potential lethality of alternating currents. One is the time for which they are applied, with the threshold decreasing as the time increases. The other is frequency. 50 Hz current is particularly dangerous, since the stimulation thresholds of excitable tissues are higher at both lower and higher frequencies. As the frequency is increased the threshold increases until, finally, a point is reached at which the tissue will not respond however great the intensity. Thus at very high frequency (>100 kHz) the heating effects of a current may be used (as with surgical diathermy) without risk of electrocution.

Mains supply

Electrical power usually enters the hospital site as a three-phase, 11 kV supply. This means that there are three supply conductors, so phased that each sinusoidal voltage is 120° out of phase with the other two. This supply is transformed down to three 240 V supplies by a local transformer (Fig. 11.1). These can either be used singly, or, when supplying heavy electric motors, all three phases can be used with 415 V between lines.

All three secondary windings are connected together as they emerge from the substation transformer, and then bonded firmly to ground. This point is known as the *star point* and forms the neutral connection. The current used by a machine or instrument passes between one of the live 240 V lines and the neutral.

Since each 240 V supply is 120° out of phase with the other two, some very odd things could happen if interconnected electrical devices were powered from different phases. Accordingly, the regulations

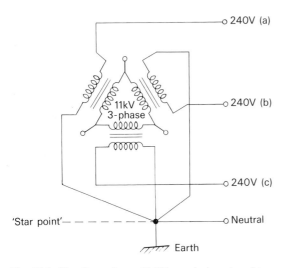

Fig. 11.1. The three-phase, 11 kV supply is reduced to three 240 V supplies by the local substation transformer. The neutral carries current returning from all three 240 V supplies.

governing the wiring of operating theatres or intensive care units specify that all the outlets must be connected to the same phase supply.

The earth bond is an essential safety feature, since it limits the voltages which could develop in the secondary circuit if the transformer were to be struck by lightning or the insulation between transformer windings were to fail.

The 240 V power supply to each theatre is distributed by one or more *ring main* circuits which are simply loops of cabling to which a number of outlets are connected. Each loop contains ground, neutral and live conductors, the latter containing a fuse to protect against overload (Fig. 11.2).

Since each outlet terminal connects with the supply by two routes, the current in the circuit will automatically distribute itself according to the relative loads on the outlets in the ring. The number of permissible outlets in each ring is determined by an assessment of the number of outlets which are likely to be in simultaneous use, together with the likely loads presented by the devices to be used. The neutral connection goes back to the earthed transformer star point and the earth connection goes to a local earth point. It is important to remember that the current returns to the transformer along the neutral wire, not the earth, which is for protective purposes only.

User devices

Any machine or instrument connected to one of the power outlets contains a *load* which is, of course, electrically live (Fig. 11.3). In most cases the load is insulated from the conductive metal enclosure, to which an earth connection is made. This earth connection is the key to the safety of the device. If the insulation deteriorates or is compromised by a short-circuit so that a connection is made between load and enclosure, current will return to the star point via both neutral and earth wires. The current thus produced is called the *leakage current* and its magnitude depends upon the resistance of the load-to-enclosure connection, and also the source potential. If the leakage current is large (several amperes) the line current will exceed the rating of the fuse, causing it to blow and

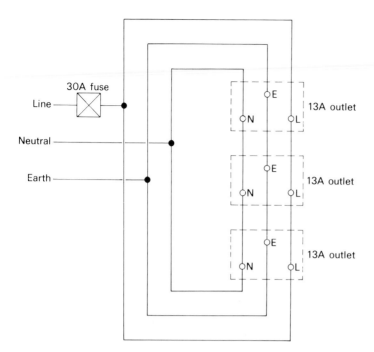

Fig. 11.2. One 30 A ring circuit supplying three 13 A outlets.

so breaking the circuit. Therefore the fuse protects the system from the effects of significant short-circuits between live parts and the enclosure. In the case of smaller leakage currents, the device may continue to operate. However, no hazard exists because the earth connection keeps the casing potential down to 0 V.

Faulty earthing of user devices

If, however, the earth connection is faulty (Fig. 11.4) a very different situation exists. Since there is no pathway to the star point via the earth connection, current does not flow, the protective fuse does not blow and the enclosure remains at the same potential as the leakage source, which may be any potential between ground and 240 V.

Anyone touching the enclosure provides a conductive pathway for the leakage current, which will flow through the body to ground and thence back to the star point. The magnitude of that current will depend upon the electrical resistance of the body.

If the person is standing on an antistatic floor but touching nothing else, the resistance to ground should be in excess of 20 kΩ, so that by Ohm's Law, the maximum current which can flow is 240/20 = 12 mA. The shock would certainly be painful, but the subject should survive.

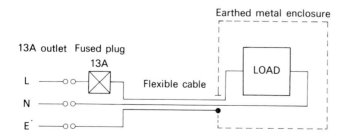

Fig. 11.3. A 'user device' connected to the mains supply.

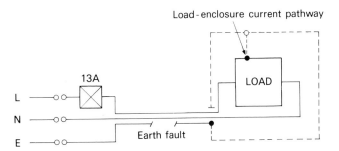

Load-enclosure current pathway

13A

L

N

E

LOAD

Earth fault

Fig. 11.4. With a load-enclosure current pathway and an earth fault, the device is now highly dangerous.

However, if the subject touches the enclosure with one wet hand while contacting an earthed conductor (such as a cold water tap) with the other, the resistance to earth might not exceed 2 kΩ. In that circumstance, the subject will sustain a lethal electrocuting current of 120 mA. Furthermore, since this current is small, the fuse will remain intact, so that the enclosure remains a hazard until the mains supply is switched off.

Gross electrocution can, of course, occur without earth faults. If a person simultaneously touches some live part and the enclosure at the same time such that the ensuing current flows through the thorax, a lethal accident is to be expected. For this reason, it is extremely dangerous to remove any part of the protective shielding from an instrument without first disconnecting it from the mains supply.

Designing for safety

It is essential that all measurement devices are designed with safety as a prime consideration. The designer is aided greatly by the provisions of our British Standard (BS 5724). This gives clear advice on all aspects of design pertinent to safety.

Patient safety depends upon three fundamental principles: over-current protection, insulation and isolation. The first two have been considered, but the third needs some explanation. That part of an instrument which comes into direct contact with the patient is known as the *applied part*. In the case of an electrocardiograph (ECG) or similar instrument the applied part is the electrode assembly, which connects directly to the *patient circuit*. Since the contact resistance may be very low, it is essential that the maximum permissible current passing between the applied part and the patient

should be very small indeed. In order to prevent such currents, the patient circuit must be designed in such a way that currents cannot flow to the grounded parts of the circuit. This is usually achieved by designing the patient circuit so that there is no direct electrical continuity whatever with ground. The signal is passed from the *isolated patient circuit* to the main instrument circuit by encoding it into a stream of pulses (often by voltage-to-frequency conversion), passing the encoded pulse train to the grounded circuitry as an optical signal and then decoding it back to the original form. This widely-practised technique is known as *opto-isolation*. Such is the effectiveness of patient isolation that the subject, connected to such an instrument, can be raised to mains voltage (by connection to another, live circuit) *without more than a few microamperes flowing to ground through the patient circuit*. Indeed, BS 5724 describes a specific test to ensure that this is possible.

Preventive maintenance

Electrical accidents can be minimized by careful maintenance, since the three-wire mains system is fundamentally safe unless leakage and earth faults occur. To avoid them, both current leakage and earth continuity need to be checked.

EARTH LEAKAGE

All mains-powered devices in patient-care areas should be checked regularly for excessive earth leakage currents. To do this, the engineer removes the earth connection and connects an alternating current (a.c.) ammeter between the enclosure and a good quality earth. The leakage current which then flows must never exceed 0.5 mA. He then reverses the live and neutral connections, and repeats the test. Any device with excessive leakage should not be used until this is corrected, except in dire emergency. This test should never be carried out by anybody but a qualified electrical engineer, who then accepts responsibility for the safety of the device.

It is possible to detect the presence of leakage currents by a device which detects the difference between the currents flowing in the live and neutral wires. This difference current is, by definition, leakage. The detected current can be made to operate a relay which switches off the supply to that electrical outlet or group of outlets. Set at a threshold of, say, 30 mA, such a contact breaker will operate very quickly and may prevent electrocution by otherwise lethal currents. However, it is not very useful to have a theatre power outlet which refuses to deliver current to a device with high but not immediately dangerous leakage, since a patient's life may depend upon it. For this reason, and despite their popularity in some other countries (notably Australasia), contact breakers are not used in British operating theatres.

EARTH CONTINUITY

The engineer tests the earth continuity of the device itself by measuring the resistance between the earth pin on the mains plug and the main earth terminal on the instrument. This is usually externally accessible to facilitate testing. The measured resistance should never exceed 0.1 ohm. It is of course possible for the flexible power cable to be badly frayed, with one single strand of wire maintaining the earth continuity, such that the resistance test will not detect any abnormality. To guard against this eventuality, the engineer employs the *surge test*. A 25 A current is passed through the earth pathway for at least 5 s. If then, any part of the pathway is limited to one or two stands, they will rapidly overheat and 'blow' like a fuse. This simple test ensures that all earth conductors entering service are capable of taking substantial currents for a few seconds without melting. The combination of surge and resistance tests guards against all likely earth faults, *but is only of value if carried out at frequent intervals.*

The earth pathway does not, of course, stop at the mains plug, but continues to the local earth point within the building. The continuity of this earth conductor must also be checked periodically. After switching the power off this is done by measuring the resistance between earth and neutral connections on the mains socket (earth-neutral loop test) and, as before, passing a surge current to detect any badly frayed or corroded connections.

A code of practice for safety in the operating theatre

Although most hazards can be prevented by regular testing and preventive maintenance, the user can easily *create* hazards by sheer carelessness. Only when all the staff in patient-care areas are aware of electrical hazards can accidents be prevented.

All staff members should be aware of the following simple rules:

1 If anyone reports a shock or even a 'tingle' from a device, do not touch it to see if they are right: switch off at the wall and call for an engineer.
2 If mains cables are seen to be knotted or frayed, insist on their replacement.
3 Do not allow electrical equipment into a patient-care area which does not satisfy the requirements of BS 5724.
4 Keep mains cables as short as practicable, to discourage long lengths of cable coiled on the floor.
5 Never push wheels or castors over mains cables.
6 Do not handle electrical equipment with wet hands.
7 Do not use portable distribution boxes unless you are certain that they are included in the engineers' earth continuity checks.
8 Ensure that preventive electrical maintenance is carried out regularly.

Earth-free mains supplies

The conventional live–neutral–earth system, as used in the UK, is relatively inexpensive and is, if properly maintained, associated with very few fatal accidents (Fig. 11.5a). In some countries, however, the mains supply specified for use in operating theatres and intensive care areas is 'earth free'.

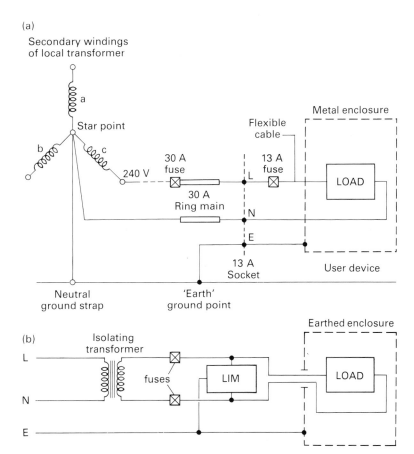

Fig. 11.5. (a) Normal mains supply system (connections to phase (a) and (b) are not shown). (b) An earth-free mains power supply. The isolating transformer supplies a single 13 A outlet socket. LIM = line isolation monitor. (From Hull, 1978.)

With this system the safety margin for all mains-powered devices can be considerably enhanced. A 1:1 isolating transformer is added to the normal system so that no voltage change occurs. The primary winding of this transformer is connected to live and neutral conductors from the main supply, while the secondary winding feeds one or more power outlets. The secondary circuit is not connected to ground, and is therefore earth-free (Fig. 11.5b). The advantage of this system lies in the fact that leakage currents do not seek earth since they no longer return to the star point, but to the isolating transformer secondary winding, which cannot be reached via an earth pathway. In fact, in the event of a live earth short-circuit, stray capacitances in the transformer do allow very small leakage currents to flow. So, for added protection, the outlet socket has an earth terminal which

connects to the device enclosure in exactly the same way as a normal live–neutral system. This is essential, because if such a fault does occur, the whole system reverts to the conventional situation where an earthed case is the first line of defence!

Consider an instrument whose earth is disconnected and has an 'earth-live' short-circuit. As we have seen, this would present a hazard if connected to a conventional supply and an earthed person touches the instrument enclosure. However, in the case of an earth-free supply, that person would no longer provide a pathway for the leakage current unless, simultaneously, *another* fault had earthed the secondary circuit. Therefore, the safety margin is very much greater. It is, however, necessary to provide a monitoring circuit, called the *line isolation monitor (LIM)*, which warns when earthing occurs even though no direct hazard is present.

Microshock

In experiments in both dogs and man, it has been shown that ventricular fibrillation can be induced by minute currents when applied to a small area of the ventricular endocardium (see Hull, 1978). The actual site of contact is important, since it has been shown that currents in the $100\,\mu$A range will only induce fibrillation if applied to the ventricular endocardium; atrial contacts require substantially larger currents. The threshold is proportional to the surface area and also related to the time for which the current is passed. As the duration of the stimulus increases the threshold decreases. The threshold is also dependent on frequency and it is unfortunate that 50 Hz is almost the most lethal frequency. Fibrillation by very small currents has come to be known as *microshock*, as distinct from gross electrocution by externally applied current.

Because of the need to have the necessary current density at a particular site, the microshock hazard only applies to a very few specialized situations. It is necessary to have an electrical contact of low surface area in or on the surface of the heart such as could be achieved by a transvenous pacemaker wire, a cardiac catheter with a terminal electrode, a catheter filled with conductive material such as radio-opaque dye, an implanted but exteriorized pacemaker wire, or a saline-filled central venous catheter. The smallest a.c. current which can produce ventricular fibrillation when applied to a small area of the right ventricular endocardium is probably about $50\,\mu$A (Watson *et al.* 1973). Devices which are to be connected directly to the patient's heart are covered by a leakage standard of $10\,\mu$A under normal working conditions, rising to a permissible $50\,\mu$A if a single fault occurs (see BS 5724). Leakage currents may also arise from faults in other equipment and reach the endocardium via a cardiac catheter.

For example, in one reported accident, a patient undergoing cineangiography developed ventricular fibrillation when the motorized syringe pump connected to the cardiac catheter was switched on (Bousvaros *et al.* 1962). From the published account it is evident that the motor of the syringe was poorly insulated and the injector not earthed (Fig.

11.6). The patient, on the other hand, was earthed by a 'right leg' electrode to the grounded chassis of a (now obsolete), non-isolated ECG. Leakage current flowed along the cardiac catheter, through the patient's heart and right leg electrode to ground.

Of course, a leakage current can flow *out* of the endocardial lead, rather than *into* it. Thus if the ECG had had a faulty earth and an excessive leakage current, but the syringe pump a perfect earth, the outcome would have been exactly the same as soon as the syringe pump was connected to the catheter. It is quite likely that the motorized injector would have passed a leakage test for equipment of its type (0.5 mA) although it would have failed an earth test.

Therefore, it follows that the stringent leakage limits must be applied to *all* equipment making contact with the patient when an endocardial lead is present. It should in fact be applied to *all* equipment in the immediate vicinity of patients who are especially electrically susceptible by virtue of intrathoracic conductors, since lethal leakage currents in the microampere range can be carried by skin contact with staff members. They need only to have one hand on a leakage source and the other holding a pacemaker wire to carry such a current without even being aware of having done so, since the current is below the threshold of sensation.

Prevention of microshock

For the special case of the electrically-susceptible patient a stringent code must be observed:
1 All electrical equipment in the vicinity of the patient must conform to a leakage specification of less than $10\,\mu$A under normal working conditions.
2 Whenever possible, such equipment should be battery operated and fully isolated from earth, thus avoiding 50 Hz leakage currents altogether.
3 All electrical circuits making contact with the patient must be electrically isolated from earth.
4 All electrical equipment in the susceptible zone should, wherever possible, be coated with resistive material, so as to limit earth pathways produced by hand to hand contacts.
5 Pacemaker leads or catheters must only be handled with gloved hands. Never hold the lead in

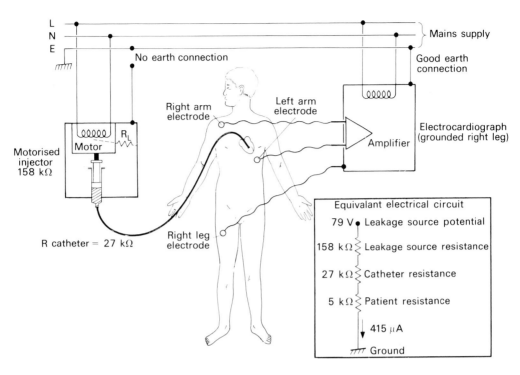

Fig. 11.6. Microshock (based on data from Bousvaros *et al.* 1962). The equivalent electrical circuit is shown on the right.

one hand while contacting an oscilloscope or any other mains powered equipment with the other.

6 Earth-free mains supplies will not in themselves provide sufficient protection against microshock, but will greatly reduce the magnitude of any leakage current, and therefore increase the safety margin.

Thermal injuries associated with clinical measurement

Injuries caused by electrical devices are not limited to electrocution. Just as likely are thermal injuries. These may be caused by high currents passing through living tissues, thereby generating heat faster than it can be dissipated, or by external heat sources such as fires and explosions.

INJURIES CAUSED BY SURGICAL DIATHERMY

Most diathermy machines are of the unipolar type; that is, the current passes from an active electrode

to a 'plate' electrode on the patient's thigh. This is not grounded, but is coupled to ground by a capacitor in order to prevent stray radiofrequency currents. This arrangement allows the current to pass from one electrode to the other by any combination of earth pathways, with the individual path currents related to their respective impedances. Normally, the plate electrode offers the easiest pathway to ground. However, if some other contact with the patient, such as a grounded ECG electrode, provides an alternative pathway, some current will return by that route. The likelihood of causing a burn depends upon the current density at the point of contact with the body; the smaller the area, the more probable will be a burn. Thus a subminiature electrode is more dangerous than a 'plate' electrode, and a needle electrode even more so.

Although ECG electrodes present the greatest problem, other devices have been reported to provide grounding pathways for radiofrequency currents. These include temperature probes, ultra-sound transducers and even a stainless steel electrode placed in the anal sphincter for the purpose of monitoring EMG activity in the sphincter muscle (Brock-Utne & Downing, 1984).

BURNS FROM NERVE STIMULATORS

Some devices are capable of causing burns un-aided. For instance, although many peripheral nerve stimulators are not capable of delivering supramaximal stimuli through surface electrodes, surface burns have been reported. Several incidents have followed use of the ball electrodes provided with the 'Wellcome' stimulator (Lippmann & Fields, 1974). Some newer devices have alternative settings for surface or needle electrodes, and it is likely that tetanic stimulation of needle electrodes while using the 'surface' setting will cause burns.

BURNS CAUSED BY HEATED 'APPLIED PARTS'

Thermal damage has been reported to follow the use of a simple photoelectric plethysmograph (Lebowitz, 1970). It was suggested that heat from the small light bulb may have been at least partly responsible. While the bulb generated little heat, this could easily cause a burn when the underlying skin is unable to conduct heat away from the site because of poor circulation.

The transcutaneous oxygen electrode has found wide application in monitoring neonates as well as older patients (see Chapter 18). In order that the measured oxygen tension may reflect that of arterial blood, the skin adjacent to the membrane is 'arterialized' by heating the electrode to 42–45 °C. At the upper end of this range there is a risk of causing thermal burns if the skin is poorly perfused. In fact, Lofgren and Jacobson (1979) showed that the optimal temperature is 44.5 °C and noted that a transient red mark always developed under the electrode. More severe lesions, such as the appearance of vesicles, have been reported in pre-term infants while shocked infants have developed frank blisters (Voora et al. 1981). Such minor lesions are of no great import when the very survival of the patient is at stake, but the margin of

safety is narrow and serious damage may follow any fault in the heating control system. There are reported cases of full-thickness burns following overheating of transcutaneous electrodes.

Explosion hazard

Electrical sparks are a major potential source of ignition for explosive anaesthetic mixtures. They may be due to the discharge of static electrical charges or to the make or break of electrical circuits which are carrying voltages well below those of the mains supply. The energy of the spark which will cause ignition depends on the particular mixture. Heated surfaces are a potent source of ignition, since temperatures as low as 200 °C can ignite ether vapour (Mushin & Jones, 1987).

Likely instrumental sources of hazard include the heated stylus of some pen recorders and, of course, sparking in mains on/off switches themselves.

The principal safety factor is distance. The explosive components of anaesthetic mixtures rapidly become diluted by diffusion so that at a distance of only 10 cm from the expiratory valve or other major leak from a breathing circuit, mixtures are not ignitable. A distance of 25 cm is therefore recommended as a safe distance for siting equipment which might ignite a flammable mixture. Vapours which are much heavier than air may pool on horizontal surfaces in special circumstances; for example, when liquid ether is spilled. The very rich mixture close to the liquid may burn with a cool, propagating flame which is unlikely to do much damage *per se*, but may cause a leaner mixture to detonate at a considerable distance from the point of ignition.

Where high concentrations of oxygen are being employed, not only are inflammable anaesthetic mixtures much more dangerous, but other materials will ignite and burn furiously. Fires have been attributed to the plastic components in ultrasonic nebulizers, to plastic masks and tubing, and to drape materials. The same hazard arises in connection with hyperbaric oxygen.

Where electrical current components are in, or within 5 cm of, a gas path which contains an anaesthetic or oxygen-enriched mixture, BS 5724 insists that construction must be of such a standard that surface temperatures do not exceed 150 °C, or 200 °C when provided with unrestricted vertical air circulation. Such equipment is to be marked APG (Anaesthetic Proof G). A less stringent standard (AP) can be adopted for equipment which can be operated between 5 and 25 cm of anaesthetic circuits (BS 5724).

References

Bousvaros, G.A., Don, C. & Hopps, J.A. (1962) An electrical hazard of selective angiocardiography. *Canadian Medical Association Journal* **87**, 286–288.

Brock-Utne, J.G. & Downing J.W. (1984) Rectal burn after the use of an anal stainless steel electrode/transducer system for monitoring myoneural junction. *Anesthesia and Analgesia* **63**, 1141–1142.

BS 5724 (1979) *Safety of medical electrical equipment. Part I: general requirements.* British Standards Institution, London.

Hull, C.J. (1978) Electrocution hazards in the operating theatre. *British Journal of Anaesthesia* **50**, 647–657.

Lebowitz, M.H. (1970) Gangrene of a thumb following use of the photoelectric plethysmograph during anaesthesia. *Anesthesiology* **32**, 164–167.

Leeming, M.N. (1973) Protection of the electrically susceptible patient. *Anesthesiology* **38**, 370–383.

Lippmann, M. & Fields, W.A. (1974) Burns of the skin caused by a peripheral nerve stimulator. *Anesthesiology* **40**, 82–84.

Lofgren, O. & Jacobson, L. (1979) The influence of different electrode temperatures on the recorded transcutaneous Po_2 level. *Pediatrics* **64**, 892–897.

Mushin, W.W. & Jones, P.L. (1987) *Physics for the anaesthetist*, 4th edn, Blackwell Scientific Publications, Oxford. pp. 501–585.

Voora, S., Wilks, A.K. & Lilien, L.D. (1981) Transcutaneous Po_2 electrode malfunction resulting in a third-degree burn. *American Journal of Diseases in Childhood* **135**, 271–212.

Watson, A.B., Wright, J.S. & Loughman, J. (1973) Electrical thresholds for ventricular fibrillation in man. *Medical Journal of Australia* **1**, 1179–1182.

Further reading

Dobbie, A.K. (1971) Electricity in hospitals. *Biomedical Engineering* **7**, 12–18.

Hahn, C.E.W. (1980) Electrical hazards and safety in cardiovascular measurements. In Prys-Roberts, C. (ed.), *The circulation in anaesthesia*, p. 605. Blackwell Scientific Publications, Oxford.

Part 2
Specific Measurements

12: The Measurement of Pressure

This chapter deals with the general principles of devices used to measure pressure, the specific applications being dealt with in subsequent chapters.

Units used in pressure measurement

Pressure is defined as force per unit area. The SI unit of pressure is the newton per square metre ($N \cdot m^{-2}$) or pascal (Pa). However, this unit is too small for most physiological applications. The kilopascal (kPa) which is 1000 times larger has therefore been adopted for most physiological measurements. In meteorology and many commercial applications it has been agreed that a still larger unit, the bar, should be used. The bar is a derivative of the CGS system in which the unit of pressure was dynes per square centimetre ($dyne \cdot cm^{-2}$). A bar was 10^6 $dyne \cdot cm^{-2}$. The newton ($kg \cdot m \cdot s^{-2}$) is 100 000 times larger than a dyne ($g \cdot cm \cdot s^{-2}$), but the square metre is 10 000 times larger than a square centimetre. Thus, the pascal ($N \cdot m^{-2}$) is 10 times as big as the dyne per square centimetre. Therefore, 10^5 Pa is equal to 10^6 $dyne \cdot cm^{-2}$, or 1 bar; 10^5 Pa is 100 kPa and, since a standard atmosphere is 101.325 kPa, this is equivalent to 1.013 bar or 1013 mbar. The bar is obviously more convenient for the measurement of pressures in compressed gas cylinders.

These units have now officially replaced the older units of pressure which related the measurement to the pressure exerted by the atmosphere or to the height of a column of fluid which the pressure would support. The pressure exerted by the atmosphere will support a column of mercury 76 cm (approximately 30 in) high. Since the density of mercury is 13.6 times the density of water, this is equivalent to a column of water 76 × 13.6 = 1033 cm (34 ft) high. If the cross-sectional area of the water column is 1 cm², the pressure is 1033 $g \cdot cm^{-2}$ or 1033 $kg \cdot m^{-2}$. This is equivalent to 14.7 pounds per square inch ($lb \cdot in^{-2}$ or psi). Since weight is the product of mass times the acceleration due to gravity (981 $cm \cdot s^{-2}$ or 32 $ft \cdot s^{-2}$) and since the latter varies slightly in different parts of the world, the height of the liquid column supported by one standard physical atmosphere will also vary with the site of measurement. Furthermore, the density of the liquid will vary with temperature, so that the height of a fluid column supported by a given pressure will be temperature-dependent as well. It is for these reasons that an attempt is being made to replace the older units with SI units which are not affected by such factors. Conversion factors between old and new units are shown in Table 12.1.

When measuring large pressures it is customary to refer them to atmospheric pressure. Such measurements are usually termed *gauge* pressures, as the reading on the gauge will be zero when the measured pressure is atmospheric and the reading on the gauge at other pressures will define how much the pressure is above or below atmospheric. In certain applications it is desirable to measure the pressure with respect to a true zero pressure (i.e. a vacuum). Such measurements are termed *absolute* pressures. Thus atmospheric pressure is zero gauge pressure or 1 atmosphere absolute (1 ATA) whilst a gauge pressure of 1 atmosphere (101.325 kPa or 760 mmHg) is 2 atmospheres (202.65 kPa or 1520 mmHg) absolute (2 ATA). Absolute pressures are most commonly used in hyperbaric medicine and in vacuum technology. However, in the latter application a *vacuum* pressure is often quoted (Fig. 12.1).

Table 12.1. Conversion factors relating the most commonly used units of pressure

	dynes·cm^{-2}	kPa	g·cm^{-2}	kg·m^{-2}	lb·in^{-2}
1 atmosphere (physical)	1 013 250	101.325	1033.227	10 332.27	14.696
1 bar	1 000 000	100	1019.716	10 197.16	14.504
1 kPa	10 000	1	10.197	101.972	0.145
1 mmHg 0 °C (Torr)	1 333.224	0.133	1.359	13.595	0.019
1 cmH$_2$O 20 °C	980.638	0.091	0.998	9.98	0.014
1 lb·in^{-2}	68 947.58	6.895	70.307	703.07	1

	mmHg 0 °C(torr)	inHg 0 °C	cmH$_2$O 20 °C	inH$_2$O 20 °C	mbar
1 atmosphere (physical)	760	29.921	1035.08	407.513	1013.250
1 bar	750.062	29.530	1021.545	402.18	1000
1 kPa	7.501	0.295	10.215	4.022	10
1 mmHg 0 °C (Torr)	1	0.039	1.362	0.536	1.333
1 cmH$_2$O 20 °C	0.734	0.029	1	0.394	0.979
1 lb·in^{-2}	51.715	2.036	70.433	27.73	68.948

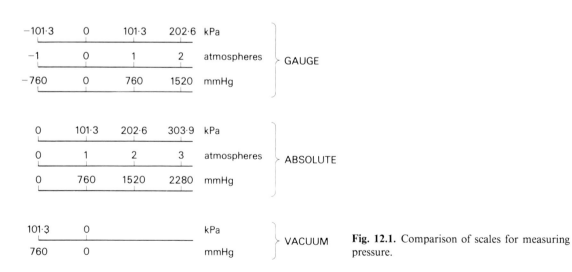

Fig. 12.1. Comparison of scales for measuring pressure.

Instruments used for measuring pressure

LIQUID MANOMETERS

The principle of the liquid manometer is best illustrated by considering the simple physics involved. The force exerted by a column of fluid is the product of mass times the acceleration due to gravity (g). However, the mass of the liquid column is the product of the volume of the fluid times its density. Therefore the force produced by a column of fluid.

= volume × density × g

= height × cross-sectional area of liquid × density × g.

Since pressure = force per unit area, the pressure exerted by a column of fluid

$$= \frac{\text{height} \times \text{cross-sectional area} \times \text{density} \times g}{\text{cross-sectional area}}$$

= height × density × g.

The pressure is thus independent of the *width* of the fluid column. It is equally true, therefore, that pressure is independent of the *shape* of the fluid column.

There are two main types of liquid manometer. An example of the first type is the mercury barometer (Fig. 12.2). In this device there is a virtual vacuum above the mercury so that the height of the mercury column indicates *absolute* pressure. In the second type the tube is open at both ends (Fig. 12.3). Since the top is open to atmosphere the height of the fluid column indicates the amount by which the pressure exceeds atmospheric, i.e. *gauge* pressure.

When using U-tube manometers it is important to remember that the pressure is given by the difference in height between the two menisci, and not the distance between each meniscus and the zero point. In single tube manometers the height of the column is measured from the meniscus in the reservoir. This falls as the fluid is forced up the tube so that a fixed scale graduated in millimetres will not accurately reflect the true difference between the two menisci. The error can be minimized by making the cross-sectional area of the reservoir large in relation to the cross-sectional area of the tube. Alternatively the scale length can be shortened to allow for the fall in reservoir level. Both methods of correction are commonly employed in mercury sphygmomanometers.

An error in the measurement of pressure by liquid manometers may arise from the surface tension of the liquid. With most liquids, the curvature of the meniscus is concave upwards. The surface tension thus causes the position of the meniscus to be higher than it should be. If the two limbs of a liquid manometer are of equal diameter, surface tension forces are the same in each limb and so cancel each other. However if the diameters differ an error may be introduced because surface

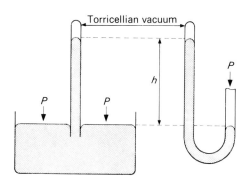

Fig. 12.2. Mercury manometer yielding measurements of absolute pressure (e.g. barometer). P = applied pressure; h = pressure measured.

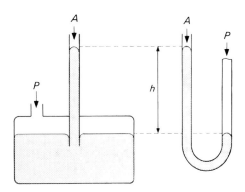

Fig. 12.3. Mercury manometer yielding measurements of gauge pressure (e.g. sphygmomanometer). P = applied pressure; A = atmospheric pressure; h = measured pressure.

forces exert a greater effect in a narrow tube than in a wide one.* Surface forces become important if the tube is less than about 1 cm in diameter. With most liquids, surface forces cause the meniscus to be higher than it should be. However, the meniscus of mercury is concave downwards and this causes a negative error in the reading in narrow tubes. In a tube 6 mm in diameter surface forces cause a water meniscus to be 4.5 mm too high whilst a mercury meniscus would be 1.5 mm too low.

The sensitivity of liquid manometers can be increased in a number of ways. The most obvious method is to use a liquid of low density, such as alcohol or liquid paraffin. Another method is to incline the tube so that the vertical movement of the meniscus is amplified (Fig. 12.4). In such an *inclined plane* manometer great care must be taken to level the baseplate accurately before taking a reading. Yet another way of increasing sensitivity is to use a *differential liquid manometer* (Fig. 12.5). Two non-miscible liquids of slightly different density are placed in opposing limbs of a U-tube, the quantities of each liquid being adjusted so that a meniscus is formed close to the top of one limb of the U. If the pressure to be measured is now applied to this limb the meniscus will be displaced downwards.

If the two reservoirs at the top have a large diameter compared with the diameter of the connecting tube a large movement of the boundary meniscus between the two liquids can occur without there being much difference in height between the fluid levels in the two reservoirs. If this slight difference in height is ignored it can be seen that the movement of the boundary meniscus will be inversely related to the difference in density between the two liquids.

$$P = h(d_1 - d_2)g$$

where P is the pressure to be measured, h is the

* The height (h) to which a liquid of surface tension σ and specific weight w is raised in a tube of diameter d is

$$\frac{h = 4\sigma \cos \theta}{wd}$$

where θ is the angle of contact between liquid and solid.

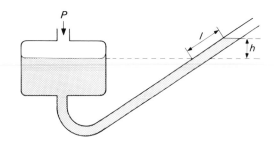

Fig. 12.4. Inclined plane manometer. The small pressure P produces a small difference in height between the two menisci (h) but this is amplified on the scale (l).

movement of the meniscus, and d_1 and d_2 are the densities of the two liquids. Therefore:

$$h = \frac{P}{(d_1 - d_2)g} \, .$$

Hence, sensitivity can be increased by using two liquids of very similar density. By an extension of this analysis, which takes into account the difference in height between the liquid in the reservoirs, it is possible to show that sensitivity is also

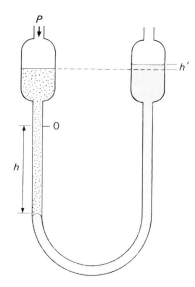

Fig. 12.5. Differential liquid manometer. P = applied pressure; h = measured pressure. h' is small in relation to h because of the difference in diameter between the manometer tube and reservoirs.

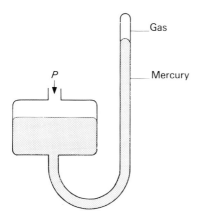

Fig. 12.6. Liquid manometer containing gas for measurement of high pressures.

increased by making the reservoir large in relation to the diameter of the connecting tube.*

The sensitivity of a manometer can be decreased by filling the closed end of the U-tube with a gas (Fig. 12.6). The movement of the meniscus is then governed by the height and density of the liquid

---

* The full equation is

$$P = wh\left[d_1\left(1 + \frac{a}{A}\right) - d_2\left(1 - \frac{a}{A}\right)\right]$$

where $w = 9.81 \times 10^3\,\mathrm{N \cdot m^{-3}}$, whilst a and A are the cross-sectional areas of the narrow and wide sections of tube (Douglas, 1975).

column and the balancing pressure exerted by the compressed gas. The latter can be calculated by the application of Boyle's law. This type of manometer is used for measuring such high pressures that the length of the mercury column would become unmanageable.

MECHANICAL PRESSURE GAUGES

Bourdon gauge

This type of manometer is usually used for measuring high pressures. However it can also be adapted for the measurement of temperature (p. 279) and flow (p. 199).

The gauge consists of a coiled tube which is flattened in cross-section (Fig. 12.7). One end of the coil is anchored to the case and connected to the source of pressure, whilst the other end is closed and attached to a mechanism which drives the pointer across the dial. The application of pressure to the inside of the tube causes the cross-section to become more circular. This causes the coiled tube to straighten. Since one end is fixed, the other unwinds, and so moves the pointer across the dial.

Aneroid gauge

A metal bellows is often used to sense smaller pressures. Expansion of this bellows is detected by

Fig. 12.7. Bourdon gauge. The increase in pressure causes the tube to become more circular in cross-section. This tends to straighten the coiled tube and so moves the needle across the dial.

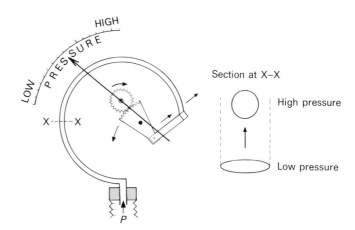

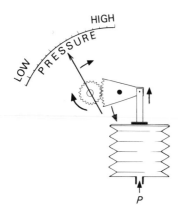

Fig. 12.8. Aneroid gauge.

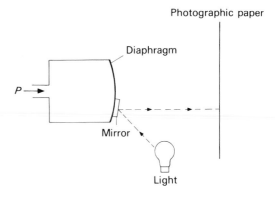

Fig. 12.9. Use of a mirror to sense the movement of a transducer diaphragm.

a lever mechanism which amplifies the movement and drives the pointer across the scale (Fig. 12.8). Aneroid gauges are commonly used for measurement of blood pressure or for monitoring the pressures developed by mechanical ventilators.

DIAPHRAGM GAUGE

Most physiological pressure measurements are now made by sensing the movement of a flexible diaphragm. This movement can be sensed directly or converted into electrical energy for subsequent processing and display.

Methods of sensing diaphragm movement are as follows:
1 Direct. The movement can be detected by attaching a thread or lever to the centre of the diaphragm, the other end being connected to a pointer or writing arm. This arrangement is not very sensitive and possesses marked inertia.
2 Optical. An improved method of sensing the movement of the diaphragm (used by many of the early physiological workers) is shown in Fig. 12.9. A small mirror is attached to one side of the diaphragm. When the diaphragm is stretched by the application of pressure it becomes curved and the mirror is rotated. The displacement of the mirror is recorded by causing it to reflect a beam of light onto moving photographic paper. Great sensitivity is possible since the light path can be lengthened by reflecting it back and forth between

fixed mirrors. However, the relationship between the applied pressure and the movement of the diaphragm is only linear over a narrow range so that the diaphragm must be sufficiently stiff to limit the degree of curvature produced by the applied pressure.
3 Electromechanical. In most diaphragm gauges used for sensing dynamic pressures the movement of the diaphragm is sensed by a device which converts the mechanical energy imparted to the diaphragm into electrical energy. The resulting electrical output has the enormous advantage that it may be processed in many different ways to yield signals which are suitable for recording or display. Thus, it may be amplified to increase the sensitivity of the instrument; it may be differentiated to give the rate of change of pressure; or it may be digitized to facilitate subsequent processing by a digital computer. Any device which converts energy from one form to another is known as a *transducer*; since a pressure transducer converts pressure energy into electrical energy it is often called an *electromanometer*.

*Physical principles of
electromechanical transducers*

Some electromechanical transducers are designed to convert electrical energy into mechanical energy. Examples are the electric motor, the loudspeaker or the piezo-electric crystal used in the generation of ultrasound. However, in the present application we are concerned with transducers which convert mechanical energy into electrical energy. The mechanical energy may cause movement which may then be sensed by a *displacement* transducer. If the tendency to movement is opposed by the transducer, a force is generated so that the instrument becomes a *force* transducer. In the case of a *pressure* transducer it is the force per unit area which is sensed by the movement of the diaphragm. The relationship between the applied pressure and the movement of the diaphragm is governed by the stiffness of the diaphragm. A relatively stiff diaphragm is necessary because undue distortion of the diaphragm causes the response to become nonlinear and because the frequency response of the transducer is intimately related to the stiffness of the diaphragm. Although many methods have been developed for sensing diaphragm movement the following are those most commonly employed in commercially available pressure transducers.

Optical

The movement of the diaphragm is sensed by reflecting a beam of light off the silvered back of the diaphragm onto a photoelectric cell. As the diaphragm is pressurized the silvered surface becomes convex. This causes the reflected light beam to diverge so that the intensity of light sensed by the photoelectric cell decreases and its electrical output falls. If both sides of the diaphragm are silvered and two light beams are reflected on to opposing photoelectric cells, the sensitivity can be greatly increased. This forms the basis of the optical defocusing manometer (Fig. 12.10).

The reflection technique has been exploited successfully for intravascular pressure measurement. The diaphragm is situated at the end of the fibre-optic bundle contained within a cardiac catheter. Light is transmitted down one section of the fibre-optic light path and transmitted back via another, the intensity of the reflected beam being sensed by a photoelectric cell placed at the external end of the fibre-optic bundle. Such a transducer has a high frequency response and completely eliminates the risk of microshock for there are no electrical components within the catheter (Lekholm & Lindström, 1969).

Wire strain gauge

When a wire is stretched or compressed it undergoes a change of electrical resistance, the change in resistance being produced by changes in the length and diameter of the wire and by changes in the atomic structure of the metal (Baldwin, 1979). In the *unbonded* wire strain gauge (now almost uniquely respresented by the Statham range of strain gauges) the resistance wire is stretched between a fixed point

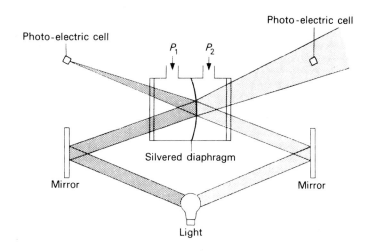

Fig. 12.10. Optical defocusing manometer. The curvature of the diaphragm produced by the difference between pressures P_1 and P_2 causes one beam of reflected light to converge and the other to diverge, thus altering the relative intensities of the light beams sensed by the two photoelectric cells.

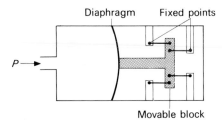

Fig. 12.11. A strain gauge using wire resistance elements.

and a moveable block attached to the diaphragm. The resistance wires are arranged in two sets so that the application of pressure stretches one set and compresses the other (Fig. 12.11). The difference in resistance between the two sets is measured by a Wheatstone bridge system, so that the output voltage is proportional to the displacement of the diaphragm (p. 42). The actual output voltage depends on the voltage used to energise the bridge but a typical output voltage would be $150\,\mu V \cdot kPa^{-1}$ $(20\,\mu V \cdot mmHg^{-1})$ at 10 volts excitation. In some strain gauges the resistance wires are formed into a zig-zag pattern and cemented to the back of the diaphragm to form a *bonded* strain gauge (Fig. 12.12). The resistance elements in this type of gauge may

also be etched out of a sheet of foil and bonded to the diaphragm by cement. Bonded gauges are considerably more robust but are subject to hysteresis and often have an inferior frequency response.

Since the resistance of the strain gauge element is affected by temperature it is important to choose a metal which possesses a low temperature coefficient of resistance. The effects of temperature can also be cancelled by using two gauges of equal dimensions in the opposite arms of the Wheatstone bridge. For example, if two gauges are bonded onto opposite sides of the diaphragm both will be equally affected by changes in temperature but one will be stretched and the other compressed, thus providing a difference in resistance which is proportional to the deflection of the diaphragm. By putting two gauges on each side and incorporating them in a 'full bridge' arrangement sensitivity can be doubled (Fig. 12.13).

Silicon strain gauge

In recent years other types of strain gauge have been developed. In one of these, the silicon bonded strain gauge, an extremely thin slice of a silicon crystal is bonded onto the back of the diaphragm. The silicon crystal changes resistance as it is

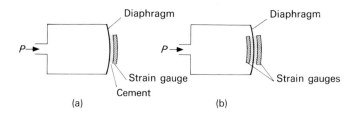

Fig. 12.12. Bonded strain gauges. (a) Single. (b) Double. Increasing the curvature of the diaphragm stretches one gauge and compresses the other.

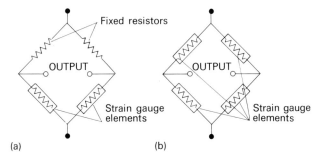

Fig. 12.13. (a) Strain gauge half-bridge circuit. (b) Full-bridge circuit.

compressed or expanded when the diaphragm changes shape. By suitably 'doping' the silicon crystal with elements such as phosphorus or boron it is possible to produce gauges with either positive or negative change in resistance characteristics. If these are mounted in parallel and incorporated in all four arms of a Wheatstone bridge great sensitivity can be achieved. Although such gauges may be 50 times more sensitive than comparable wire strain gauge elements they are very temperature-sensitive and also tend to suffer from nonlinearity. However, improvements in technology have now reduced these disadvantages.

Another type of silicon strain gauge utilizes a silicon diaphragm with a number of silicon gauges etched into the back of the diaphragm. Although the gauge elements are temperature sensitive they are mounted beside temperature-sensitive elements of opposing coefficient so that the thermal effects are fully compensated. Such gauges have a high sensitivity and can produce an output of $2 \, mV \cdot kPa^{-1}$ (or $25 \, mV \cdot 100 \, mmHg^{-1}$). The diaphragm is very stiff so that the gauge has a high natural frequency and is very resistant to the application of excess pressure. These transducers can be made very small and have been incorporated in the tip of a cardiac catheter.

Capacitance

The diaphragm of the pressure transducer is used as one plate of a capacitor, the second plate being fixed. Movement of the diaphragm varies the distance between the plates, and this varies the charge which can be carried by the capacitor. This is sensed by a bridge circuit energized by an

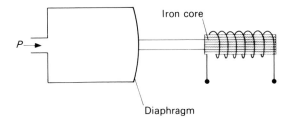

Fig. 12.14. Variable inductance transducer.

alternating current. This type of transducer can be made very sensitive with a high frequency response but it is also much affected by ambient temperature variation. This renders it relatively unstable.

Inductance

The inductance of a coil can be varied by changing the position of a core of magnetic material lying within the magnetic field of the coil (Fig. 12.14). The magnetic core is attached to the diaphragm and the inductance of the coil is measured by making it part of a bridge circuit which is energized by an alternating current.

A more common form of inductance transducer is that employing a differential transformer (Fig. 12.15). The core is placed between the two secondary windings of a transformer. These are wound in opposite directions so that when the core is situated symmetrically between them the a.c. voltage induced in the secondary coils is equal in magnitude but opposite in phase. There is therefore zero output. If the core is now displaced by movement of the diaphragm the voltage in one coil will exceed that in the other and an output voltage will appear at the terminals. If the core is moved in the

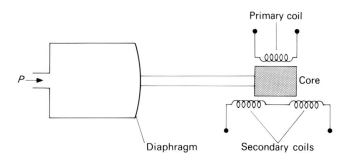

Fig. 12.15. Differential transformer transducer. The output signal appears across the secondary coils.

opposite direction the output will be equal in voltage but opposite in phase. By using a phase-sensitive rectifier (which changes the a.c. signals to d.c.) an appropriate d.c. voltage will be produced.

Single-ended and differential
pressure transducers

Most pressure transducers are designed to measure a pressure applied to one side of a diaphragm, the other side of the diaphragm being at atmospheric pressure. These are termed *single-ended* transducers. However, there are a number of occasions on which it is necessary to measure the difference between two pressures. This is most conveniently done by applying the two pressures to the opposite sides of the diaphragm. A transducer which is designed for this mode of operation is known as a *differential* transducer. Most differential pressure transducers are designed to measure the difference in pressure between two gases (for example the difference between airway and oesophageal pressure or the difference in pressure between the two sides of a pneumotachograph screen (p. 201). Some transducers are designed to accept liquid on one side but can only tolerate gas on the opposite side

because liquid would damage the sensing mechanism. Such transducers may be used for measurements of transmural pressure differences within the thorax (i.e. the difference between intravascular and oesophageal pressure). In some circumstances (e.g. the differential pressure method of measuring cardiac output, p. 211) it is necessary to compare two liquid pressures. This can usually only be achieved by using two carefully-matched single-ended liquid pressure transducers.

References

Baldwin, A. (1979) Transducers. *British Journal of Clinical Equipment* **4**, 32–36.
Douglas, J.F. (1975) *Solution of problems in fluid mechanics.* Part 1, p. 14. Pitman Publishing, London.
Lekholm, A. & Lindström L. (1969) Opto-electric transducer for intravascular measurements of pressure variations. *Medical and Biological Engineering* **7**, 333–335.

Further reading

Geddes, L.A. & Baker, L.E. (eds) (1989) *Principles of applied biomedical instrumentation*, 3rd edn. John Wiley & Sons, New York.
Mushin, W.W. & Jones, P. (1987) *Physics for the anaesthetist*, 4th edn. Blackwell Scientific Publications, Oxford.

13: Direct Measurement of Intravascular Pressure

Although non-invasive methods of measuring arterial pressure may be satisfactory in routine clinical practice they often prove inadequate in the acute situation. Direct measurements of arterial pressure are usually indicated when sudden, large changes of blood volume are anticipated (aortic graft or other major surgery); when rapid and extreme changes of pressure are likely (operation for phaeochromocytoma or controlled hypotension during surgery); when the shape of the arterial wave form can provide useful information (assessment of cardiac contractility or aortic valve disease); when myocardial function is disturbed by dysrhythmias, myocardial infarction or open-heart surgery; and when non-invasive methods are likely to be inaccurate (gross obesity, cardiopulmonary bypass).

Direct measurements of central venous or pulmonary artery wedge pressures are of use during transfusion in patients with severe anaemia, haemorrhage or other forms of shock; in patients with acute heart failure and in those undergoing cardiac surgery; and when deciding whether the sudden onset of hypotension is caused by a decreased venous return or cardiac failure.

Although liquid manometers have been used for measuring mean arterial pressure they are now only employed in central venous pressure measurement. However, even in this application there is a tendency to replace them by electromanometers, for the display of the venous waves and respiratory fluctuations provides a continuous confirmation of the patency of the catheter and may also provide diagnostic information (e.g. tricuspid incompetence).

Liquid and aneroid manometers

CENTRAL VENOUS PRESSURE

Catheters may be inserted into central veins through the median cubital, axillary, subclavian, internal or external jugular, or femoral routes, and are then connected to the sensing system with a bridge of saline. The simplest sensing system is a saline manometer. This is connected to an intravenous infusion set by a three-way tap so that the patient can be connected directly to the manometer, to a flushing solution, or to both. It is an advantage to add 1000 international units (10 mg) of heparin to each litre of flushing solution to minimize clotting in the catheter. There should always be a dependent loop of tubing between the manometer and the patient to minimize the risk of air embolus.

The zero on the manometer scale should first be adjusted to lie on the same horizontal plane as the

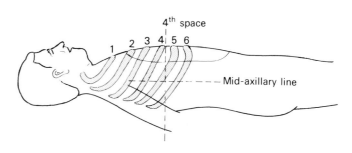

Fig. 13.1. Zero reference point for central venous pressure measurement.

163

patient's right atrium. The surface marking for the right atrium (Fig. 13.1) is the junction of a line running in the coronal plane half-way between the xiphoid and the dorsum of the body, and a line drawn at right angles to the fourth interspace where it meets the sternum (Winsor & Burch, 1945). In some circumstances it is simpler to use an alternative fixed point such as the manubriosternal junction (angle of Louis) but in these circumstances due allowance must be made for the difference in level. When the manubriosternal junction is used the measured pressure will be 0.5–1.0 kPa (5–10 cmH$_2$O) lower than that recorded using the true reference point at atrial level (Debrunner & Buhler, 1969). Since the normal venous pressure is 0–0.6 kPa (0–6 cm H$_2$O) when referred to the atrium, negative values will often be obtained when the manubriosternal junction is used as the reference point.

There are several methods of aligning the zero of the scale with the right atrium. The simplest is to use a hinged arm which is permanently fixed to the manometer stand (Fig. 13.2). When this arm is lowered it impinges on a stop which maintains it at right angles to the stand and which thus ensures that the tip of the arm is aligned with the manometer zero. The stand is then raised or lowered until the tip of the arm is opposite the reference

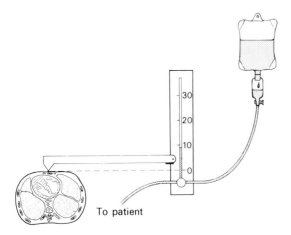

Fig. 13.2. Use of a hinged arm to set the manometer zero. The arm folds back into the stand when not in use. The manubriosternal junction is being used as a reference point.

point and clamped in position to the drip pole. To avoid errors the manometer stand must be kept vertical. An alternative method is to align the two zero points by means of a spirit level. Optical sights on the manometer stand have also been used but again these must be kept horizontal by means of a spirit level. For greatest accuracy a hydrostatic method should be used. One method utilizes a closed loop of intravenous drip tubing which is half filled with liquid containing a small quantity of dye. One side of the loop is fixed to the manometer stand parallel to the lower part of the manometer tube whilst the other side of the loop is held opposite the zero point on the patient. The menisci within the loop remain at the same horizontal level and thus provide a clear and accurate indication of the true zero level (Fig. 13.3).

When the zero position has been set and the central venous line has been flushed through, the manometer is filled from the reservoir. The three-way tap is then turned to connect the manometer to the vein. The saline meniscus should fall fairly rapidly and should stabilize at the venous pressure. It is normally possible to see a small respiratory fluctuation (up to several cm H$_2$O with a deep breath) and, under some circumstances, venous pulsations in time with the heart beat are also visible. The absence of a respiratory swing indicates that the catheter is situated peripherally or is blocked, and that the measurement is not acceptable. Occasionally the recorded pressure is found to be higher than expected or marked cardiac pulsations are observed. This may be due to passage of the catheter into the right ventricle or pulmonary artery and may be corrected by withdrawing the catheter. Another little recognized error used to occur when the cotton-wool plug at the top of the manometer tubing became wet, restricting the free movement of air in and out of the measuring limb. This error has now been overcome by the replacement of this plug by a non-wettable air filter.

In order to check the patency of the catheter it is advisable to fill the manometer tube before each reading and then to observe the fall of the saline when the flushing line is excluded from the circuit. This ensures that the cannula is patent. An alternative method is to set the three-way tap so that

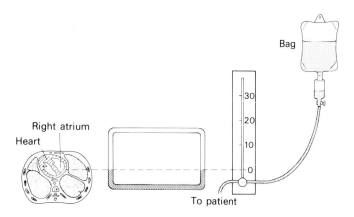

Fig. 13.3. Use of a closed loop of coloured liquid to set manometer zero. The two menisci remain at the same horizontal level.

the flushing line, manometer and venous catheter are all interconnected. A slow drip of flushing solution is then maintained throughout the period of measurement. This does not affect the manometer reading if the flushing rate is in the region of 10 drops per minute and the resistance of the catheter is in the normal range.

An aneroid blood pressure manometer gauge may also be used for monitoring mean arterial pressure, providing the bellows is sterilized and no liquid is allowed to enter the gauge (Fig. 13.4) (Zorab, 1969). This is a useful technique, particularly in an emergency and in unsophisticated surroundings, and for monitoring during transfer of a patient from one electronic recording system

to another. However, the fluid level must be aligned with the right atrial zero.

Electromanometers

Although catheter-tip pressure transducers are now available they are expensive and their use is restricted to situations in which a high frequency response is essential. For routine measurements the lumen of the vessel is connected to the pressure transducer by a fluid-filled catheter. The fluid and the diaphragm of the transducer then constitutes a system which will oscillate in simple harmonic motion. The fluid and the mass of the diaphragm represent the oscillating mass, while the compliance

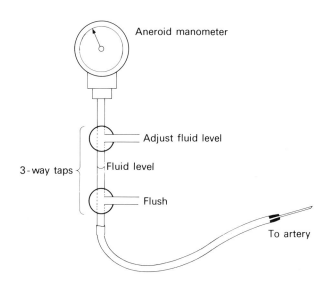

Fig. 13.4. Aneroid gauge used for recording mean arterial pressure. The fluid level should be aligned with the zero reference point.

of the diaphragm, the tubing and any air bubbles in the system represent the spring. Such a system can only record the pressure and waveform accurately if certain physical conditions are satisfied.

The problem is that the waveform is a complex one and not a sine wave as would be the case for simple harmonic motion. Fourier showed, however, that all complex waves can be analysed as a mixture of simple sine waves of varying amplitude, frequency and phase. These consist of a fundamental wave (at the pulse frequency) and a series of harmonics. Since the lower harmonics tend to have the greatest amplitude, a reasonable approximation to the arterial pressure waveform can often be obtained by accurate reproduction of the fundamental and the first eight to ten harmonics. In the case of the arterial waveform at 70 beats per minute this would require a frequency response which is undistorted up to (70 × 10/60) = 11.7 Hz. In order to reproduce pulse rates up to 140 beats per minute a flat frequency response up to 20 Hz is required. However, for extremely accurate recording of complex waveforms it is necessary to be able to record a greater range of harmonics. Thus, to record the maximum rate of rise of left ventricular pressure (dP/dt_{max}) it may be necessary for the transducer system to respond accurately up to 30 Hz or even higher. In general the sharper the waveform (i.e. the more rapid the rate of change in pressure) the greater the number of harmonics and the higher must be the frequency response.

FREQUENCY RESPONSE

A recording system must accurately reproduce both the *amplitude* and *phase difference* of each harmonic present in the waveform. To achieve this it is necessary to design a system with a high *undamped natural frequency* (resonant frequency) and then to apply the correct amount of *damping* (Kleinman, 1989).

Undamped natural frequency

A simplified measuring system together with its mechanical analogue is shown in Fig. 13.5. If the mass is set in motion by suddenly applying a force

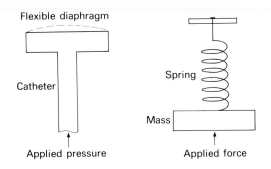

Fig. 13.5. Principle of electromanometer recording system with its mechanical analogue.

to its under surface it will oscillate up and down in simple harmonic motion, the frequency of oscillation being governed by the mass and the stiffness of the spring. The undamped natural frequency of this oscillation (f_0) is given by the general formula:

$$f_0 = \frac{1}{2\pi}\sqrt{\frac{S}{M}}$$

where S is the stiffness of the spring (applied force/displacement) and M is the mass of the oscillating body. From this formula it can be seen that the natural frequency of oscillation will be highest when the spring is stiff and the mass is small.

This formula can also be applied to a catheter–transducer system; S still refers to the stiffness of the diaphragm of the transducer but the mass implied by M is a more complex concept.

The essence of any oscillating system is the continual interchange between energy in two forms; in this case it is between the kinetic energy of the mass in motion and the potential energy of the deformed spring. Now the kinetic energy of the mass in motion is related to the square of the velocity ($e = 1/2\ mv^2$). It thus takes more energy to make any given mass of fluid oscillate in a narrow tube than in a wider tube, because it has to reach a higher velocity in the narrow tube. Since the velocity of the fluid in the catheter exceeds that of the fluid in contact with the diaphragm its effective (or equivalent) mass is greater; the narrower the catheter the higher the velocity and the higher the effective mass. This larger 'effective mass' lowers the natural frequency of the system below the figure which would be deduced from the actual mass.

Thus the undamped resonant frequency of a catheter–transducer measuring system is highest when the velocity of movement of fluid in the catheter is minimized. This is achieved when the diaphragm is stiff and when the catheter is short and wide. In the manufacturer's literature the stiffness of the diaphragm is usually given in terms of the volume displacement in $mm^3 \cdot kPa^{-1}$ or $mm^3 \cdot 100\,mmHg^{-1}$. This is the reciprocal of stiffness.

An additional factor which must be considered is the frictional resistance to fluid flow through the catheter. This is the principal factor producing damping. If laminar flow is assumed, Poiseuille's equation indicates that the resistance to flow is directly proportional to the length of the tube and to the viscosity of the fluid, and inversely proportional to the fourth power of the radius. Thus the minimal hindrance to the flow of fluid in the catheter will occur when the catheter is short and wide and when the viscosity is low. It is therefore apparent that the least amount of damping will be obtained when the velocity of fluid movement is reduced by a low volume displacement transducer and a wide catheter. However, it is very important that the catheter has rigid walls for any elasticity in the catheter will increase the compliance of the whole system and so decrease f_0.

Determination of resonant frequency and damping

If a catheter–transducer system is artificially oscillated by applying a sinusoidal pressure of constant amplitude but gradually increasing frequency (e.g. with a sinusoidal pump) it yields an electrical signal similar to that shown in Fig. 13.6. At low frequencies the amplitude of the output signal remains constant indicating that the system accurately follows the input pressure waveform. However, as frequency is increased further the output signal increases in amplitude, the peak of the response occurring at the resonant frequency of the catheter–transducer system. At still higher frequencies the amplitude of the response declines towards

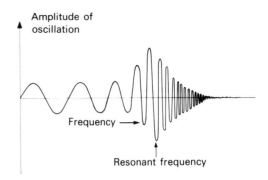

Fig. 13.6. Amplitude of oscillation of a diaphragm in a catheter–transducer system as the applied frequency is increased. The amplitude is maximal at the resonant frequency of the system but at higher frequencies the diaphragm fails to follow the applied pressure.

zero due to the increasing magnitude of the viscous and inertial forces already described. It is apparent that errors in the amplitude of the recorded waveform will be minimal if the resonant frequency of the system is well above the significant harmonics in the input waveform, but that the amplitude of a waveform will be exaggerated when any of its contained frequencies are close to the resonant frequency of the system. When the resonant frequency is less than any of the important harmonics there will be attenuation of the waveform due to damping.

The effects of damping are best illustrated by applying a single step change in pressure to the catheter–transducer system and recording the response. This is conveniently done by pressurizing a thin rubber balloon to about 6–7 kPa (50 mmHg) and then bursting it with a red-hot wire (Fig. 13.7). The various possible responses are shown in Fig. 13.8. In a system with no damping the system would oscillate at the undamped natural frequency and there would be no decrease in the recorded oscillations with time ($D = 0$). In a system with minimal damping ($D = 0.2$, say) the recorded signal falls rapidly, overshoots the base line and is then followed by a series of oscillations of decreasing amplitude. The frequency of oscillation is close to the undamped natural frequency of the system and the rate at which the amplitude decreases gives a measure of the amount of damping. If damping

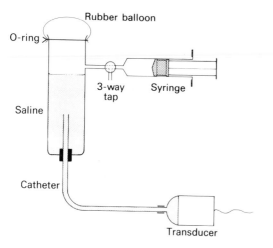

Fig. 13.7. Generation of a square wave fall in pressure for testing catheter–transducer system ('pop test'). The pressurized balloon is burst with a red-hot needle or lighted match.

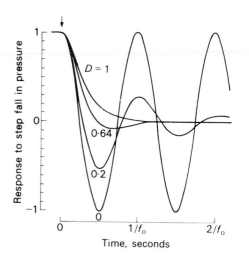

Fig. 13.8. The response of a catheter–transducer system to a step fall in pressure generated by the apparatus shown in Fig. 13.7. Results are shown for four values of the damping factor (D): undamped ($D = 0$); slightly damped ($D = 0.2$); critically damped ($D = 1$); damping 64% of critical ($D = 0.64$). The time-scale is the reciprocal of the undamped natural frequency. (After Gabe, 1972.)

is excessive the recorded signal falls slowly and takes some time to reach the baseline. However, there is no overshoot. With care it is possible to adjust the damping so that the output signal falls more rapidly but overshoot is just avoided. In this state the system is said to be *critically damped* ($D = 1$).

All of these situations are obviously undesirable, for on the one hand the system responds rapidly but overshoots, and on the other hand the amplitude of response is correct but the speed of response is too slow. In the underdamped state

pressures with a frequency close to the resonant frequency will be exaggerated whilst in the over-damped state high frequency oscillations will be damped out so that the true pressure change will be underestimated (Fig. 13.9). However, it is found that if the damping of the system is carefully adjusted a recording can be achieved in which overshoot is minimal and yet the speed of response

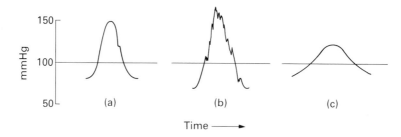

Fig. 13.9. Errors in arterial pressure waveform caused by inadequate frequency response of catheter–transducer system. (a) Correct waveform: optimally-damped system with adequate frequency response. (b) Underdamped system with low resonant frequency resulting in exaggeration of high frequency transients. Systolic pressure overestimated and diastolic pressure underestimated. (c) Overdamped system due to presence of air bubble or partial blockage of catheter. This results in underestimation of systolic pressure and overestimation of diastolic pressure. Note that the mean pressure is the same in all recordings (13.3 kPa or 100 mmHg).

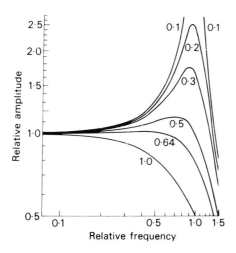

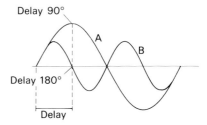

Fig. 13.11. Waveform B has twice the frequency of waveform A. To ensure that an equal time delay is applied to both waveforms the phase lag must be 90° with waveform A and 180° with waveform B, i.e. phase lag must be proportional to the frequency of the harmonics.

Fig 13.10. Effect of damping on the amplitude of the recorded signal. The horizontal axis indicates the signal frequency expressed as a fraction of the natural resonant frequency of the system. The figures by each curve indicate the damping factor (D). $D = 0.1$ indicates gross underdamping whilst $D = 1$ indicates critical damping. When the damping factor is 0.64 there is less than 2% distortion in the recorded amplitude of the signal up to about two thirds of the resonant frequency. (After Gabe, 1972.)

is only slightly reduced. This point is reached when the overshoot is 7% of the original deflection. The damping is then 64% of critical ($D = 0.64$, Fig. 13.8). This represents the best compromise that can be obtained between speed of response and accuracy of registration of the amplitude of the pressure trace. When the damping is adjusted in this manner and the response to a sinusoidal pressure signal of increasing frequency is measured, it is found that the amplitude of the recorded oscillation remains within 2% of the input signal up to a frequency which is about two-thirds that of the undamped resonant frequency of the system. At higher frequencies the amplitude of response gradually decreases, there being no resonant zone. With underdamped or overdamped systems amplitude distortion occurs at much smaller fractions of the natural resonant frequency (Fig. 13.10). Optimal damping thus ensures that the maximum use is made of the natural resonant frequency of the system.

Phase shift

The accurate registration of a pressure wave depends not only on the correct reproduction of the amplitude of the harmonics but also on the reproduction of the correct *phase difference* between them.

Since all recording systems possess inertia they impose a time delay on the recorded signal. This delay is not important as long as it is applied equally to all the components of the wave so that the original phase relationships between the harmonics are maintained. It is only possible to achieve an equal time delay for each harmonic if the phase lag is directly proportional to the frequency of the wave (Fig. 13.11). However, in recording systems the phase lag is a function not only of the frequency of the wave but also of the amount of damping present in the system (Fig. 13.12). All waves having a frequency equal to the undamped natural frequency of the system are delayed by 90° whatever the degree of damping, but at other frequencies the phase lag is only linearly related to the frequency when damping is about 64% of critical. It is thus apparent that both amplitude and phase distortion are minimal when damping is adjusted to this figure. However, it must be remembered that although the shape of the waveform is accurately reproduced when damping is 64% of critical, the whole waveform is slightly delayed. This delay is only of importance in certain specialized measurements, for example, when the

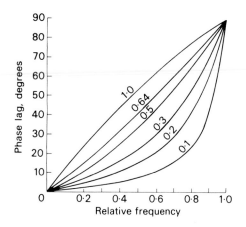

Fig. 13.12. Relation of phase shift to damping. Phase shift is directly related to frequency when damping is about 64% of critical ($D = 0.64$). Relative frequency is the ratio of the applied frequency to the undamped natural frequency of the system. (After Gabe, 1972.)

pressure measurement is being related to an electrophysiological event in the cardiac cycle.

Practrical considerations

It will be apparent that one way of overcoming the problems inherent in arterial pressure measurement is to choose a pressure recording system with an extremely high undamped natural frequency. The only transducer with these characteristics is the catheter-tip transducer which may have an undamped natural frequency of 25–40 kHz. Since this is many times greater than the frequency of the 10th harmonic of an arterial pressure waveform, amplitude and phase distortion will be minimal. However, such transducers are still somewhat delicate and expensive so that for most applications it is necessary to use a standard catheter–transducer system.

Although a standard pressure transducer may, by itself, have an undamped natural frequency of 100 Hz or more, the addition of the catheter, tap and arterial cannula will reduce the resonant frequency very considerably. Moreover, the frequency response which may be achieved in a laboratory is not often reproduced under clinical conditions. The most frequent reason is the presence of air

bubbles. As the arterial pressure changes from systolic to diastolic the bubbles are compressed and expanded and with even quite a small bubble the volume of saline that flows in and out of the catheter in response to this volume change in the bubble may be greater than the volume change due to the displacement of the transducer diaphragm. Since this extra flow has to take place during the same period, the velocity of the flow is increased, thus increasing the effective mass. This has two effects. It lowers the resonant frequency of the system, and may bring it below the frequencies which are being measured, and it increases the damping. These effects do not depend on the bubble being in the catheter, and are just the same if it is in the transducer. It is of the greatest practical importance, therefore, to avoid bubbles anywhere in the system. In the most stringent applications the catheter–transducer system is flushed with boiled saline for several hours before use to promote absorption of all the bubbles.

A second cause of damping is any elasticity of the walls of the catheter. Soft catheters distend in response to the pulse wave and so have the same effect as an air bubble. Attaching the transducer directly to the arterial cannula greatly improves the reproduction of the waveform.

A further cause of excessive damping is clotting in the arterial cannula which reduces the lumen and increases the velocity of the saline flow, thus increasing the effective mass. This is minimized by maintaining a slow flow ($3 \text{ ml} \cdot \text{h}^{-1}$) of flush solution through the catheter using a pressurized reservoir and fine capillary or by flushing with 0.5 ml aliquots of solution at hourly intervals. It must also be remembered that the narrowest parts of the catheter–transducer system are usually the arterial cannula and the orifices inside taps and that the use of a relatively wide bore cannula (minimum size 20 standard wire gauge (SWG) for adults) and wide bore taps greatly improves the frequency response of the system (Shapiro & Krovetz, 1970).

Finally, it must be remembered that the display or recording system must have a frequency response which exceeds that of the catheter–transducer system. A good heated-stylus recorder is usually adequate for the routine monitoring of arterial and venous pressure. However, for adequate registration of left ventricular end-diastolic pressure or left ventricular dP/dt_{max} it is necessary to employ a photographic, ultravoilet or ink-jet recorder.

Adjustment of damping

Damping of the system can be increased both hydrostatically and electrically. It can be increased hydrostatically by inserting an additional constriction in the line (Gabe, 1972) or by allowing the velocity of flow in the catheter to rise by inserting a compliant tube into the system (Latimer & Latimer, 1974). Electrical damping is used more commonly and is achieved by passing the electrical signal arising from the moving diaphragm through frequency-selective circuits. It must be emphasized, however, that manipulation of electronic controls cannot put back frequencies that were lost on their way to the transducer. Regular flushing to prevent clotting and to remove air bubbles is essential.

Correct damping is less important when the natural frequency of the transducer is high in relation to the frequencies being recorded. With a number of modern transducers which have a very small compliance and with catheter-tip transducers, correct damping is of relatively little im-portance since the undamped natural frequency is very much higher than the frequencies of interest. However, when the natural frequency is closer to the applied frequencies, only a critically-damped system will be accurate. When the natural frequency is so low that important harmonics of the pressure wave correspond with it, over-damped systems produce a smaller error than under-damped ones. Since it is difficult to measure, still less control, the damping, it is common practice to increase the damping if the record looks 'spiky', the assumption being that this is due to the higher frequency harmonics being near the resonant frequency.

This approach, while pragmatic, is making the best of what may be a very bad job. If accuracy is important one must make some evaluation of the frequency reponse in the prevailing conditions. This can be done by observing the response to a sudden stepwise change (Gabe, 1972) or to a sweep frequency sine-wave generator as already described (McCutcheon *et al.* 1972; Asmussen *et al.* 1975). Providing the undamped response is adequate, further damping can then be added electronically.

Unfortunately, the response of a catheter–transducer system tested under laboratory conditions may not be reproduced when the system is used clinically. It is therefore necessary to test the system when connected to the patient (Schwid, 1988). The most practical way of assuring accurate

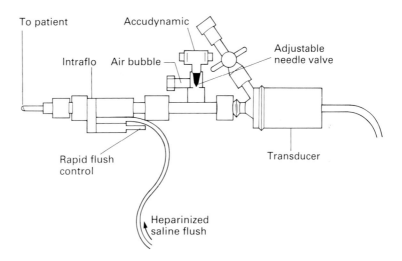

Fig. 13.13. Device for adjusting damping. The resistance of the passage between the air bubble and manometer line is adjusted by altering the position of the needle valve until an optimal response to a square wave of pressure is obtained. The 'Accudynamic' and 'Intraflo' are commercially available devices that facilitate these manoevres.

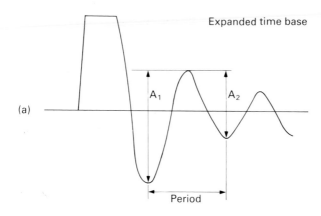

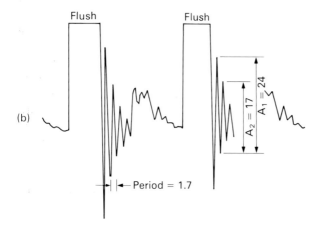

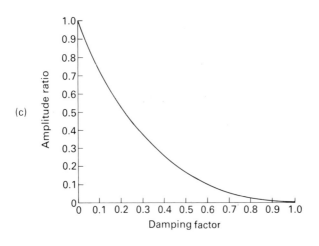

Fig. 13.14. Measurement of damping factor from dynamic response to square wave change of pressure produced by cessation of fast flush. (a) Expanded time base to show measurements required. (b) Dynamic trace of arterial pressure with two short flushes. The undamped natural frequency is obtained by dividing the paper speed (in $mm \cdot s^{-1}$) by the period (the distance between successive periods in mm). The damping factor is determined by taking the ratio of the amplitudes of successive oscillation peaks (A_2/A_1) and reading the value from the graph (c). (After Gardner, 1981.)

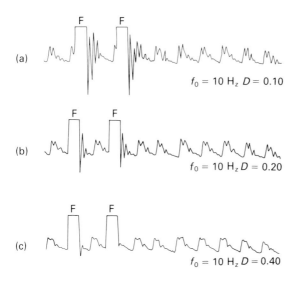

(a)

$f_0 = 10$ Hz $D = 0.10$

(b)

$f_0 = 10$ Hz $D = 0.20$

(c)

$f_0 = 10$ Hz $D = 0.40$

(d)

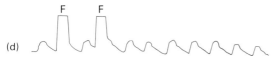

Fig. 13.15. Adjustment of damping by observing response to square wave of pressure produced by intermittent flush device (F). (a) Natural frequency 10 h Hz, damping factor 0.1. Note overshoot and 'ringing' arterial pressure waveform. (b) Damping increased to 0.2 by adjustment of needle valve. Oscillation from flush dies away more quickly. (c) Damping increased to 0.4. Small overshoot shows damping is almost optimal. Arterial waveform accurate. (d) Damping excessive. There is no overshoot after the flush and the arterial waveform appears damped. (After Gardner, 1981.)

pressure measurements is to incorporate a fast flush and damping system in the line between the catheter and manometer. A system which has been used clinically consists of a small air bubble connected to the pressure line via a saline-filled needle valve (the Accudynamic) (Fig. 13.13). The effective cross sectional area of the needle valve, and hence its resistance, can be adjusted by rotating the control knob so that the impedance of the device can be matched to the characteristic impedance of the catheter–transducer system. When this is accomplished damping is optimal (Allan *et al.* 1988).

To use the device, a square wave of pressure is produced by activating a continuous flush device such as the 'Intraflo' and then suddenly releasing the plug. The square wave is followed by oscillations which progressively decrease in amplitude. The undamped natural frequency of the system is calculated from the period between successive peaks (Fig. 13.14) whilst the damping factor is determined by measuring the amplitude of successive peaks. The factor may then either be calculated by the formula of Gabe (1972) or read off a graph (Gardner, 1981). To ensure accurate results it is necessary to record the oscillations at a fast paper speed. Then:

$$f_0 = \frac{\text{paper speed (mm} \cdot \text{s}^{-1})}{\text{distance between peaks (mm)}} \, .$$

In practice it is possible to adjust damping by observing the overshoot in response to a flush. When damping is optimal there is one undershoot followed by a small overshoot, with the pressure then following the patient's waveform (Fig. 13.15). However, it must again be emphasized that the device is no substitute for the utmost care in setting up the pressure recording system. The cannula and taps should have as large a diameter as possible, the catheter should be short, rigid and at least 1–2 mm in diameter, the transducer should have a low volume displacement and all air bubbles should be rigorously excluded from the system.

Choice of apparatus for intravascular pressure measurement

In order to obtain a high natural frequency, designers of transducers for arterial pressure recording have developed stiffer and stiffer diaphragms with smaller volume displacements.

Most of the standard strain gauge transducers have a volume displacement of $1–5 \times 10^{-5}$ mm^3 $\cdot$ kPa^{-1} (0.01–0.04 mm$^3 \cdot$ 100 mmHg^{-1}) whilst the internal volume of the transducer dome is about 1 ml. When a pressure of 13.3 kPa (100 mmHg) is applied to this volume of saline it reduces its volume by about 0.006 mm^3. Since this represents about half the volume displacement of the transducer it is apparent that the only way to secure a further reduction in volume displacement is to decrease the volume of fluid in the dome. Volumes as low as 0.2 ml have now been achieved in some silicon strain gauge transducers. Since these devices give a high electrical output for a given deflection it has been possible to reduce the volume displacement to 1.3×10^{-7} mm$^3 \cdot$kPa^{-1} (0.0001 mm$^3 \cdot$100 mmHg). This results in an undamped natural resonant frequency of 5 kHz. A still higher undamped natural frequency (25–40 kHz) is obtained with catheter-tip transducers where the diaphragm is very small and is in direct contact with the blood.

In general, a stiffer diaphragm has to be paid for by a reduced sensitivity of the system. A stiff diaphragm must result in a smaller movement for a given pressure change, and no matter what method is used to sense the movement, a smaller change of that quantity will result. A high frequency response, and a sensitive system, are therefore mutually incompatible characteristics.

Venous pressure measurements require high sensitivity but very little high frequency capability, and transducers with a higher volume displacement may be used. When the shape of the waveform is of importance, as in arterial tracings, one needs a high frequency response, and for this a low volume displacement is essential. If the shape of the waveform is not of crucial importance, and it is only desired to record the systolic and diastolic pressures, a flat response up to 10 Hz will give figures within 5% of the correct figure, despite amplitude and phase distortion.

It is important to ensure that the gauge is aligned with the right atrium and that the zero and gain of the transducer–amplifier–recorder system are checked at regular intervals using a saline or mercury manometer. Drift is usually not a problem with modern pressure recording systems when measuring arterial pressure, but may become significant when using higher gain settings to measure venous pressures. Although many recording systems incorporate an electrical calibration signal, this may become inaccurate. It should only be used as an interim standard if it has previously been checked against a known hydrostatic pressure.

References

Allan, M.W.B, Gray W.M, & Asbury, A.J. (1988) Measurement of arterial pressure using catheter–transducer systems. Improvement using the Accudynamic. *British Journal of Anaesthesia* **60**, 413–418.

Asmussen, M., Lindström, K. & Ulmsten, U. (1975) A catheter manometer calibrator — a new clinical instrument. *Biomedical Engineering* **10**, 175–180.

Debrunner, F. & Buhler, F. (1969) 'Normal central venous pressure', significance of reference point and normal range. *British Medical Journal* **3**, 148–150.

Gabe, I.T. (1972) Pressure measurement in experimental physiology. In Bergel, D.A. (ed.), *Cardiovascular fluid dynamics*, Chapter 2. Academic Press, London.

Gardner, R.M. (1981) Direct blood pressure measurement—dynamic response requirements. *Anesthesiology* **54**, 227–236.

Kleinman R. (1989) Understanding natural frequency and damping and how they relate to the measurement of blood pressure. *Journal of Clinical Monitoring* **5**, 137–147.

Latimer R.D. & Latimer K.E. (1974) Continuous flushing systems. A critical review. *Anaesthesia* **29**, 307–317.

McCutcheon, E.P., Evans J.M. & Stanifer, R. (1973) In McCutcheon, E.P. (ed.), *Evaluation of miniature pressure transducers in chronically implanted cardiovascular instrumentation*. Academic Press, New York.

Shapiro, G.G. & Krovetz, L.J. (1970) Damped and undamped frequency responses of underdamped catheter manometer systems. *American Heart Journal* **80**, 226–236.

Schwid H.A. (1988) Frequency response evaluation of radial artery catheter–manometer systems: sinusoidal frequency analysis versus flush method. *Journal of Clinical Monitoring* **4**, 181–185.

Winsor, T. & Burch, G.E. (1945) The phlebostatic axis and phlebostatic level, reference levels for venous pressure measurements in man. *Proceedings of the Society for Experimental Biology and Medicine* **58**, 165–169.

Zorab, J.S.M (1969) Continuous display of the arterial pressure. A simple manometric technique. *Anaesthesia* **24**, 431–437.

Further reading

Gersh B.J. (1980) Measurement of intravascular pressures. In Prys-Roberts, C. (ed.) *The circulation in anaesthesia*, p. 511. Blackwell Scientific Publications, Oxford.

14: Indirect Methods for Measuring Arterial Pressure

Most indirect methods are based on the occlusion of a major artery by the Riva-Rocci type of cuff (Riva-Rocci, 1896). In the standard clinical technique, systolic and diastolic end-points are detected by auscultation of the Korotkoff sounds (Korotkoff, 1905). Although there are many alternative techniques for recognizing the systolic point the only other methods which provide a reliable indication of diastolic pressure are those which detect sound energy at lower than audible frequencies, those which detect the movement of the arterial wall by the use of ultrasound, and the plethysmographic method.

Before discussing the techniques available it is important to consider how the accuracy of any indirect method may be assessed. Readings obtained must be compared with some standard, which in this case is a direct measurement of arterial pressure. However, as was pointed out in Chapter 13, direct pressure measurements are themselves prone to error, but such errors are rarely considered when assessing an indirect method. The site of indirect measurement may cause difficulties, because arterial pressure cannot be assumed to be identical in every artery. For instance, it is well established that as the pulse wave travels from the ventricle to peripheral arteries the velocity increases, so leading to greater pulse pressures (Bruner *et al.* 1981). Furthermore, it is well known that arterial pressure may differ in the two arms, and it has been suggested that comparisons should be made between the cuff pressure and the direct pressure recorded from the subclavian artery in the same arm. However, even this comparison may be invalid since inflation of the cuff may cause pressure wave reflections and so increase the pressure in the artery proximal to the cuff. Yet another problem is that most indirect methods are, by their very nature, intermittent, with the systolic and diastolic readings reflecting conditions in the artery at two instants at which the end-points are detected. The direct pressure, however, is a continuously changing waveform from which the systolic and diastolic pressures are determined by averaging a number of cycles. Small wonder that estimates may differ, however precise the methods themselves. Comparisons of indirect and direct methods of recording arterial pressure should therefore be assessed critically, and conclusions drawn only from those in which the accuracy of direct pressure measurement has been properly considered (Bruner *et al.* 1981).

Riva-Rocci cuff and auscultation of Korotkoff sounds

Although this technique is generally believed to correlate reasonably well with direct measurements in the majority of patients, there are a number of occasions on which there are gross discrepancies between the two methods, particularly in the determination of the diastolic point (Berliner *et al.* 1960).

PROCEDURE

The cuff is wound closely round the upper arm (which should be at heart level) and the site of the brachial artery is identified by palpation. The cuff is inflated to 250–300 mmHg and then deflated at a rate of about 10 mmHg·s^{-1} so that a rough estimate of the systolic point is obtained by palpation (this precaution is necessary because in some hypertensive patients there is a 'silent zone' between systolic and diastolic points, and inadequate cuff inflation might cause the observer to

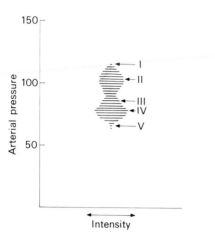

Fig. 14.1. Diagrammatic representation of the Korotkoff sounds.

mistake the return of the sounds for the systolic point). The cuff is then inflated to about 30 mmHg above the estimated systolic point and deflated at a rate of about 2 mmHg·s⁻¹ whilst the observer listens over the brachial artery. The systolic point is marked by the sudden appearance of clear, tapping sounds which are synchronous with the heart beat (Fig. 14.1; Phase I). As cuff deflation continues a palpable pulse appears at the wrist (usually about 5–10 mmHg below the audible systolic point) and the sounds then become somewhat quieter (Phase II). In some patients the sounds disappear completely (the 'auscultatory gap') whilst in other patients there may be little reduction in the intensity of the sound. As the diastolic point is approached the sounds usually become louder and develop a tapping quality (Phase III). They then suddenly become muffled (Phase IV) and usually disappear altogether at some 5–10 mmHg below the point of muffling (Phase V), although in high output states and in exercise, the sounds may not disappear until cuff pressures approach zero.

THE PHYSICAL BASIS OF THE METHOD

Riva-Rocci described the idea of using an inflatable cuff to occlude the artery in two papers published in 1896, but he used a cuff which was only 5 cm wide. The pressure in such a narrow cuff was often not transmitted fully to the underlying artery and it

was von Recklinghausen (1901) who suggested that the cuff should be 12 cm wide. However, at this time the systolic pressure was determined by palpation of the pulse distal to the cuff and the only method of determining diastolic pressure was to use an aneroid gauge to observe the pulsations transmitted to the cuff between the systolic and diastolic points (Hill & Barnard, 1897). It was in December 1905 that N. C. Korotkoff, a Russian surgeon, first reported the auscultatory method of measuring blood pressure (Booth, 1977).

The mechanism by which Korotkoff sounds are generated is still not fully agreed but a reasonable conceptual model is that turbulent flow makes the arterial wall vibrate excessively and that this vibration is amplified by resonance of the tissue in the arm. When the cuff pressure lies between systolic and diastolic pressure and the arterial pressure rises during systole, the transmural pressure difference (across the vessel wall) is greatly reduced. Under these conditions turbulent flow can readily induce gross vibrations in the vessel wall. Just below the systolic point the sounds have both low and high frequency components although the former predominate. The high frequency components become particularly marked during Phase III and disappear abruptly as Phase IV is reached leaving only the low frequency components.

ACCURACY OF THE KOROTKOFF METHOD

The sudden appearance of the Korotkoff sounds during cuff deflation corresponds closely with directly-measured systolic pressure, although the indirect measurement usually gives values which are slightly lower than direct measurements. Unfortunately, correlation between the two measurements of diastolic pressure is not so good. In the UK the diastolic pressure is generally assumed to correspond with Phase IV, and a similar recommendation was made by the Postgraduate Education Committee of the American Heart Association. However, a number of important epidemiological studies both in the USA and the UK have since utilized Phase V (Hunyor *et al.* 1978), and the most recent recommendation of the American Heart

falling at a rate of about $2 \, \text{mmHg} \cdot \text{s}^{-1}$. Small oscillations of the pointer are observed as the pressure falls. These are due to pulse waves striking the upper occluding cuff, producing pressure transients across the diaphragm of aneroid A. Since the occluding cuff does not allow the pulse wave to reach the lower, sensing cuff, the lever fulcrum on aneroid B remains still, so the observed oscillations are small. When the pressure in the occluding cuff falls to just below systolic pressure, the pulse wave passes under the occluding cuff, and strikes the larger sensing cuff. The resulting pressure transient in aneroid (B) raises the fulcrum simultaneously with compression of aneroid A, whilst the fine bore interconnections prevent rapid equalization of pressure. At this point the pressure swings in aneroid B are larger than those in the main chamber because of the relative disparity between the volumes of the two cuffs and the two chambers, the small occluding cuff discharging through a narrow tube into the large main chamber whilst the larger sensing cuff discharges through a wide tube into the relatively small volume of aneroid (B). Furthermore aneroid (B) has a higher compliance than aneroid (A) thus further amplifying the pressure swings displayed by the pointer. Systolic pressure is usually taken as the cuff pressure at which the needle swings show an abrupt increase in amplitude. However, Hutton and Prys-Roberts (1982) showed that the changes occurring at the systolic end-point are quite complex, and can be indicated by several different patterns of needle response. They recommended that the systolic end-point be taken as the cuff pressure at which the needle swings show a definite change in character.

Partial or complete occlusion of the small holes in the valve by dirt or valve lubricant may cause the pressure in the main chamber or in aneroid (B) to be much higher than it should be. This results in wild swings of the pointer when the lever is released and is a frequent source of error with this instrument. Similar errors may occur if the occluding cuff pressure is reduced too quickly, for this also results in a gross imbalance in pressure between the occluding and sensing systems.

To measure diastolic pressure the lever is once again pulled forward and the deflation of the occluding cuff continued. The oscillations of the pointer usually increase slightly and then suddenly decrease when the diastolic point is reached. This indicates that the artery is remaining open throughout the pulse cycle, so that the impact of the pulse wave is greatly diminished. The lever is released and diastolic pressure read from the scale. Both cuffs are then completely deflated by opening the discharge valve on the inflating bulb. In their study, Hutton and Prys-Roberts (1982) found no definite end-point for diastolic pressure, making estimation most uncertain.

It has been suggested that the relative position of the cuffs is of little importance. Corall and Strunin (1975) found that positioning the sensing cuff proximal to the occluding cuff did not produce an error in the reading if the cuffs were old, but it did produce an error if the cuffs were new. However, most experienced anaesthetists would agree that there are enough sources of error in blood pressure measurement without adding yet one more!

It can be seen that the instrument utilizes the same underlying mechanisms as other indirect methods of blood pressure measurement. It is therefore prone to the same sources of error. In their careful comparison with directly measured arterial pressure, Hutton and Prys-Roberts (1982) found a very close correlation between the two methods when considering systolic pressure ($r = 0.986$, 95% confidence interval $\pm 13.7 \, \text{mmHg}$). However, they showed that such precision can be achieved only with slow deflation of the cuff; rapid deflation leads to a much wider confidence interval ($\pm 27.8 \, \text{mmHg}$). Similarly, mean arterial pressure showed close agreement ($r = 0.956$, 95% confidence interval $\pm 17.3 \, \text{mmHg}$). However, diastolic pressure estimations showed poor agreement ($r = 0.642$, 95% confidence interval $\pm 38.1 \, \text{mmHg}$); this is not surprising when the authors commented that they could not establish a satisfactory end-point. They concluded that the instrument provides a good method for estimating systolic and mean pressures, but for diastolic pressure it is useless.

OSCILLOMETRIC MEASUREMENT OF
BLOOD PRESSURE

Observations by Van Bergen (1954) and Posey *et al.* (1969) showed that blood pressure can be estimated by analysis of the pressure oscillations in a standard sphygmomanometer cuff as it is slowly deflated.

A number of automatic, non-invasive devices have been introduced, operating on this oscillometric principle of measurement. In each case, a single cuff of standard dimensions is applied to the upper arm and inflated to at least 30 mmHg above systolic pressure. During slow deflation, each pulse wave leads to a pressure transient in the cuff which is transmitted along the connecting tube and can be detected by a suitable transducer. Above systolic pressure the transients are small, but when the cuff pressure reaches the systolic point they quickly increase in magnitude. As the cuff pressure decreases further, the amplitude reaches a peak and then starts to diminish. The mean arterial pressure correlates closely with the lowest cuff pressure at which the maximum amplitude is maintained. As the cuff pressure reaches diastolic pressure, the transients abruptly diminish in amplitude.

The first instrument to make use of this principle was the 'Dinamap' (Critikon Ltd), based on a design by Ramsey (1979). This fully automatic device inflates the cuff and then deflates it in small increments, whilst the pressure fluctuations within the cuff are sensed by an electronic transducer and analysed by a microprocessor (see Fig. 14.3).

At each pressure plateau successive pulses are compared, and accepted only if their amplitudes are similar. In the presence of mechanical noise, the pressure is maintained until an 'acceptable' pair of pulses are detected. Heart rate, systolic, diastolic and mean arterial pressures are displayed digitally. Ramsey claimed a high correlation between mean arterial pressure readings from his prototype device and direct arterial pressure ($r = 0.979$), with an average mean difference between direct and indirect estimates of only -0.23 mmHg with a standard deviation of 4.21 mmHg.

In their assessment of the commercially built 'Dinamap' applied to 10 patients undergoing surgery, Hutton et al. (1984) found a less impressive correlation with direct arterial pressure. Systolic pressure showed a good correlation ($r = 0.95$), but with a bias towards overestimation at low pressures and underestimation at high pressures (similar to the Korotkoff sounds method). Overall, the 95% confidence interval for systolic pressure was ± 16.4 mmHg. Mean arterial pressure showed a less satisfactory correlation ($r = 0.87$), with a similar systematic bias and confidence interval. Diastolic pressure showed a similar relationship ($r = 0.85$, 95% confidence interval ± 15.3 mmHg).

Studies in neonates and infants have reached similar conclusions (Kimble et al. 1981).

Other devices operate according to similar principles (Johnson & Kerr, 1985). Newer devices deflate the cuff continuously rather than in steps, thus achieving a shorter measurement cycle. For

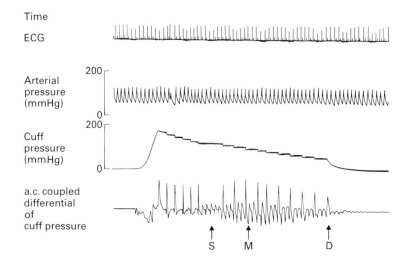

Fig. 14.3. Blood pressure estimation using the 'Dinamap', compared with directly measured ipsilateral brachial artery pressure. The lower trace shows the signal derived from cuff pressure oscillations, used by the 'Dinamap' in determining systolic mean and diastolic endpoints. (Reproduced with permission from Hutton et al. 1984.) (S = systolic pressure, M = mean pressure, D = diastolic pressure.)

instance, the 'Accutorr' (Ohmeda) analyzes the whole 'cuff pressure: pulse amplitude' relationship. The systolic, mean and diastolic values are determined from the computed pulse amplitude profile, thereby avoiding the need for individual pulses to be validated at each pressure.

All automatic oscillometric instruments have one major limitation; they rely heavily upon a regular cardiac cycle, with no great differences between successive pulses. It is often impossible to obtain consistent or even satisfactory readings in patients with atrial fibrillation.

Continuous non-invasive measurement

An entirely new technology has emerged, based upon what Penaz called 'the unloaded artery principle' (Penaz, 1973). In fact, it is an example of the force balance: the force exerted by a body may be measured by determining the counter force which must be applied to stop the original force from causing some physical event. The virtue of this principle is that the counter force can be measured very precisely, and the detection system does not need to be linear for it must only be capable of detecting the null condition.

A small cuff is placed around the finger, and can be inflated and deflated by a high-speed servo-system. Inside the cuff a light-emitting diode (LED) transilluminates the finger, and on the opposite side a photodiode detects the light intensity after it has passed through the finger. The principle is similar to that of a simple pulse monitor and its derivative, the pulse oximeter. The detected light intensity is a crude indicator of blood volume in the finger, but a very precise indicator of any change in that volume. The servo-system inflates the cuff to above systolic and then deflates in the traditional manner. As soon as the pulse wave is sensed by the optical detector, the servo increases the pressure so as to diminish the flow and so maintain a constant signal. Then, because the servo-system can operate very quickly, the pressure waveform applied to the finger by the cuff exactly mirrors the pressure waveform within the arteries.

By this means the device is able not only to determine systolic and diastolic pressure, but also to reproduce the actual arterial pressure waveform.

The 'Finapres' (Ohmeda) monitor is a commercial implementation of this principle (Smith *et al.* 1985). The small number of reports on the performance of this system suggest that it is highly effective in the normal or vasodilated finger, showing a high correlation with directly measured arterial pressure even during hypotensive anaesthesia (Kurki *et al.* 1987). Other reports have found unreliable results in some patients with poor peripheral blood flow, and suggest caution in interpreting results in poor-risk patients until the performance of the device is more thoroughly evaluated (Gibbs *et al.* 1988).

Although the device appears to provide an accurate record of rapidly changing trends in blood pressure in an individual patient, it is less satisfactory as a method of measuring absolute pressures. The differences between 'Finapres' and directly measured arterial pressures show marked inter–patient variability and small differences in the positioning and tightness of the cuff produce significant differences in recorded pressure in the same patient. The maintained pressure in the cuff leads to discomfort after 20–30 min, but this can be overcome by periodic deflation of the cuff.

References

Berliner, K., Fujiy, H., Ho Lee D., Yildiz M. & Garnier, B. (1960) The accuracy of blood pressure determinations: a comparison of direct and indirect measurements. *Cardiologica* **37**, 118–128.

Booth, J. (1977) A short history of blood pressure measurement. *Proceedings of the Royal Society of Medicine* **70**, 793–799.

Bruner, J.R.M., Krenis L.J., Kunsman, J.M. & Sherman A.P. (1981) Comparison of direct and indirect methods of measuring arterial blood pressure. *Medical Instrumentation* **15**, 11–21.

Burch, G.E. & Shewey, L. (1973) Sphygmomanometric cuff size and blood pressure recordings. *Journal of the American Medical Association* **225**, 1215–1218.

Cohn, J.N. (1967) Blood pressure measurement in shock. *Journal of the American Medical Association* **199**, 972–976.

Conceicao, S., Ward, M.K. & Kerr, D.N.S. (1976) Defects in sphygmomanometers: an important source of error in blood pressure recording. *British Medical Journal* i, 886–888.

Corrall, I.M. & Strunin, L. (1975) Assessment of the Von Recklinghausen oscillotonometer. *Anaesthesia* **30**, 59–66.

Gibbs, N.M., Larach, D.R. & Derr, J.A. (1988) The performance of the FINAPRES continuous blood pressure monitor during the peri-induction period in high-risk patients. *Anesthesiology* **69**, A324.

Greenfield, A.D.M., Whitney R.J. & Mowbray, J.F. (1963) Methods for the investigation of peripheral blood flow. *British Medical Bulletin* **19**, 101–109.

Hill, L. & Barnard, H. (1897) A simple and accurate form of sphygmomanometer or arterial pressure gauge contrived for clinical use. *British Medical Journal* ii, 904.

Holland, W.W. & Humerfelt, S. (1964) Measurements of blood pressure: comparison of intra-arterial and cuff values. *British Medical Journal* ii, 1241–1243.

Hunyor, S.N., Flynn, J.M. & Cochineas, C. (1978) Comparison of performance of various sphygmomanometers with intra-arterial blood pressure readings. *British Medical Journal* iii, 159–162.

Hutton, P., Dye, J. & Prys-Roberts, C. (1984) An assessment of the Dinamap 845. *Anaesthesia* **39**, 261–267.

Hutton, P., & Prys-Roberts, C. (1982) The oscillotonometer in theory and practice. *British Journal of Anaesthesia* **54**, 581–591.

Johnson, C.J.M., & Kerr, J.M. (1985) Automatic blood pressure monitors. A clinical evaluation of five models in adults. *Anaesthesia* **40**, 471–478.

Kazamias, T.M., Gander, M.P., Franklin,D.L. & Ross, J. (1971) Blood pressure measurement with Doppler ultrasonic flowmeter. *Journal of Applied Physiology* **30**, 585–588.

Kimble, K.J., Darnell, R.A., Yelderman, M., Ariagno, R.L. & Ream, A.K. (1981) An automated oscillometric technique for estimating mean arterial pressure in critically ill newborns. *Anesthesiology* **54**, 423–425.

King G.E. (1967) Errors in clinical measurement of blood pressure in obesity. *Clinical Science* **32**, 223–237.

Kirby, R.R., Kemmerer, W.T. & Morgan, J.L. (1969) (1969) Transcutaneous Doppler measurement of blood pressure. *Anesthesiology* **31**, 86–89.

Kirkendall, W.M., Feinleib, M., Freis, E.D., & Mark, A.L. (1980) Recommendations for human blood pressure determination by sphygmomanometers. Subcommittee of the AHA Postgraduate Education Committee, American Heart Association. *Circulation* **62**, 1146A–1155A.

Korotkoff, N.S. (1905) *On methods of studying blood pressure, vol. 2, p. 365.* Izvestiya Imperatorskoi Voenno-Meditsinskoi akademii, St. Peterburg.

Kurki, T., Smith N.T., Head, N., Dec-Silver, H. & Quinn, A. (1987) Noninvasive continuous blood pressure measurement from the finger: optimal measurement conditions and factors affecting reliability. *Journal of Clinical Monitoring* **3**, 6–13.

Moss, A.J., Liebling, W., Austin, W.O. & Adams, F.H. (1957) An evaluation of the flush method for determining blood pressures in infants. *Pediatrics* **20**, 53–62.

Pederson, R.W. & Vogt, F.B. (1973) Korotkoff vibrations in hypotension. *Medical Instrumentation* **7**, 251–256.

Penaz, J. (1973) Photoelectric measurement of blood pressure, volume and flow in the finger. *Digest of the 10th International Conference on Medical and Biological Engineering* p. 104.

Pereira, E., Prys-Roberts, C., Dagnino, J., Anger, C., Cooper, G.M. & Hutton P. (1985) Auscultatory measurement of arterial pressure during anaesthesia: a reassessment of Korotkoff sounds. *European Journal of Anaesthesiology* **2**, 11–20.

Posey, J.A., Geddes, L.A., Williams, H. & Moore, A.G. (1969) The meaning of the point of maximum oscillations in cuff pressure in the indirect measurement of blood pressure. *Cardiovascular Research Center Bulletin* **8**, 15–25.

Ramsey, M. (1979) Noninvasive automatic determination of mean arterial blood pressure. *Medical and Biological Engineering and Computing* **17**, 11–18.

Riva-Rocci, S. (1896) Un sfigmomanometro nuovo. *Gazetta Medica di Torino* **47**, 981–988.

Sara, C.A. & Shanks, C.A (1978) The peripheral pulse monitor — a review of electrical plethysmography. *Anaesthesia and Intensive Care* **6**, 226–233.

Simpson, J.A., Jamieson, G., Dickhaus, D.W. & Grover, R.F. (1965) Effect of size of cuff bladder on accuracy of measurement of indirect blood pressure. *American Heart Journal* **70**, 208–215.

Smith N.T., Wesseling, K.H. & de Wit B. (1985) Evaluation of two prototype devices producing non-invasive, pulsatile, calibrated blood pressure measurement. *Journal of Clinical Monitoring* **1**, 17–29.

Stegall, H.F., Kardon, M.B. & Kemmerer, W.T. (1968) Direct measurement of arterial blood pressure by Doppler ultrasonic sphygmomanometry. *Journal of Applied Physiology* **25**, 793–798.

Taguchi J.T. & Suwangool, P. (1974) 'Pipe-stem' brachial arteries — a cause of pseudo-hypertension. *Journal of the American Medical Association* **228**, 733.

Van Bergen, F.H., Weatherhead, D.S., Treloar, A.E., Dobkin A.B. & Buckley, J.J. (1954) Comparison of indirect and direct methods of measuring arterial blood pressure. *Circulation* **10**, 481–490.

Von Recklinghausen, H. (1901) Uber Blutdruckmessung beim Menschen. *Archiv für experimentelle Pathologie und Pharmakologie* **46**, 78–132.

Von Recklinghausen, H. (1931) *Neue Wege zur Blutdruckmessung.* Springer Verlag, Berlin.

Wallace, C.T., Carpenter, F.A. & Evins S.C. (1975) Acute pseudohypertensive crisis. *Anesthesiology* **43**, 588–589.

Whitcher C.E. (1968) Stethoscope performance in transduction of human Korotkov blood pressure sounds. *Anesthesiology* **29**, 215–216.

World Health Organization (1962) *Arterial hypertension and ischaemic heart disease: preventive Aspects.* Technical Report Series No. 231:4. World Health Organization, Geneva.

Zahed, B., Sadove, M.S., Hatano, S. & Wu, H.H. (1971) Comparison of automated Doppler ultrasound and Korotkoff measurements of blood pressure of children. *Anesthesia and Analgesia Current Researches* **50**, 699–704.

15: Measurement of Gas Flow and Volume

The SI unit of volume is the cubic metre (m^3), but it has been agreed that the more convenient unit, the litre ($\simeq 1000$ cm^3) may be retained as an alternative. Since flow rate is defined as the volume passing a fixed point in unit time, it is measured in cubic metres (or litres) per second. This concept must be clearly differentiated from the velocity of gas flow. Velocity is the distance moved by a gas molecule in unit time. For a given flow rate, velocity will therefore be higher when the gas is flowing through a narrow tube rather than a wide one. For example, if gas flows at a rate of 1 $L \cdot s^{-1}$ through a cylindrical tube having a radius of 2 cm and a cross-sectional area (πr^2) of $3.14 \times 2^2 = 12.6$ cm^2, then the average velocity of the gas molecules (v) is given by the flow rate divided by the cross-sectional area:

$$v = \frac{1000 \text{ cm}^3 \cdot \text{s}^{-1}}{12.6 \text{ cm}^2} = 79.6 \text{ cm} \cdot \text{s}^{-1}.$$

If the tube has a radius of 4 cm then:

$$v = \frac{1000 \text{ cm}^3 \cdot \text{s}^{-1}}{50.2 \text{ cm}^2} = 19.9 \text{ cm} \cdot \text{s}^{-1}.$$

The reverse conversion of velocity to flow rate is accomplished by multiplying the velocity by the cross-sectional area through which the gas passes.

The concept of velocity is important in the context of flow measurement because a number of instruments measure the velocity of flow and not flow rate. If the velocity of all the molecules in the gas or liquid were to be the same there would be no problem in converting the measured velocity to flow rate. Unfortunately this is rarely the case. For example, when flow is laminar, the velocity of particles in the central part of the stream is higher than that of particles situated more peripherally,

those next to the wall of the tube being virtually static. This creates a parabolic profile of velocities within the moving gas stream (Fig. 15.1). However, when converting this velocity profile to flow it is not sufficient to average the velocities and then multiply by the cross-sectional area of the tube since the more peripherally-situated layers of gas or fluid have a larger volume than the same thickness of gas or fluid situated more centrally. They therefore contribute proportionately more to the total flow than their velocities would suggest.

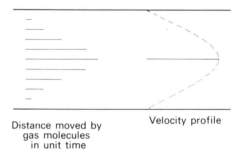

Distance moved by gas molecules in unit time

Velocity profile

Fig. 15.1. Velocity profile during laminar flow in a parallel-sided tube with a constant driving pressure. The axial stream has a higher velocity than the more peripheral stream.

Flowmeters are standardized by measuring the volume of gas which passes through the meter in unit time, so that methods of measuring gas volumes will be detailed first.

Volume measurements

Volumes of gas entering or leaving the lungs are usually measured directly by connecting the lungs to the measuring instrument. However, there is an increasing interest in indirect methods of measurement which do not require a connection between the measuring device and the patient's airway.

Measurements of gas volume are accomplished by collecting the gases in a calibrated spirometer or by passing the gases through some type of gas meter. Most metering devices are suitable for both continuous or intermittent flows of gas but if the device is only suitable for use with a continuous flow the gas must first be collected in a Douglas bag and then driven through the device at a steady rate.

Spirometers

Spirometers may be wet or dry, the wet using a liquid seal between the static and moving parts of the instrument and the dry achieving a seal by a folded bellows or a rolling diaphragm.

The *wet spirometer* (such as the 300 L Tissot or the 6 L Benedict–Roth) consists of a light but rigid cylinder which is suspended inside a larger double-walled container (Fig. 15.2). The space between the walls is filled with water to produce a seal and the bell is counter-balanced by a suitable weight. The movement of the bell is recorded by a pen or by a

simple electronic circuit which senses the rotation of the pulley wheel which is part of the bell suspension. The main advantage of the wet spirometer is that the relationship between an added volume of gas and the linear displacement of the bell can be calculated from the measured cross-sectional area of the bell. This type of spirometer can thus be used to provide a standard for calibrating flow meters or other volume measuring devices. However, a wet spirometer becomes inaccurate at high respiratory rates or during the performance of a forced vital capacity manoeuvre since a large pressure must be generated within the bell to overcome the inertia of the moving parts. The change in pressure produces fluctuations in the water level and compression of gas within the bell, thus causing a lag in the excursion of the pen. These problems can be overcome by using a light-weight bell of large diameter (which minimizes the acceleration during rapid breathing) and a large volume of water to minimize the oscillations (Bernstein *et al.* 1952).

The *dry spirometer* is more convenient for clinical work. One type consists of a large diameter, light-weight piston moving horizontally within a cylinder, a low friction seal between the two being

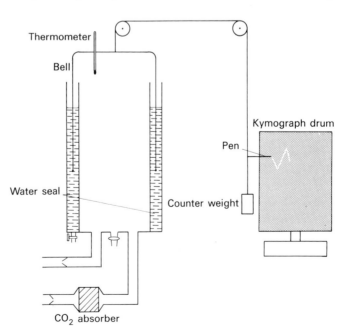

Fig. 15.2. Wet spirometer. The CO_2 absorber is inserted when closed-circuit spirometry is used for the measurement of oxygen consumption. The bell is then filled with O_2.

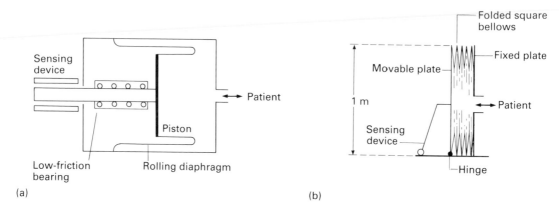

Fig. 15.3. (a) Piston-type of dry spirometer. (b) Wedge spirometer.

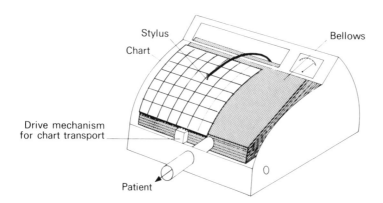

Fig. 15.4. Principle of the 'Vitalograph' spirometer.

achieved with a rolling diaphragm (Fig. 15.3a). A second type consists of two vertically mounted end-plates (about 1 m²) joined by a square folded bellows (Fig. 15.3b). One end-plate is fixed and the other is attached to the base plate by a hinge so that the bellows becomes wedge shaped when fully expanded. In both these devices the change in pressure within the chamber (and hence the resistance to airflow) is minimized by making the cross-sectional area large.* Since this results in a small horizontal displacement of the end plate the movement must be detected electronically. The resulting signal can be amplified to produce a volume recording of appropriate scale or differentiated to produce a trace of flow rate.

*The force moving the end-plate is the product of pressure × area.

A more specialized type of bellows spirometer used for lung function testing is exemplified by the 'Vitalograph' (Fig. 15.4). This is used for measuring forced vital capacity (FVC), forced expiratory volume in 1 s (FEV$_1$) or other indices of airway resistance such as peak expiratory flow rate (PEFR) or maximum mid-expiratory flow rate (MMEF). The patient makes a maximal forced exhalation into the spirometer through a wide-bore tube, the expansion of the wedge-shaped bellows being recorded on a pressure-sensitive chart by a pointed stylus. To conserve chart space, the movement of the chart along the x (time) axis only commences when gas begins to flow into the bellows. The resultant trace represents a volume/time plot of the patient's expiration. The FVC is the maximal volume expired. The slope of the line at any point represents the instantaneous relationship between

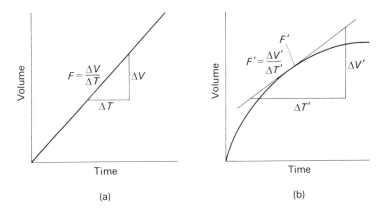

Fig. 15.5. (a) Flow (F) is derived from the volume measured in unit time. (b) Where flow rate varies rapidly, instantaneous flow rate at any point (F') is derived from the tangent of the volume curve at that point.

volume and time (i.e. flow) and can be derived by drawing a tangent to the line at that point (Fig. 15.5). Some of the more popular measurements used to provide information about airways resistance are shown in Fig. 15.6.

There is a small lag between the onset of expiration and the movement of the stylus due to preliminary expansion of the bellows. This is offset by ensuring that the stylus is aligned with the 'stylus start' position on the chart before making the measurement. It is extremely important to ensure that the patient makes an airtight seal with the mouthpiece and that the nose is occluded with a noseclip. The patient must be actively encouraged to breath out as forcibly and as rapidly as

possible, and the best of three or four attempts should be recorded.

When bronchospasm is present the measurement should be repeated after the administration of a bronchodilator. The linearity and accuracy of this machine is remarkably good and its impedance is quite small (Drew & Hughes, 1969). Another type of dry spirometer for lung function testing using a square-shaped bellows has been described by Collins et al. (1964).

Gas meters

Gas meters may be wet or dry. *Wet* meters are now rarely used since they need to be kept filled with water and carefully levelled: furthermore, the maximum flow rate which can be tolerated during measurement is limited to about $2.5 \, L \cdot min^{-1}$. Such a meter consists essentially of a paddle-wheel, the lower half of which rotates under water. Gas is admitted to the space between two paddle blades and this causes the paddle-wheel to rotate. The gas then passes out through the exit tube. Since the volume of gas isolated in each section of the paddle-wheel is constant, the degree of rotation of the paddle-wheel is proportional to the volume which has passed. The paddle-wheel is connected to a gear chain which drives a pointer on a dial so that a direct reading is obtained.

Dry gas meters are widely used in the gas industry and have proved useful in medicine since they are portable, accurate and relatively cheap. The meter consists of a box divided into three by

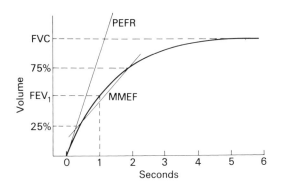

Fig. 15.6. Information which can be derived from forced vital capacity trace. FVC = forced vital capacity; PEFR = peak expiratory flow rate at beginning of expiration; FEV_1 = volume expired in 1 s; MMEF = average flow rate between 25 and 75% of FVC.

two partitions: one partition is horizontal and separates an upper gas inlet and valve compartment from two identical measurement compartments below (see Fig. 15.7). Each of the measurement compartments is further functionally divided by a plastic or leather bellows. Two compound rotary or sliding valves, mounted in the top compartment, direct the gas flow into and out of the four gas chambers thus created. These valves are activated by the movements of the bellows and are linked together so that the bellows themselves move in fixed relationship to each other. Within each pair of measuring chambers, movement of gas into or out of the inside of the bellows is exactly balanced by an equal volume of gas moving out of or into the chamber surrounding the bellows. Thus, at no time is the gas in the measuring compartments

under pressure. The connection between the valves and the bellows ensures that each bellows and its related valves is always 90° out of phase with the other. Thus, apart from the instants when either bellows is at the extreme end of its travel, gas is flowing into or out of all four compartments simultaneously. The movement of the bellows is activated by the pressure of the inlet gas, which need be only 2–3 cm of H_2O (0.2–0.3 kPa): when either of the bellows is at the point of reversal, there is an instant when there is no inlet pressure to that bellows or the surrounding chamber (like top dead centre in the cylinder of an internal combustion engine). A mechanism which relied on a single pair of chambers would be liable to stick at this point: having a second pair, 90° out of phase, mechanically linked to the valve mechanism en-

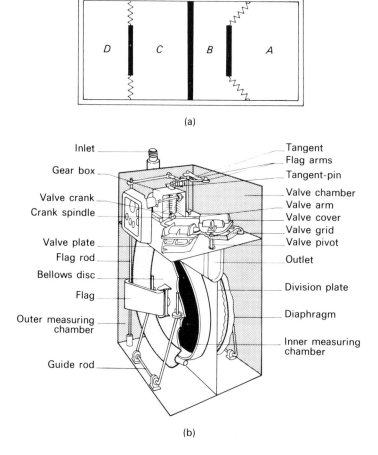

(a)

(b)

Fig. 15.7. (a) Coronal section of a dry gas meter. (b) Details of mechanism. (From Adams et al. 1967.)

sures that when one bellows is reversing at either end of its travel, the other bellows is moving with maximum velocity. This ensures smooth running and reasonably accurate measurements even at low flow rates. In addition to driving the valve mechanism, the movement of the two bellows is linked to a common mechanism which drives a pointer round a scale or provides the motive power for a sequence of clockwork-linked dials. The calibration is accurately adjusted to match the excursion of the bellows by altering the length of a tangent arm on the valve mechanism.

The volume which is passed during a complete cycle of a gas meter depends on the size of the meter and this depends on the flow which the meter is expected to handle. Between 2 and 2.5 L is a common volume for domestic-sized meters which are suitable for use on mechanical ventilators or in laboratories. This volume, of course, bears no relationship to a complete rotation of the indicator dial. Within the cycle, there may be gross inaccuracies due, for example, to irregular unfolding of a bellows. Once the meter has returned to the same position in the cycle, however, these temporary irregularities have evened out. The greatest accuracy is therefore obtained when the volume to be measured is a multiple of the meter volume. When large volumes are measured, any 'within cycle' inaccuracies are averaged over a large number of cycles. For example, a serious 200 ml irregularity within a cycle would amount to only a 0.44% error in measuring 50 L and 0.004% in 500 L. This increasing accuracy over large volumes has, of course, been the feature which enabled commercial undertakings to sell gas at a profit for over a hundred years. The flow rate also has an influence on accuracy, but even the smallest meters likely to be encountered can be accurate to ±1% over a range of flow rates from 0 to 100 L·min^{-1} if properly adjusted and maintained (Adams *et al.* 1967).

The Dräger volumeter

This instrument is somewhat larger than the Wright respirometer (see below) and responds to airflow in either direction (Fig. 15.8). The registra-

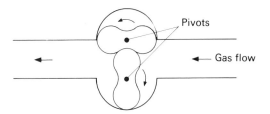

Fig. 15.8. Dräger volumeter.

tion of volume flow is accomplished by two light, interlocking, dumb-bell-shaped rotors. The meter is more accurate than the Wright respirometer but also more expensive. It is affected by moisture but regains its accuracy when dried out.

Wright respirometer

This device contains a light mica vane which rotates within a small cylinder (Fig. 15.9). The wall of the cylinder is perforated with a number of tangential slits so that the air stream causes the vane to rotate. Flow in the reverse direction impinges on the bottom edge of the vane and so produces no rotational movement. The instrument is therefore unidirectional.

The rotation of the vane activates a gear chain, which in turn drives the pointer round the dial. By adjusting the relation between the number of rotations of the vane and the volume of gas which has passed through the meter, it has been possible to arrange that the recorded volume approximates closely to the volume of gas which has actually passed through the meter. This calibration is performed with a sinewave pump and is valid for normal tidal volumes and breathing rates, but the

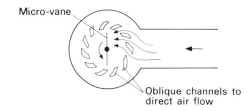

Fig. 15.9. Wright respirometer. Cross-section (viewed from above).

meter over-reads at high tidal volumes and under-reads at low tidal volumes due to its inertia. The meter tends to over-read when there is a high peak flow at the beginning of expiration (e.g. during mechanical ventilation) and also overestimates steady flows (Byles, 1960; Nunn & Ezi-Ashi, 1962; Bushman, 1979). A paediatric version of this instrument is now available (Hatch & Williams, 1988).

In a recent version of this instrument the rotation of the vane is detected electronically. The elimination of the gear chain minimizes inaccuracies due to inertia, renders the head less liable to damage from external shocks and reduces inaccuracies due to water condensation (Cox *et al.* 1974). The accuracy of this and two other electronic respirometers has been evaluated by Conway *et al.* (1974).

Integration of the flow signal

The flow signal from a pneumotachograph (p. 201) or any other rapidly-responding flowmeter may be electronically integrated with respect to time to yield a volume signal. Although digital methods of integration have greatly increased the accuracy of the procedure there are always problems with baseline drift. This arises from several sources. Firstly, under zero conditions it is difficult to achieve and maintain a zero output from a very sensitive differential pressure transducer because the balance is affected by changes in ambient temperature and by electronic drift. Whilst a small electronic signal resulting from a slight imbalance may not produce any detectable difference in the zero flow baseline, this signal is continually integrated by the integrator and may thus produce significant baseline drift on the volume signal. A second cause of baseline drift in clinical practice is a difference between the inspired and expired volume signals. This arises not only from the actual difference between inspired and expired volumes (due to the unequal volume exchange of oxygen and carbon dioxide and to the uptake or elimination of anaesthetic gases) but also to the difference in composition between inspired and expired gases.

These factors cause the inspired and expired signals to differ by about 6% (Grenvik *et al.* 1966).

These problems together with changes in resistance of the pneumotachograph head due to the deposition of water vapour or lung secretions, greatly reduce the usefulness of this technique for prolonged monitoring. However, it is possible to overcome these difficulties by resetting the integrator to zero at the end of each expiration, by heating the head and by applying repeated calibrations.

INDIRECT METHODS OF MEASURING TIDAL VOLUME

All the devices outlined in the previous sections need to be connected directly to the patient's airway. It is often difficult to secure a leak-free connection in the absence of an endotracheal tube, even with the use of a physiological mouth piece, and connection to the measuring apparatus often results in a change in the pattern of breathing (Gilbert *et al.* 1972). Since it is often desirable to monitor ventilation over long periods various devices have been developed which enable tidal volume to be derived from measurements of chest wall movement. These devices measure changes in the diameter, circumference or cross-sectional area of the thorax and abdomen. To relate these measurements to tidal volume it is necessary to establish the relative contributions of the chest and abdominal signals to the volume change and then to compare the summed signal with the actual tidal volume measured by spirometry.

One method of establishing the relative contribution of the two signals is for the subject to perform an iso-volume manoeuvre by occluding the upper airway and then alternately contracting and relaxing the abdominal and chest muscles. Since no overall lung volume change occurs this provides signals from the chest and abdominal sensors which are exactly out of phase. By adjusting the gains until the sum of the outputs equal zero, one can match the contributions of the two components and compare the sum to the actual tidal volume measured during breathing into a spirometer (Sackner *et al.* 1989).

Many patients find the iso-volume manoeuvre difficult to perform and calibration is therefore achieved by the use of the least squares regression technique. This is best performed by a computer which continuously compares the sum of the chest and abdominal signals with the output from the spirometer during a period of spontaneous breathing. By repeatedly solving two simultaneous equations the computer is able to derive the appropriate gain to be applied to each channel. Once this relationship is established, the calibrations can remain stable for several hours providing the position of the sensors and the patient is unchanged. However, a change in position often results in a change in the relative contribution of chest and abdominal components or a change in the position of the sensors, and so necessitates a repeat calibration.

Magnetometers

These devices have been used to measure changes in the diameter of the chest and abdomen in studies of chest wall mechanics. A magnetic field is generated by small electromagnets attached to the chest wall and abdomen, and the strength of the magnetic field sensed by small coils diammetrically opposite. Although changes in diameter can be measured accurately these are not well correlated with changes in volume. The devices have therefore not been used widely in clinical practice.

Pneumographs

Several instruments have been used to sense changes in chest and abdominal circumference. A non-elastic tape is placed around the chest and another around the abdomen. The ends of each tape are then connected to a sensor which measures the distance between them. A simple sensor which has been extensively used in physiological studies is a small bellows (usually made from corrugated rubber tubing) the interior of which is connected to a pressure transducer (Fig. 15.10). If the bellows are made from the appropriate material and are tensioned correctly the change in pressure is linearly related to the change in length (Morel *et al.* 1983). Commercially produced linear displacement transducers may be used in a similar manner.

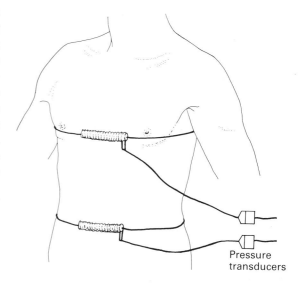

Fig. 15.10. Bellows pneumograph showing two transducers measuring the pressure in short lengths of corrugated tubing which are connected to non-elastic bands encircling the chest and abdomen.

Another device is the mercury-in-rubber strain gauge. This consists of a narrow silicon rubber tube containing mercury with electrical contacts at each end. Elongation of the tube narrows and lengthens the mercury column and so changes the resistance to the passage of an electrical current.

An alternative method of following circumference changes is to measure the change in electrical impedance when a high frequency oscillating current is passed through the chest wall. Since this technique only requires the application of four electrodes to the chest wall it provides a simple non-invasive method of monitoring chest wall movement. It has found wide application in paediatric intensive care units but is not suitable for quantitative measurements.

All the above techniques can be calibrated to provide a tidal volume signal but, since they are position-sensitive, frequent recalibration is required.

Capacitance spirometry

Changes in tidal volume can be detected by measuring the change in capacitance between two plates placed in front and behind the subject. This technique has been used for monitoring apnoeic periods in infants but has not found wide acceptance.

Respiratory inductance plethysmograph

Each sensing element consists of a wire coil which is sewn into an elasticated strap in a zig-zag pattern (Fig. 15.11). Expansion of the chest and abdomen increases the space between the coils and so alters the inductance generated by a high frequency alternating current (a.c.) current. The change in inductance is directly related to the cross sectional area of the body enclosed by the coil and so is closely related to the change in volume. Changes in body position generally have less effect on the calibration than with other devices, but recalibration should be performed if the body position is changed (Sackner *et al.* 1980).

The commercial instrument (Respitrace) provides a choice of a.c. or direct current (d.c.)

coupling. The former minimizes baseline drift and so facilitates long-term monitoring. Coupling can be switched to d.c. when it is desired to record acute changes of lung volume e.g. the response to the application of positive end-expiratory pressure (PEEP). The inductance plethysmograph has been used for various types of physiological studies and has also been used to monitor the respiratory effects of drugs given during the post-operative period. In this type of study apnoeic periods due to central depression can be differentiated from obstructive episodes by the presence of paradoxical movement between the chest and abdominal bands (Catley *et al.* 1985).

MEASUREMENTS OF LUNG VOLUME

Body plethysmograph

The patient sits in a sealed box and breathes through a tube connected to a pneumotachograph. The change in volume of the lungs can then be measured by one of two different methods. In the *constant pressure* plethysmograph the volume of gas displaced by the breathing movements is measured by a small wedge-shaped spirometer which is connected directly to the interior of the box. In the *constant volume* plethysmograph the change in lung volume creates a change in pressure in the box which is sensed by a sensitive pressure transducer. The relationship between volume and pressure change can then be established by pumping known volumes of air in and out of the box whilst the patient is in the box (Fig. 15.12).

The body plethysmograph can be used for measuring airflow rates and changes in lung volume and can also be used to measure thoracic gas volume. This is a particularly valuable attribute since airway resistance is critically dependent on lung volume and a knowledge of the lung volume at which airway resistance is measured greatly helps the interpretation of the results.

To measure thoracic gas volume (V) the patient makes inspiratory and expiratory efforts against a closed shutter whilst the change in mouth pressure (ΔP) and change in box volume (ΔV) are recorded. During the panting procedure the gas in the lungs is alternately compressed and expanded by the

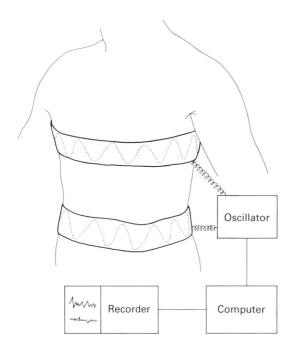

Fig. 15.11. Respiratory inductance plethysmograph showing detector bands placed around chest and abdomen.

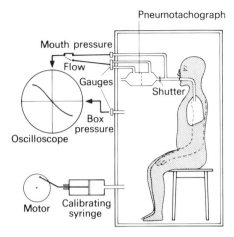

Fig. 15.12. A constant-volume box plethysmograph. To measure thoracic gas volume the patient pants against the closed shutter whilst changes in mouth pressure (= alveolar pressure) and box pressure (= change in gas volume) are recorded on the oscilloscope. The box pressure signal is then calibrated against the known volume injected by the calibrating syringe. Thus the relationship between the changes in alveolar pressure and thoracic gas volume can be established. To measure airway resistance the patient pants through the pneumotachograph whilst flow and box pressure are recorded, and then pants against the closed shutter to establish the relationship between changes in alveolar pressure and box pressure. From these two relationships it is possible to relate flow rate to the pressure drop across the airways and so to derive airway resistance.

action of the chest muscles. Since there is no flow of gas through the airways, changes in mouth pressure accurately reflect the changes in the pressure of the intra-thoracic gas in response to the changes in chest wall volume. The change in volume of this gas is measured by the body plethysmograph.

By applying Boyle's law ($PV = k$) the following equation can be derived:

$$PV = (P + \Delta P)(V - \Delta V).$$

Since P is barometric pressure minus water vapour pressure, and ΔP and ΔV are measured, V can be calculated. Thoracic gas volume measured by this technique equals that measured by inert gas dilution techniques in patients with normal lungs, but in patients with airways obstruction the dilution methods yield lower values because of the volume

of trapped gas which does not equilibrate with the inert gas (DuBois *et al.* 1956a).

The body plethysmograph can also be used to measure airway resistance by causing the patient to pant through a pneumotachograph which is situated within the box. During panting the alveolar pressure rises and falls during expiration and inspiration because of the resistance to airflow within the airways. There is a simple inverse relationship between the changes in alveolar pressure and the changes in volume recorded by the plethysmograph which can be determined by panting against the closed shutter. When this has been determined the resistance of the airways (R_A) can be calculated from the equation:

$$R_A = \frac{\Delta P}{\Delta V} \times \frac{\Delta V}{v}$$

where v is the instantaneous flowrate recorded by the pneumotachograph. The advantage of this technique is that it yields a measure of airway resistance which is unaffected by tissue resistance. It also obviates the need to swallow an oesophageal balloon for measurement of oesophageal pressure (DuBois *et al.* 1956b).

In practice the change in box volume is displayed on the x-axis of an oscilloscope screen and mouth pressure or flow on the y-axis (Fig. 15.12) so that the inter-relationships can be derived directly from the slope of the resulting trace.

Washout and dilution methods

These techniques are most frequently used for measurements of functional residual capacity (FRC) but can also be used to measure other gas volumes which cannot be derived by water displacement. The principle can be illustrated by the nitrogen washout method of determining FRC. The patient breathes air through a non-rebreathing valve. At the end of a normal expiration two additional valves are turned so that the inspired gas is abruptly changed to pure oxygen, whilst the expired gas is directed into an empty Douglas bag. The patient continues to expire into the bag until the nitrogen has been washed out of the lungs (about 7 min in those with normal lungs) and the volume of the expired gas and its nitrogen concentration are measured. Since the gas in the lungs initially contained approximately 80% nitrogen the FRC must have been 100/80 times the volume of nitrogen collected in the bag. In practice corrections must be applied for the volume of nitrogen eliminated into the lungs from the tissues during the washout period, and for the small quantity remaining in the alveoli at the end of the washout.

The other common technique to determine FRC is the closed-circuit method. A measured volume of an insoluble gas, such as helium, is added to a spirometer containing oxygen. The gases are mixed by recirculating around the closed circuit of the spirometer and the volume of the spirometer circuit derived from the volume of helium added and its final concentration. The spirometer is then connected to the patient at the end of expiration and rebreathing continued until the gases in the lung and spirometer are thoroughly mixed. If He_1 and V_1 represent the initial concentration of He and the volume of gas in the spirometer and He_2 is the final concentration of helium after dilution by the volume of gas in the lung (FRC) then

$$He_1 \times V_1 = He_2 \times (V_1 + FRC).$$

Thus FRC can be calculated.

Measurement of steady gas flow rate

Two basic principles are employed. In the first, flow rate is calculated from the volume of gas collected in unit time. This principle is of limited application but is widely used to standardize other methods. The second, which is the basis of most clinical methods of measuring flow, depends on the relationship between the pressure drop and flow rate across a resistance. In one application the pressure drop is maintained constant and flow is assessed by measuring the size of the orifice required to transmit the flow (variable orifice flowmeter). In the second method the size of the orifice is kept constant and the flow rate is determined by measuring the pressure drop across the orifice (fixed orifice flowmeter).

VOLUME/TIME METHODS

The volume of gas is determined by collecting it in a container of known size or by some other measuring device. The simplest clinical application of this method is the measurement of rotameter or oxygen bypass flow on an anaesthetic machine by measuring the time taken to fill the 2 L reservoir bag. If this takes 5 s the flow rate is 2/5 = $0.4 \, L \cdot s^{-1}$ or $24 \, L \cdot min^{-1}$. A similar principle is used in soap film flowmeters where the gas flow rate is derived from the time taken for a soap film bubble to ascend through a vertical glass tube of known dimensions. Most accurate flowmeters are calibrated by spirometers, appropriate corrections being made for any changes in pressure and temperature between the flowmeter and spirometer.

PRESSURE DROP/ORIFICE METHODS

Variable orifice (constant pressure drop) flowmeters

In these devices the orifice through which gas flows enlarges with flow rate so that the pressure difference across the orifice remains constant.

Rotameter. This type of flowmeter has now displaced most of the other types of flowmeter previously used in anaesthesia. Although it was patented in Aachen in 1908 and first used in anaesthesia in 1910 it was not fitted to the Boyle's machine until 1937.

A rotameter consists of a vertical glass tube inside which rotates a light metal alloy bobbin. The flow of gas is controlled by the fine-adjustment flow control valve at the bottom of the rotameter and when this is opened the pressure of the gas forces the bobbin up the tube. The inside of the tube is shaped like an inverted cone, so that the cross-sectional area of the annular space around the bobbin is greater at the top end of the tube than it is at the bottom. Since the weight of the bobbin is constant, the bobbin will rise until the pressure drop across the cross-sectional area of the annular space exactly opposes the downward pressure resulting from the weight of the bobbin. The pressure drop therefore remains constant throughout the range of flows for which the tube is designed and the bobbin floats freely in the stream of gas. Friction between the bobbin and tube wall is avoided by adding vanes to the bobbin so that it rotates in the stream of gas, and additional stability at low flow rates is achieved by modifying the shape of the bobbin (Fig. 15.13).

Each rotameter has to be calibrated for a specific gas. The reason for this becomes apparent when the physical principles are considered (Fig. 15.14). At the bottom of the rotameter the length of the bobbin is much greater than the distance between the bobbin and glass. The channel therefore approximates to a tube and, providing flow is laminar, Poiseuille's formula is applicable. In this situation viscosity is an important determinant of pressure drop:

$$\text{pressure difference} \propto \frac{\text{viscosity} \times \text{length} \times \text{flow rate}}{(\text{radius})^4}.$$

As the bobbin rises, the distance between bobbin and tube increases, so that the space around the bobbin approximates more to an orifice than to a tube. Under these circumstances the density becomes an important factor. Since the transition from a tubular space to an orifice is not clearly defined and since a certain amount of turbulence must occur even at low flow rates, it is apparent that each rotameter must be calibrated specifically for one gas. Furthermore, since viscosity and density vary with temperature and pressure, the calibration must be carried out under the appropriate conditions.

The flow rate is indicated by the position of the top of the bobbin. Under ideal conditions the indicated flow rate should be within ±2% of the true flow rate. However, as indicated later (p. 199)

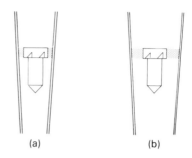

Fig. 15.14. Physical principles underlying measurement of flow by rotameter. (a) At the bottom of the tube the length of the annular space is greater than the distance between tube and bobbin. (b) At the top of the tube the annular space approximates to an orifice.

this accuracy is rarely retained under clinical conditions (Waaben *et al.* 1978).

Further complexities in calibration have resulted from the introduction of rotameters in which portions of the scale are expanded so that increased accuracy of reading is available over specific ranges of flow. This feature is made possible by varying the taper of the cone in different parts of the tube. However, if the scale is read carelessly or the marking is not clear, serious errors can result from incorrect gas flow settings. It is essential therefore to observe where the deviations from linearity occur, before using the flowmeter (Fig. 15.15).

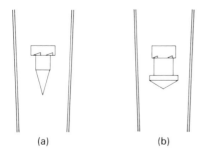

Fig. 15.13. Rotameter tubes. (a) Original shape of bobbin. (b) Bobbin modified to increase stability at low flow rates.

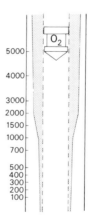

Fig. 15.15. Non-linear scale on rotameter. The shaded area illustrates how the annular space between bobbin and tube increases as the bobbin moves up the tube.

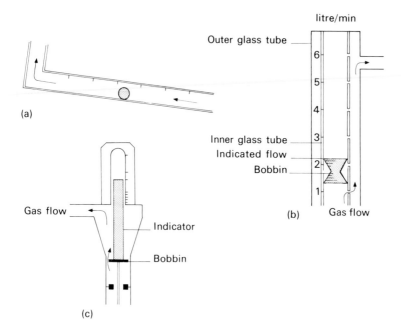

(a)

(b)   Gas flow

(c)

Fig. 15.16. Other forms of variable orifice constant pressure drop flowmeters used in the past. (a) Ewing (two balls were used for stability in the inclined tube flowmeter on the Connell 'stratosphere' anaesthetic machine). (b) Coxeter. (c) Heidbrink.

Other variable orifice flowmeters. A number of other types of variable orifice flowmeters have been used in the past but are now only of historical interest. The main types are illustrated in Fig. 15.16.

Variable pressure drop (fixed orifice) flowmeters

In these flowmeters the resistance is maintained constant so that changes of flow are accompanied by changes in pressure drop across the resistance element.

Water-depression flowmeter. This type of flowmeter was widely used in the USA on Foregger anaesthetic machines. There were two basic designs (Fig. 15.17). In one the gas was caused to flow through an orifice and the pressure drop across the orifice was measured with a water manometer. Since the pressure drop across an orifice is proportional to the square of the flow rate, the scale was non-linear, being crowded at the lower readings and expanded at the higher readings. This was obviously undesirable for anaesthesia and so parallel-sided tubes were substituted for the orifice. This ensured that flow was laminar, and consequently the pressure

drop was proportional to flow rate: a linear scale could therefore be obtained. It was, however, necessary to provide a number of flowmeters in parallel to obtain accuracy over a wide range of flow rates and there was always the danger of blowing water into the patient circuit when the cylinders were suddenly opened.

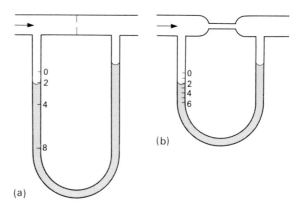

(a)   (b)

Fig. 15.17. (a) Orifice-type water depression flowmeter with non-linear scale. (b) Laminar flow type with linear scale.

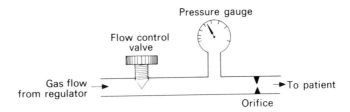

Fig. 15.18. Bourdon gauge flowmeter.

Bourdon gauge flowmeter. In this instrument a Bourdon gauge is used to sense the pressure drop across an orifice so that the scale is nonlinear (Fig. 15.18). The meter is rugged, not affected by changes in position, and useful for metering the flow from gas cylinders when transporting patients from one place to another. It is however, affected by back pressure, and complete occlusion of the outlet will cause the meter to record maximum flow. In some types of meter an aneroid system is used instead of the Bourdon gauge to detect the pressure difference.

Variable orifice and variable pressure drop flowmeters

Water-sight flowmeter. This type of flowmeter was used in the earlier models of the Boyle's machine (Fig. 15.19). Both the pressure drop and the cross-sectional area of the orifices increased as flow increased. The gas was passed through a tube which was immersed in water and escaped through one or more holes bored in the side of the tube. The pressure drop across the hole was balanced by

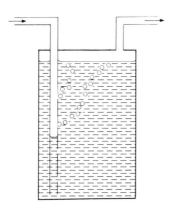

Fig. 15.19. Water-sight flowmeter.

the hydrostatic pressure of the external water column. If flow rate was increased the pressure drop across the hole was increased and the water in the flowmeter was forced down until the gas could escape through a lower hole. Observation of the lowest hole through which the gas was bubbling yielded a measure of flow rate. The height of water in the reservoir had to be kept constant and high flows of gas could not be used since the resultant excessive bubbling prevented proper observation of the tubes.

SOURCES OF ERROR WHEN USING BOBBIN FLOWMETERS

Errors most commonly occur as the result of sticking of the rotameter bobbin. This may be caused by the tube not being vertical, by the presence of dirt in the tube or by the attraction between bobbin and tube produced by electrostatic charges. Errors from the latter source are particularly common when the bobbin is being regularly depressed by the use of intermittent positive pressure ventilation and at low flow rates may result in an inaccuracy of up to 35% of the reading (Hagelsten & Larsen, 1965; Greenbaum & Hesse, 1978).

Sticking of the bobbin was at one time very common in cyclopropane flowmeters. The trouble developed when manufacturers started to fit flowmeter control valves which isolated cyclopropane under pressure in the tube connecting the cylinder to the flowmeter control valve. When the ambient temperature fell at night the gas liquified and dissolved small quantities of grease and debris from the connecting tube. These impurities were carried into the flowmeter when flow was next restored (Russell, 1961). This problem was overcome by changing the type of grease used in the flowmeter control valve and by connecting the cylinder to the rotameter with metal instead of rubber tubing.

Errors in delivered gas concentration may be caused by factors other than flowmeter inaccuracy. The most common causes are a leak from a cracked rotameter tube, a deficient sealing washer between the tube and the rotameter block or a leak from the tube connecting the top of the flowmeters (Thompson, 1976). To reduce the risk of hypoxia caused by a leak between the oxygen and nitrous oxide flowmeters Eger *et al.* (1963) suggested that the oxygen flowmeter should be situated nearest the outlet from the flowmeter bank. In the UK the oxygen flowmeter has traditionally been sited on the left (input) side of the flowmeter bank so it has been decided to retain this position to prevent confusion. However, in recent years manufacturers have moved the outlet pipe from the right (nitrous oxide) side to the left (oxygen side) so that the oxygen now enters downstream from the nitrous oxide. Finally, it is important to remember that the position of the bobbin may not be noticed if it is driven to the top of the rotameter tube by a high gas flow. This complication can only be prevented by checking that all flowmeter control valves are at the off position before the flowmeters are put into service.

EFFECT OF PRESSURE ON FLOWMETERS

The pressure within a flowmeter may be altered by a variation in ambient pressure or by a change in the resistance to outflow. The effects of changes in ambient pressure are seen at altitude or when the flowmeter is used in a hyperbaric chamber. Alterations in outflow resistance are more commonly encountered and may be caused by the attachment of anaesthetic vaporizers, nebulizers or gas-driven ventilators (e.g. the Manley).

Under hyperbaric conditions the density of the gas is increased so that at a given flow rate a larger orifice will be necessary to maintain the same pressure difference. In other words a rotameter will read high in a pressure chamber. McDowall (1964) found that the actual flow (F_A) is given by the equation:

$$F_A = F_1 \times \sqrt{\frac{\rho_0}{\rho_1}}$$

where F_1 is the indicated flow under hyperbaric conditions whilst ρ_0 and ρ_1 are the densities of the gas at atmospheric and hyperbaric pressures, respectively. Thus, if pressure is increased to 2 ATA density is doubled and

$$\sqrt{\frac{\rho_0}{\rho_1}} = \sqrt{\frac{1}{2}}$$

so that F_A is 71% of F_1. It should be noted that F_A is the volume flow rate which is actually occurring under the hyperbaric conditions existing in the chamber. Similar reasoning indicates that with a constant orifice meter (e.g. Bourdon gauge meter) the pressure difference for a given flow rate will be greater under hyperbaric conditions so that this too will read high.

When back pressure is exerted on a rotameter by attaching a nebulizer or ventilator to the outlet the circumstances are different, for the gas issuing from the nebulizer or expired by the patient on a ventilator is at atmospheric pressure. It is necessary therefore to consider both the effect of the back pressure on the rotameter reading and the change in gas volume resulting from the transition to atmospheric pressure. As has already been shown, increasing the pressure in the rotameter increases the density so that the actual flow is less than the indicated flow. However, the density of a gas is proportional to its absolute pressure so that if P_F represents the pressure in the flowmeter and P_B represents atmospheric pressure

$$F_A = F_1 \sqrt{\frac{P_B}{P_F}}.$$

However, F_A represents the actual flow measured under the pressurized conditions in the flowmeter. When the pressure of this gas becomes atmospheric its volume will increase in the ratio P_F/P_B so that the flow, if measured at atmospheric pressure (P_B), will be:

$$F_H = F_1 \sqrt{\frac{P_B}{P_F}} \times \frac{P_F}{P_B} = F_1 \sqrt{\frac{P_F}{P_B}}.$$

Thus, the flow at atmospheric pressure will be larger than the flow indicated on the flowmeters. If the back pressure is of the order of 13 kPa (100 mmHg or 860 mmHg absolute), the actual flow is about 7% greater than indicated flow (Conway, 1974).

There is a further error in the flow measurement arising from the effect of increased outlet pressure on flow through the flow control valve. This also depends on the pressure drop across it, normally about 4 bar (400 kPa). If the outlet pressure rises by 13 kPa, there is a 3.25% fall in the pressure drop across the orifice of the fine-adjustment needle valve and a corresponding real drop in the flow. Thus, a 7 L flow of N_2O will fall by about 0.25 L.

The problems introduced by back pressure on rotameters can be easily overcome by placing the fine-adjustment flow control valve on the outlet side of the rotameter instead of the inlet side. The gas in the tube is thus constantly pressurized to regulator-outlet pressure, and back pressure effects are reduced to the effect on the flow through the flow control valve. Special precautions have to be taken to prevent leaks from the rotameter, and the flowmeter must be calibrated under the correct pressure conditions, but such pressure-compensated flowmeters are now being widely used.

Measurement of unsteady gas flow rates

The instruments so far described possess marked inertia so that they respond relatively sluggishly to rapid changes in flow rate. Furthermore, they are essentially direct reading instruments which cannot be connected easily to a recording system. More sophisticated instruments are therefore required to record flow rates which vary rapidly with time.

PRESSURE DROP/ORIFICE METHODS

Variable pressure drop (fixed orifice) flowmeters

Pneumotachograph. This instrument measures flow rate by sensing the pressure drop across a laminar resistance. The pressure difference across the resistance is kept small (usually less than 0.1 kPa or 10 mmH$_2$O), so that the flow of gas is minimally affected by the resistance, and the pressure tappings are carefully designed to ensure that the differential manometer senses the true lateral pressure exerted by the gas on each side of the resistance element.

Two types of pneumotachograph head are in common use (Finucane *et al.* 1972). In the Fleisch head (Fig. 15.20a) the resistance consists of a bundle of parallel-sided tubes each tube having a diameter of 1–2 mm. Since reducing the diameter of a tube increases both the pressure drop and the critical velocity, this arrangement yields the biggest possible pressure drop whilst conserving laminar flow. The number of tubes is matched to the desired range of flow rates. The resistance unit is made by rolling strips of corrugated and plain foil into a cylinder and then enclosing the unit within an electric coil. The coil is heated to prevent

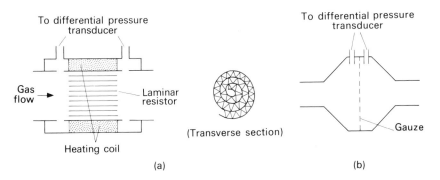

Fig. 15.20. Pneumotachograph. (a) Longitudinal section and transverse sections of Fleisch head showing corrugated foil wound into a spiral to form a series of parallel laminar resistors. (b) Longitudinal section of Lilly-type head.

condensation when the instrument is being used with moist gases. The pressure tappings consist of a series of holes in the casing at each end of the resistance unit. These lead into two annular chambers ('piezometer rings') which are connected to the differential manometer by flexible tubes.

In the Lilly type of head (Fig. 15.20) the resistance unit consists of a layer of metal or plastic gauze, the pressure tappings being taken from each side of the gauze. When metal gauze is used it may be heated to prevent condensation. A plastic mesh causes less condensation and does not require heating if used for a short period. Recently, it has been suggested that the problem of condensation can be overcome by using a resistance unit which consists of a diaphragm with a V-shaped incision in it (Osborne, 1978). The resulting flap opens progressively as flow is increased and so maintains a linear relationship between pressure and flow (Fig. 15.21). This type of head is now used in several mechanical ventilators. When using pneumotachographs it is important to ensure that the gas flow is spread evenly across the resistance unit. It is also essential to adjust the size of head to the expected flow rates, for turbulence causes non-linearity if the specified flow is exceeded. On the other hand the use of too large a head results in a very small pressure signal and an unnecessarily large dead space. A Fleisch No. 2 head, for example, has a dead space of 16 ml, is linear to within ±5% from 0-60 L·min^{-1}, and gives a pressure of about 0.1 kPa (10 mmH$_2$O) at the maximum rated flow rate. The size of the pressure drop depends not only on the characteristics of the resistance but also on the viscosity of the gas. This in turn, is temperature and, to a small extent, pressure dependent (Grenvik et al. 1966; Hobbs, 1967). Thus, whilst it is relatively easy to achieve an output signal which does not deviate by more than ±5% of the actual flow when a single gas is being measured at atmospheric temperature and pressure, it is much more difficult to compensate for the differences in pressure, temperature, humidity and composition between the inspired and expired gas during mechanical ventilation (Yeh et al. 1984). (Humidity is a particular problem since water vapour has a markedly lower viscosity than dry air.)

The differential manometer needs to be very sensitive to record the small changes in pressure across the resistance. Furthermore, since this signal may be integrated to give volume, the manometer must have very good zero and gain stability. It is important to ensure that the geometry of the gas path from each side of the transducer diaphragm to the head is similar so that abrupt changes of pressure within the head (e.g. from intermittent positive pressure ventilation) do not produce transient pressure artefacts from the transducer (Kafer, 1973; Churches et al. 1977). Pneumotachographs have been widely used in both respiratory and anaesthetic research. Although their principles are easy to understand their practical application is very much more difficult.

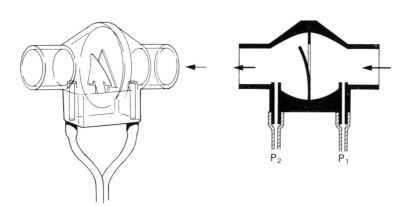

P_2 P_1

Fig. 15.21. The 'Accutach' pneumotachograph. The V-shaped flap is designed to open in a manner which ensures that the pressure drop is proportional to flow rate.

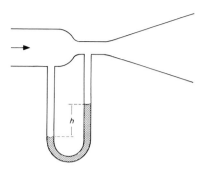

Fig. 15.22. Venturi tube flowmeter. The difference in pressure h is related to the flow rate. This would be measured by a differential transducer when dynamic measurements are required.

Two other types of variable-pressure flowmeter must be mentioned, although they have not been widely used clinically.

Venturi tube flowmeter. When gas passes through a narrowed portion of tube it accelerates. Some potential energy is thus converted to kinetic energy and the pressure recorded from a side arm in the constricted part of the tube is less than the pressure in the wider part of the tube (Fig. 15.22). Because the pressure difference is roughly proportional to the square of the flow rate, the scale is non-linear, sensitivity being least at low flow rates. Furthermore, the instrument is very sensitive to changes in the density of the gas.

Pitot tube flowmeter. This again utilizes the difference between the amount of potential and kinetic energy possessed by the gas. The potential energy is proportional to its pressure, and the kinetic energy is proportional to its velocity. In the pitot tube flowmeter (Fig. 15.23) the kinetic energy is sensed by the difference in pressure between a tube facing

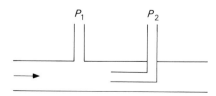

Fig. 15.23. Pitot tube flowmeter.

into the stream of gas and a tube measuring the lateral pressure exerted by the gas. This pressure difference is proportional to the square of flow rate, so that the scale is again nonlinear. Furthermore the range of flow which can be accommodated by any particular instrument is somewhat limited. These disadvantages have discouraged its use in clinical practice.

Variable orifice (constant pressure drop) flowmeters

The peak flowmeter. The peak expiratory flow rate which can be achieved by normal adults often exceeds $500\ L \cdot min^{-1}$. Peak flow can be measured by a pneumotachograph or dry spirometer but a more useful clinical instrument is the peak flowmeter (Wright & McKerrow, 1959). This is basically a variable orifice meter and is capable of measuring flows up to $1000\ L \cdot min^{-1}$ with the imposition of only a small resistance to gas flow.

The meter consists of a metal cylinder about 12 cm in diameter and 6 cm deep. The cylinder contains three compartments (Fig. 15.24). The first is shallow and contains the dial and pointer. The middle compartment contains the measuring apparatus and communicates with the third compartment via an annular orifice around the circumference of a metal partition. A mouthpiece is attached to the wall of the middle chamber and a fixed partition deflects the expired air onto a movable vane. The vane fits the inside of the cylinder closely and is free to rotate around a central axle. The air flow causes the vane to rotate against the force exerted by a light spiral spring. The movement of the vane opens up a section of the annular orifice which thus permits the air to escape through holes in the outer casing of the third compartment to the atmosphere. As the force exerted by the spiral spring is essentially constant throughout the range of movement of the vane, the position adopted by the vane depends primarily on the flow rate and on the area of the annular orifice which must be exposed to the air flow to maintain a constant pressure difference. The vane is very light and rapidly attains a maximum position in res-

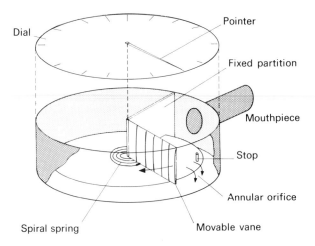

Dial

Pointer

Fixed partition

Mouthpiece

Stop

Annular orifice

Spiral spring

Movable vane

Fig. 15.24. Peak expiratory flowmeter.

ponse to the peak expiratory flow. It is then retained in this position by a ratchet which can be released after the reading has been taken. The reading is obtained from a pointer which is attached at an angle of 180° to the vane, and so balances it. The meter tends to under-read when compared with the peak expiratory flow rate recorded by a pneumotachograph, but there is a consistent relationship between the two measurements.

The patient must be encouraged to expire as rapidly as possible but the total volume expired is much less than that of an FVC manoeuvre, since peak flow rate is being measured. It is essential that the meter should be held with the axis of the mouth-piece horizontal and with the dial pointing to the right of the patient. This minimizes the effect of gravity on the position of the vane. The peak flowmeter is now tending to be replaced by various types of peak flow gauge which are cheaper and yet yield similar results (Campbell *et al.* 1974; Wright, 1978). These work on a similar principle, a light

piston being displaced down a cylinder to open up a linear orifice running down the length of the cylinder (Fig. 15.25). The piston is again opposed by a very light spring and is either held in the position of maximal displacement by a ratchet or displaces a sliding pointer which indicates the peak flow rate. The instrument must also be held horizontal when making the measurement and the breath expelled as rapidly as possible. With all these instruments the measurement is repeated 3–5 times and the maximum reading recorded. This is compared with normal values derived from a nomogram (e.g. Cotes, 1975).

Other devices for measuring gas glow

Hot wire flowmeter. There are a number of devices which measure flow rate by sensing the change in temperature of a heated wire. The rate of cooling depends on the gas flow rate and the thermal conductivity of the gas and is therefore affected by gas composition and the presence of water vapour. Some commercial flowmeters incorporate devices which minimize these effects so that the accuracy is acceptable for clinical use (Chakrabarti & Loh, 1984).

Ultrasonic flowmeter. The most successful commercial instrument is based on the vortex-shedding technique (Fig. 15.26). The gas is passed through a

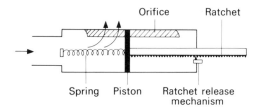

Orifice   Ratchet

Spring   Piston   Ratchet release
mechanism

Fig. 15.25. Peak flow gauge.

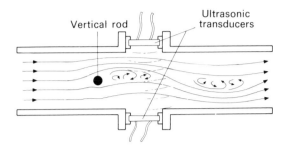

Fig. 15.26. Ultrasonic flowmeter.

tube containing a rod 1–2 mm in diameter, mounted at right angles to the direction of gas flow. Vortices form downstream from the rod, the number of vortices formed being directly related to the flow rate. The vortices are detected by an ultrasonic beam and integrated to give a volume signal. It appears that the device is not greatly affected by temperature, humidity or changes in gas composition but vortices are not formed if flow is below a critical level (about $5 \, L \cdot min^{-1}$ in one commercial instrument). The flowmeter is thus most accurate when tidal volumes are large.

Recently, an ultrasonic 'time of flight' flow transducer has been marketed. The transmitting and receiving crystals are mounted at an angle of 40° to the gas stream and the difference in transit times between the forward and reverse ultrasound beams is measured (see p. 214). The flowmeter is very accurate and has a high frequency response but is affected by gas temperature and composition (Buess *et al.* 1986).

References

Adams, A.P., Vickers, M.D.A., Munroe, J.P. & Parker, C.W. (1967) Dry displacement gas meters. *British Journal of Anaesthesia* **39**, 174–183.

Bernstein, L., D'Silva, J.L. & Mendel, D. (1952) The effect of the rate of breathing on the maximum breathing capacity determined with a new spirometer. *Thorax* **7**, 255–262.

Buess, C., Pietsch, P., Guggenbuhl, W. & Koller E.A. (1986) A pulsed diagonal-beam ultrasonic airflow meter. *Journal of Applied Physiology* **61**, 1195–1196.

Bushman, J.A. (1979) Effect of different flow patterns on the Wright respirometer. *British Journal of Anaesthesia* **51**, 895–898.

Byles, P. (1960) Observations on some continuously acting spirometers. *British Journal of Anaesthesia* **32**, 470–475.

Campbell, I.A., Prescott, R.J., Smith, I., Anderson, C., Johnson, A. & Campbell, J. (1974) Peak-flow meter versus peak-flow gauge. *Lancet* **ii**, 199.

Catley, D.M., Thornton, C., Jordan, C., Lehane, J.R., Royston, D. & Jones, J.G. (1985) Pronounced episodic oxygen desaturation in the postoperative period: its association with ventilatory patterns and analgesic regime. *Anesthesiology* **63**, 20–28.

Chakrabarti, M.K. & Loh L. (1984) Evaluation of Spirolog I volume meter. *Anaesthesia* **39**, 268–271.

Churches, A.E., Loughman, J., Fisk, G.C., Abrahams, N. & Vonwiller, J.B. (1977) Measurement errors in pneumotachography due to pressure transducer design. *Anaesthesia and Intensive Care* **5**, 19–29.

Collins, M.M., McDermott, M. & McDermott, J.T. (1964) Bellows spirometer and transistor timer for the measurement of forced expiratory volume and vital capacity. *Journal of Physiology* **172**, 39P.

Conway, C.M. (1974). Anaesthesia and measurement. *Proceedings of the Royal Society of Medicine* **67**, 1087–91.

Conway, C.M., Leigh, J.M., Preston, T.D., Walter, E.J.M. & Webb, D.A. (1974). An assessment of three electronic respirometers. *British Journal of Anaesthesia* **46**, 885–891.

Cotes, J.E. (1975) *Lung function: assessment and application in medicine*, 3rd edn. Blackwell Scientific Publications, Oxford.

Cox, L.A., Almeida, A.P., Robinson, J.S. & Horsley, J.K. (1974) An electronic respirometer. *British Journal of Anaesthesia* **46**, 302–310.

Drew, C.D.M. & Hughes, D.T.D. (1969) Characteristics of the Vitalograph spirometer. *Thorax* **24**, 703–706.

DuBois, A.B., Botelho, S.Y., Bedell, G.N., Marshall, R. & Comroe, J.H. (1956a) A rapid plethysmographic method of measuring thoracic gas volume. A comparison with a nitrogen washout method for measuring FRC in normal subjects. *Journal of Clinical Investigation* **35**, 323–326.

DuBois, A.B., Botelho, S.Y. & Comroe, J.H. (1956b) A new method of measuring airway resistance in man using a body plethysmograph. Values in normal subjects and in patients with respiratory disease. *Journal of Clinical Investigation* **35**, 327–335.

Eger, E.I., Hylton, R.R., Irwin, R.H. & Guadagni, N. (1963) Anesthetic flowmeter sequence — a cause for hypoxia. *Anesthesiology* **24**, 396–397.

Finucane, K.E., Egan, B.A. & Dawson, S.V. (1972) Linearity and frequency response of pneumotachographs. *Journal of Applied Physiology* **32**, 121–126.

Gilbert, R., Auchinloss, J.H. Brodsky, J. & Boden, W. (1972) Changes in tidal volume, frequency, and ventilation induced by their measurement. *Journal of Applied Physiology* **33**, 252–254.

Greenbaum, R. & Hesse, G.E. (1978) Electrical conductivity of flowmeter tubes. *British Journal of Anaesthesia* **50**, 408.

Grenvik, Å., Hedstrand, U. & Sjogren, H. (1966) Problems in pneumotachography. *Acta anaesthesiologica Scandinavica* **10**, 147–155.

Hagelsten, J.O. & Larsen, O.S. (1965) Inaccuracy of anaesthetic flowmeters caused by static electricity. *British Journal of Anaesthesia* **37**, 637–641.

Hatch, D.J. & Williams, G.M.E. (1988) The haloscale Infanta Wright respirometer. An *in vitro* and *in vivo* assessment. *British Journal of Anaesthesia* **60**, 232–238.

Hobbs, A.F.T. (1967) A comparison of methods of calibrating the pneumotachograph. *British Journal of Anaesthesia* **39**, 899–907.

Kafer, E.R. (1973) Errors in pneumotachography as a result of transducer design and function. *Anesthesiology* **38**, 275–279.

McDowall, D.G. (1964) Anaesthesia in a pressure chamber. *Anaesthesia* **19**, 321–326.

Morel, D., Forster, A. & Suter, P.M. (1983) Noninvasive ventilatory monitoring with bellows pneumographs in supine subjects. *Journal of Applied Physiology* **55**, 598–605.

Nunn, J.F. & Ezi-Ashi, T.I. (1962) The accuracy of the respirometer and ventigrator. *British Journal of Anaesthesia* **34**, 422–432.

Osborn, J.J. (1978) A flowmeter for respiratory monitoring. *Critical Care Medicine* **6**, 349–351.

Russell, F.R. (1961) Deposits in the cyclopropane flowmeter. *British Journal of Anaesthesia* **33**, 323.

Sackner, J.D., Nixon, A.J., Davis, B., Atkins, N. & Sackner, M.A. (1980) Non-invasive measurement of ventilation during exercise using a respiratory inductance plethysmograph. *American Review of Respiratory Disease* **122**, 867–871.

Sackner, M.A., Watson, H., Belsito, A.S., Feinerman, D., Suarez, M., Gonzalez, G., Bizousky, F. & Krieger, B. (1989) Calibration of respiratory inductive plethysmograph during natural breathing. *Journal of Applied Physiology* **66**, 410–420.

Thompson, P.W. (1976) Safety of anaesthetic apparatus. In Hewer C.L. & Atkinson R.S. (eds), *Recent advances in anaesthesia and analgesia*, vol. 12, Chapter 9. Churchill Livingstone, London.

Waaben, J., Stokke, D.B. & Brinklov, M.M. (1978) Accuracy of gas flowmeters determined by the bubble meter method. *British Journal of Anaesthesia* **50**, 1251–1256.

Wright, B.M. & McKerrow, C.B. (1959) Maximum forced expiratory flow rate as a measure of ventilatory capacity. *British Medical Journal* **ii**, 1041–1047.

Wright, B.M. (1978) A miniature Wright peak-flow meter. *British Medical Journal* **ii**, 1627–1628.

Yeh, M.P., Adams, T.D., Gardner R.M. & Janowitz, F.G. (1984) Effect of O_2, N_2 and CO_2 composition on nonlinearity of Fleisch pneumotachograph characteristics. *Journal of Applied Physiology* **56**, 1423–1425.

16: Measurement of Blood Flow

The principles of flow measurement described in the last chapter can also be applied to the measurement of blood flow. However, the much greater density and viscosity of blood necessitate a number of modifications to the apparatus. Furthermore, blood has some properties, such as electrical conductivity, which permit other measurement techniques to be used. In all these applications it is particularly important to differentiate between the measurement of flow rate and flow velocity (p. 186). Since blood flow in many vessels is not only pulsatile but also varies with respiration, the techniques described will be divided into those which average the flow over a given time and those which provide instantaneous measurements of oscillatory flow. The latter can usually be integrated to give a measure of average flow per unit time. For a useful review, see Mathie (1982).

Direct measurement of steady flow in blood vessels

VOLUME/TIME METHODS

A number of relatively simple instruments have been used in physiological research to measure mean flow. The simplest method is to divert the flow into a graduated vessel for a known time. To prevent physiological alterations due to loss of blood from the circulation the Ludwig stromuhr can be utilized (Fig. 16.1).

ROTAMETERS

Rotameters have found a wide application both in industry and medicine. The basic principle is similar to the gas rotameter but the movement of the bobbin is sensed by recording the change in inductance in a coil when a soft-iron core attached to the rotameter rises within the coil (Fig. 16.2). By

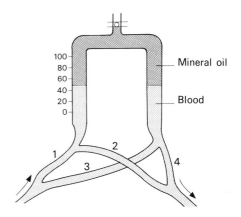

Fig. 16.1. Ludwig stromuhr. Blood normally flows in the direction shown by arrows. When tubes 2 and 3 are clamped blood flows into one chamber and out of the other. By using a stop watch it is possible to calculate the flow rate. On the next occasion tubes 1 and 4 are clamped to reverse the flow.

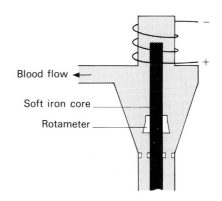

Fig. 16.2. Liquid rotameter. An increase in flow causes the rotameter to move upwards. This is sensed by the change of inductance in the coil produced by the movement of the soft iron core attached to the rotameter.

207

careful design the effect of viscosity changes in the blood can be minimized so that calibration does not change appreciably with changing haematocrit.

Another instrument utilizing a rotating vane is the Potter electroturbinometer. In this instrument the vane is built around a permanent magnet which is free to rotate in a tube inserted between the cut ends of a blood vessel. The speed of rotation of the rotor is sensed by a pick-up coil situated in the wall of the instrument. This instrument is remarkably stable and is capable of an accuracy of ± 5%. However, the resistance to flow is greater than with a good rotameter and it ceases to rotate at very low flows.

HEAT-DISSIPATION METHODS

The thermostromuhr is an example of an instrument which has been widely used. In one of the more recent modifications two thermistors are placed in close apposition to the blood vessel. The thermistors are separated by a heating coil and it is arranged that their electrical outputs oppose each other. When the heating coil is switched on the downstream thermistor will record a higher temperature than the upstream thermistor. The difference in temperature between the two thermistors is inversely related to blood flow. This instrument is reasonably accurate if flow is non-pulsatile, but may become very inaccurate when pulsatile flow is present.

Other heat-dissipation methods have been used. One of the simplest was a length of resistance wire passed down the length of the blood vessel. An electrical current was passed down the wire to heat it and the loss of heat, which was proportional to blood flow, was detected by measuring the change in resistance of the wire. A similar catheter tip flowmeter utilizing thermistors has been used more recently to measure pulsatile flow.

LIMB PLETHYSMOGRAPHY

A simple clinical technique for measuring limb blood flow is that known as plethysmography. The venous return is intermittently occluded by abruptly pressurizing a proximal cuff to a pressure

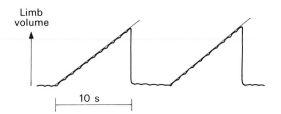

Fig. 16.3. Limb plethysmography. Recorded changes in limb volume following two occlusions of 10 s each. In this recording there was no initial occlusion artefact.

of about 6–7 kPa (50 mmHg). After allowance for an initial occlusion artefact, the rate of increase of volume of the limb during the first few seconds after occlusion is directly related to the arterial flow. A number of techniques are available for measuring the rate of change of limb volume. In air or water plethysmographs the limb is sealed into a box and surrounded with air or water at a constant temperature close to that of the skin, the increase in limb volume being transmitted directly to a small recording spirometer. Some air-filled plethysmographs have a fixed volume, and measure instead the small changes in pressure (Greenfield *et al.* 1963). Another simple form of plethysmograph is based on the demonstration by Whitney (1953) that the change in limb girth bears a direct relation to the change in limb volume. This change in girth is recorded with a mercury-in-rubber strain gauge which surrounds the limb. When the rubber tube containing the mercury is stretched it becomes longer and narrower. The electrical resistance of the column of mercury therefore increases. This change in resistance can be detected, amplified and recorded (Fig. 16.3).

The change in limb volume can also be recorded by measuring the change of electrical impedance of the limb (Geddes & Baker, 1975).

USE OF TRACERS TO MEASURE STEADY FLOW IN BLOOD VESSELS OR ORGANS

The first tracers to be used were drugs, whose concentrations could be measured spectrophotometrically, and hypertonic saline, which could be detected by a change in conductivity. Other tracers

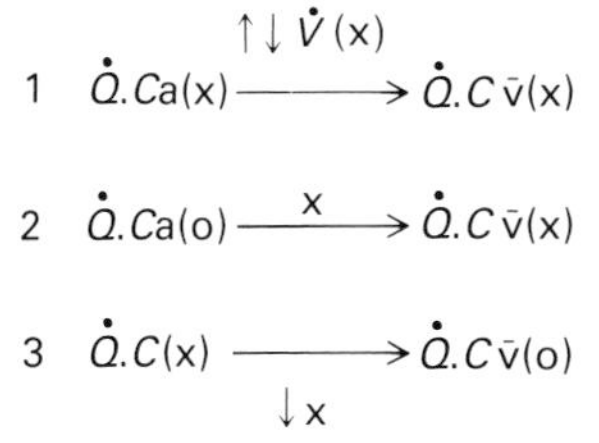

$1 \quad \dot{Q}.Ca(x) \xrightarrow{\uparrow\downarrow \dot{V}(x)} \dot{Q}.C\bar{v}(x)$

$2 \quad \dot{Q}.Ca(o) \xrightarrow{\quad x \quad} \dot{Q}.C\bar{v}(x)$

$3 \quad \dot{Q}.C(x) \xrightarrow{} \dot{Q}.C\bar{v}(o)$
$\qquad\qquad \downarrow x$

Fig. 16.4. There are three basic methods of using a tracer (x) to measure blood flow ($\dot{Q}$) where C is the concentration in arterial (a) or mixed venous (v̄) blood.

such as oxygen, CO_2 or radioisotopes are also used. All the tracer methods are based on the principle of conservation of matter, namely that the quantity of tracer entering or leaving a blood vessel must equal the flow multiplied by the difference in concentration between the input and output.

There are three basic methods of using tracers (Fig. 16.4). The first utilizes measurements of the uptake or clearance of a tracer within an organ, together with measurements of the arterio-venous difference in concentration. The second assumes that the arterial concentration is zero and derives flow from the exponential pattern of washout of tracer from a reservoir through which blood flows, whilst the third assumes complete clearance of tracer from the arterial blood so that the venous concentration is zero.

The first method is exemplified by the Fick principle used for measuring pulmonary blood flow ($\dot{Q}$). The indicator is a gas (usually oxygen or carbon dioxide, though any other soluble gas could be used). The gas is either taken up or eliminated from the blood during its passage through the lungs. If the oxygen consumption ($\dot{V}o_2$) is expressed in $ml \cdot min^{-1}$ standard temperature and pressure dry (STPD) and the arterial and mixed venous oxygen contents (Cao_2, $C\bar{v}o_2$) are in $ml \cdot L^{-1}$ STPD then:

$$\dot{V}o_2 = \dot{Q}(Cao_2 - C\bar{v}o_2)$$

or

$$\dot{Q}(L \cdot min^{-1}) = \frac{\dot{V}o_2\,(ml \cdot min^{-1}\,STPD)}{Cao_2 - C\bar{v}o_2(ml \cdot L^{-1}\,STPD)}$$

If CO_2 is used, the denominator is $C\bar{v}co_2 - Caco_2$ since the gas is excreted instead of being taken up.

The measured blood flow includes intrapulmonary right-to-left shunt but is inaccurate if large extrapulmonary right-to-left shunts are present. It is essential that the patient should be in a steady-state when the measurement is made; that the inspired oxygen concentration is maintained constant; and that the blood samples are withdrawn slowly whilst the oxygen consumption is being determined (Visscher & Johnson, 1953). The accuracy is limited by errors in $\dot{V}o_2$ measurement ($\pm 10\%$) and oxygen content measurement (± 0.2 vol.%). Attempts have been made to eliminate the need for catheterization of the pulmonary artery by measuring mixed venous Pco_2 by a rebreathing technique and calculating mixed venous CO_2 content but this results in unacceptable errors.

Another example of the application of this principle was the Kety & Schmidt (1945) technique for the measurement of cerebral blood flow. The subject inhaled 10% N_2O in air for 10 min. During this period blood samples were taken at intervals from an artery and the main venous drainage (the jugular bulb). The blood samples were analysed for N_2O and the results plotted on a graph (Fig. 16.5). The rise in venous concentration lagged behind the arterial concentration whilst N_2O was being taken

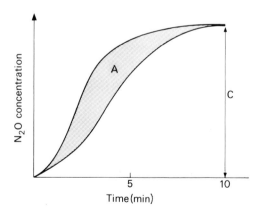

Fig. 16.5. Principle of Kety–Schmidt technique for measuring cerebral blood flow. The area (A) between the arterial and venous N_2O concentration time curves represents the quantity of N_2O taken up by the brain. At the end of 10 min inhalation the brain is fully saturated and the arterial and venous concentrations are almost equal (C).

up by the brain, but by the end of the period of breathing the venous and arterial concentrations were almost equal, indicating that the brain was fully saturated. If the mass of the brain is M, the final concentration of nitrous oxide in blood C and the brain:blood partition coefficient λ. then the quantity of N_2O in the brain is $MV\lambda$. This quantity is equal to the total blood flow during the period of inhalation, Q, multiplied by the integral of the arterio-venous concentration differences given by area A. Hence,

$$QA = MC\lambda$$

or

$$\frac{Q}{M} = \frac{C\lambda}{A}$$

In the second type of tracer application, the arterial concentration is maintained at zero throughout the period of measurement by using an indicator which is relatively insoluble in blood and so is eliminated by one passage through the lungs. If this indicator is deposited in the area of interest, blood flow can then be calculated from the exponential pattern of clearance of the indicator. Examples of clearance techniques are those used to measure cerebral or muscle blood flow.

In the early studies, a bolus of krypton-85 or xenon-133 dissolved in saline was injected into an internal carotid artery and the radioactivity over the appropriate side of the head detected with an array of scintillation counters or a gamma camera. The bolus was distributed rapidly throughout the brain tissue and then cleared by the continuing blood flow. Most of the isotope was cleared from the blood during the subsequent passage through the lungs and the remainder distributed widely throughout the body so that the arterial concentration after the bolus had been injected was effectively zero. Although the pattern of clearance would have been expected to be a mono-exponential, it was found that when human clearance curves were replotted on semi-logarithmic paper, there was an initial steep decline followed by a more gradual fall in radioactivity (Fig. 16.6). This indicates that the curve is probably representative of two tissue components, one having a relatively

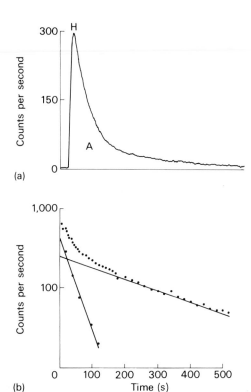

Fig. 16.6. (a) ^{133}Xe clearance curve from brain after bolus injection into carotid artery. Blood flow can be calculated from the peak height (H) and the area under the curve (A) or from the initial slope.
(b) Semi-logarithmic replot of a clearance curve showing fast and slow components.

fast washout and the other a much slower washout. These may correspond with the flows through white and grey matter. If the line drawn through the tail of the curve on the semi-log plot is now projected back to cut the y-axis it is possible to subtract the values of this slow component from the values of the original curve to define the rate constant of the fast component. This process is termed 'exponential stripping' and is now usually performed by a digital computer program.

However, it appears that for most practical purposes it is the fast component of the washout curve which is important so that it is usual to compare regional washouts by determining the initial slope. This can be obtained by measuring the $t_{1/2}$, the time taken for the curve to decline to half its initial value (McDowall, 1969). Then

$$\text{initial slope} = \frac{0.693}{t_{1/2}}.$$

Attempts have been made to render the method non-invasive by giving the patient radioactive xenon to breathe until the brain tissue is saturated and then suddenly switching the breathing circuit to room air. Unfortunately the extracerebral tissues contribute significantly to the activity recorded and it is impossible to obtain a step change in arterial radioactivity because the lung radioactivity takes some time to wash out. The analysis is therefore more complicated (McDowall, 1976; Rowan & Harper, 1982).

Muscle blood flow may be measured by a variation of this technique in which radioactive sodium or xenon dissolved in saline is injected directly into the muscle and the subsequent clearance followed with a scintillation detector positioned above the site of injection.

The third method of using tracers assumes complete clearance of the isotope by the organ so that the venous concentration is zero. One example is the injection of radioactive microspheres which impact in the capillaries and so enable the distribution of blood flow to different organs to be measured. The microspheres must be injected into a ventricle to ensure thorough mixing with the blood stream and, although there are often difficulties in measuring the concentration of microspheres in the region of interest, the technique gives a useful measure of the distribution of flow at the time of injection. For example, the injection of microspheres into the right heart has been used to study the distribution of pulmonary blood flow during conditions of zero or increased gravity whilst left heart injection has been used to study the distribution of systemic blood flow during exercise. However, the absolute flow to an organ can only be calculated if the total blood flow is known. A second example of this type of application is the measurement of plasma clearance of an indicator by an organ. In this case the rate of fall of arterial concentration provides a measure of the organ flow providing the clearance of the tracer is confined to the organ of interest and the venous concentration is zero.

A third example of this type of application is the Stewart–Hamilton technique for measurement of cardiac output. In this case, the effect of recirculation of indicator is eliminated by assuming an exponential clearance of indicator and predicting the tail of the curve from the initial down-slope recorded before recirculation occurs (see p. 216).

Direct measurement of oscillatory flow in blood vessels

METHODS BASED ON PRESSURE MEASUREMENT

In one method the difference in pressure between two points situated proximally and distally in the vessel is sensed with a double-lumen catheter and a differential electromanometer. If the diameter of the vessel can be measured by angiographic techniques and if the velocity profile is reasonably laminar, it is possible to apply Poiseuille's equation to derive instantaneous flow. Unfortunately the mathematical analysis of the pressure curves is extremely complex and very high fidelity recordings are essential.

Other methods are based on the analysis of the pulse wave contour recorded by intra-arterial pressure measurement (Wesseling *et al.* 1974). The analysis of the wave form is performed by a small bedside computer which can display beat-to-beat values for stroke volume, heart rate and cardiac output. However a preliminary calibration against some other standard technique (e.g. dye-dilution) is required to establish correction factors for each patient.

ELECTROMAGNETIC FLOWMETERS

These are the most widely-used instruments for the direct measurement of blood flow in both the experimental and clinical situation. The measurement technique is based on the laws of electromagnetic induction described by Faraday. If blood or other electrolyte flows at right angles to a magnetic field, then an electromotive force (e.m.f.) will be induced in a plane which is mutually perpendicular

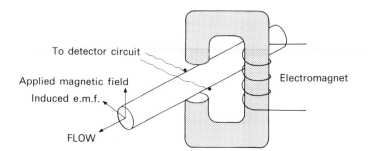

Fig. 16.7. Principle of electromagnetic flowmeter.

to the magnetic field and to the direction of fluid flow. The induced voltage can be measured by two electrodes situated in the appropriate plane and connected to a suitable detector circuit (Fig. 16.7). The induced voltage is proportional to the strength of the magnetic field and to the velocity of blood flow within the blood vessel. Since the flowmeter wraps around the blood vessel and forms a snug fit, the diameter of the vessel is held constant. By the application of a suitable calibration factor the velocity signal can therefore be read in terms of flow.

Although many of the earlier instruments used a constant electromagnetic field the method proved unsatisfactory, for the constant field generated a steady current round the detector circuit which caused polarization of the detector electrodes (p. 49). To overcome this, most modern instruments utilize an alternating magnetic field produced by an electromagnet supplied with either a sinusoidal, square wave or trapezoidal alternating current (Geddes & Baker, 1975). The use of an alternating field creates large artefactual signals in the detector circuit which result from the inductive forces generated by the rising and falling of the a.c. current. With a sine wave current the error signals are also sinusoidal, but out of phase with the flow signal and so can be eliminated by suitable electronic processing. In the case of the square wave flowmeter, the error signals appear as spikes each time the curve reverses. These can be eliminated by using a simple gating technique (Fig. 16.8).

Although sine wave flowmeters are more complex than square wave instruments they are more efficient. This is an important consideration for it means that a smaller excitation current and magnet

are required to produce any given output signal. However, many other factors must be considered when choosing an instrument for a given application.

One important factor is zero stability. In the experimental situation the zero reading can be checked by occluding the vessel with a clamp or pneumatic occluder. However, this is often impossible in the clinical situation or when flowmeters are used on the aorta or pulmonary artery. The problem has now been minimized by using a

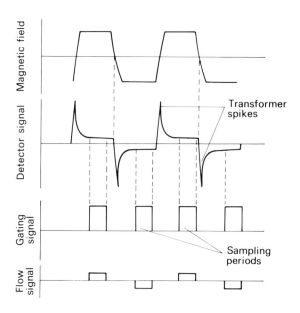

Fig. 16.8. Processing of signal from square wave electromagnetic flowmeter. The gating system causes the detector signal to be sampled when interference from the 'transformer spikes' is minimal. The flow signal is then rectified and displayed.

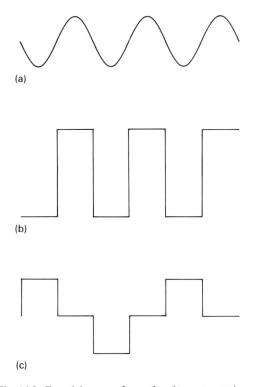

Fig. 16.9. Energizing waveforms for electromagnetic flowmeters. (a) Sinusoidal. (b) Square wave. (c) Pulsed-square wave with 'no-flow' interval which permits automatic zeroing of instrument.

pulsed energizing current as shown in Fig. 16.9. With this waveform there is a period of zero current flow; this can be used to re-zero the instrument automatically.

A second factor is the type of probe which can be used. In some types of flowmeter the probe is an integral part of a cannula which is inserted between the cut ends of a blood vessel or more commonly incorporated into an extracorporeal perfusion circuit. For most clinical and experimental applications the probe is C-shaped so that it can be slipped around the vessel. The probe must be carefully chosen so that it fits snugly round the vessel but does not compress it. This type of probe can be designed to produce a very even magnetic field, so that accurate measurements can be obtained, but it is important to ensure that changes in blood pressure or vessel tone do not impair the signal by creating a disparity between vessel and probe

diameters. This not only alters the calibration but also impairs the detection of the very small voltages which are generated by the flow. A reduction in signal will also occur if the direction of the magnetic field deviates significantly from the perpendicular plane. With very small vessels an I-type probe is used. In this the electromagnet is placed to one side of the vessel. Although the resulting magnetic field is not as even as with the C-type, the resulting errors are usually acceptable providing the vessel is small. A recent introduction is a probe which is shaped like a strap and which can be wrapped round the aorta after cardiac surgery and used to monitor left ventricular output during the post-operative period. When measurements have been completed the probe is withdrawn through the chest incision with little more difficulty than withdrawing a chest drain.

The electromagnetic principle has also been used in a catheter-tip flow probe which can be passed into the heart or large vessels. Since the resulting magnetic field is very uneven the instrument yields measurements of the velocity of blood flow in close proximity to the catheter tip (Fig. 16.10). In the aorta where the velocity profile is relatively flat the positional error is not great. However, absolute flow rates can only be measured if the aortic diameter can be determined by some other method.

Flow probes can be calibrated *in vitro* or *in vivo*. *In vitro* calibration is accomplished by collecting

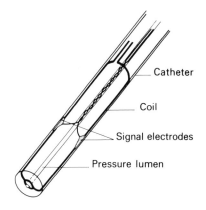

Fig. 16.10. Catheter-tip flow probe. (After Mills, 1968.)

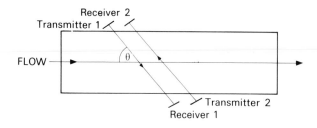

Fig. 16.11. Ultrasonic flow meter using transit time difference.

the blood in a measuring cylinder for a given time and comparing this with the integrated signal from the flowmeter. *In vivo* calibration can be performed by placing a clamp distal to the flow probe and by withdrawing a measured quantity of blood through a needle placed between the probe and clamp. Alternatively the measurement can be calibrated against some indirect method of measuring flow, e.g. the indicator-dilution technique. The calibration factor of each probe remains reasonably constant with time so that once this has been established the machine can be set to match the flow probe in use. However, the probe must be recalibrated if haematocrit changes. Flow probes are relatively robust and have been implanted for long-term experiments in animals. However, regular checks of their performance are desirable.

ULTRASONIC FLOWMETERS

These instruments detect the velocity of flow so that the actual flow rate can only be determined if the vessel diameter has been determined by an independent technique.

The fundamental requirement when using ultrasound is that the wavelength must be short compared with the dimension of the system being measured. Two different principles are used (see Chapter 9). In the first, two transmitter–receiver crystals are placed on opposite sides of the vessel

so that one lies downstream from the other (Fig. 16.11). The upstream crystal transmits a pulse of ultrasound to the downstream crystal and the process is then reversed about 800 times a second. The transit time of the pulses between the two crystals depends on the speed of transmission of ultrasound in blood and the distance between the two crystals. However, the transit time of the pulses moving downstream will be shorter than that of the pulses moving upstream because the transmitting medium is also moving downstream. This difference in transit time will depend on the angle between the transmitter–receiver axis and the direction of blood flow, and on the velocity of blood flow. Since the position of the crystals is fixed by the flowmeter the difference in transit time between the two directions can be related directly to blood velocity. An extremely sensitive and stable detecting device is required to measure the very small difference between the transit times but the method has the advantage that the direction, as well as the velocity, of flow is indicated.

The second type of ultrasonic flowmeter utilizes the Doppler principle. In this instrument a combined transmitter–receiver crystal is directed at an angle to the flowing stream (Fig. 16.12). The ultrasound beam is reflected from the moving corpuscles, the frequency of the reflected sound depending upon the direction and velocity of blood

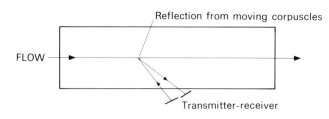

Fig. 16.12. Ultrasonic flow meter utilizing Doppler principle.

flow. Ultrasound reflected from corpuscles moving away from the transmitter will have a lower frequency than that transmitted, while that reflected from corpuscles moving towards the transmitter will have a higher frequency. The difference between transmitted and received frequencies is the *Doppler* frequency (see Chapter 9) which is directly proportional to the velocity of the reflecting surface with respect to the transmitter. Since the difference is small, the Doppler frequency is usually within the audible range, so can be monitored using a loudspeaker or headphones. The Doppler flowmeter generates a signal whose amplitude is proportional to the frequency of the Doppler signal and therefore to mean corpuscular velocity. Simple instruments cannot discriminate between blood flowing towards or away from the transmitter. If flow reversal is possible in the vessel under study, a more sophisticated device must be used, which by detecting whether the reflected signals are higher or lower in frequency than the transmitter, can be made fully directional.

Doppler instruments have proved useful in many clinical situations for the transducer can be situated some distance away from the vessel. Ultrasound is reflected by an air–tissue interface so that the transducer must be coupled to the vessel or skin with a liquid or gel acoustic coupling medium. Ultrasound is also reflected strongly by bone so that blood flow measurements within the skull are impracticable. Some attenuation of the ultrasound beam by body tissues also occurs. Since the attenuation increases with frequency, and the best resolution is only obtained at high frequencies, some compromise in respect of frequency must be made. Another problem is that the recorded velocity depends on the angle between the ultrasound beam and the direction of flow. Despite these problems, the instrument has proved useful to detect the presence of flow in peripheral arteries or in peripheral veins. Thus it has been used to detect flow in the radial artery after prolonged arterial cannulation, to detect peripheral venous thrombosis in the legs, and to localize the placenta.

THIN-FILM FLOWMETERS

Considerable advances in thermal techniques of measuring flow were made by Bellhouse *et al.* (1968). The probe consisted of a small glass bead on the end of a catheter. Three thin metallic rings about 1 μm in thickness were deposited on the bead. The central ring acted both as a resistance thermometer and as a heating element. It was incorporated in a Wheatstone bridge which was in turn connected to a high gain amplifier so that any fall in temperature of the resistance caused an increased heating current to flow through the element. Thus the temperature was maintained constant slightly above the surrounding blood temperature whatever the prevailing flow conditions. Changes in the flow velocity were then detected by measuring the fluctuations in power necessary to balance the bridge. The two end rings were used to detect the direction of flow by sensing the temperature difference produced by the central, heated ring. The instrument had minimal thermal inertia and a remarkably fast response time, but was only used in research applications.

Measurement of cardiac output and organ blood flow

CARDIAC OUTPUT

The standard by which all the other methods have been judged is the Fick technique (p. 209). However, this requires the sampling of mixed venous blood, can only be performed when the patient is in a steady state and is, at best, subject to errors of $\pm 10\%$. Measurements of equal accuracy may be obtained by indicator dilution using dye or thermal indicators but again these are invasive. Non-invasive estimates of cardiac output may be made using impedance or ultrasound techniques or ballistocardiography.

Indicator dilution

In this technique an indicator is injected as a 'slug' into the vena cava, the right heart or, preferably, the pulmonary artery. The concentration of the

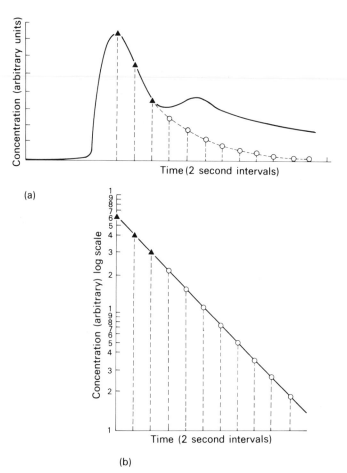

(a)

(b)

Fig. 16.13. (a) Single injection indicator dilution curve showing distortion of downslope produced by recirculation. (b) Re-plot on semi-logarithmic paper. ▲ = points taken from the downslope in (a) to establish the slope of the re-plot in (b). ○ = points taken from (b) to plot tail of curve in (a).

indicator reaching the systemic side of the circulation is then plotted against time. The flow is calculated in the following manner. Suppose that 5 mg of indicator was injected, that the duration of the curve was 30 s and that the mean concentration of the indicator on the systemic side was $2 \text{ mg} \cdot \text{L}^{-1}$ (the latter is calculated from the area under the curve divided by the duration of the curve). Then the 5 mg of indicator must have been diluted by $5/2 = 2.5 \text{ L}$ of blood during the 30 s. Hence, the cardiac output must have been $60/30 \times 2.5 = 5 \text{ L} \cdot \text{min}^{-1}$.

The general formula is:

$$\text{cardiac output (L} \cdot min^{-1})$$
$$= \frac{60 \times \text{indicator dose (mg)}}{\text{average concentration (mg} \cdot \text{L}^{-1}) \times \text{time (s)}}.$$

One of the problems with this method is that recirculation of indicator occurs before the downslope of the curve is complete (Fig. 16.13a). A number of techniques have been proposed to overcome the difficulty, but the most commonly-used method utilizes the exponential character of the down-slope. If such a curve is replotted on a semi-logarithmic scale a straight line results (Fig. 16.13b). The slope of the semi-logarithmic plot is established from the top portion of the recorded dye curve. Points from the lower portion of this slope are then replotted back onto the original curve to define the tail of the curve which would have been recorded if recirculation had not occurred (Fig. 16.13a). The area may be measured by counting squares, weighing the paper enclosed by the curve or by planimetry,* although the calculations are now usually performed by a microprocessor. Other methods of calculating the area of the curve have been devised but all involve a variable degree of approximation.

A number of indicators have been used for this technique. Of the dyes used indocyanine green (Cardio-green or Fox-green) is the most popular. It is non-toxic and has a relatively short half-life, so that repeated measurements can be made. It has a peak spectral absorption at 800 nm, which is the wavelength at which the absorption of oxygenated and reduced haemoglobin is identical. The measurement is therefore not affected by changes in arterial saturation. Indicator dilution curves have also been inscribed using radioactive tracers such as radioactive human serum albumin or chromium-labelled red cells.

In the original Stewart–Hamilton method the concentration of dye or isotope in the systemic circulation was obtained by allowing a continuous stream of blood from a peripheral artery to flow into a series of small tubes which were supported at the periphery of a rotating disc and sequentially moved under the open end of the sampling catheter. Each of the 30 or so blood samples was then analysed separately and the curve plotted by hand. Nowadays the dye concentration is recorded by spectrophotometric means, the arterial blood being sampled at a continuous rate of about 30 ml·min^{-1} through a cuvette densitometer by means of a motorized syringe. For radioactive measurements the arterial blood is drawn through a small coil situated within a scintillation detector. Baseline adjustments for both dye and radioactivity detectors are made by passing the patient's blood through the detector and calibration is then performed with blood samples containing known

amounts of the indicator. A dynamic calibration may also be used. This is achieved by drawing a sample of the patient's blood through a mixing unit consisting of a small glass tube filled with glass beads. A known amount of the indicator is injected proximal to this tube so that an indicator–dilution curve appears downstream from the mixing unit. The blood is then drawn through the densitometer or scintillation detector and the curve recorded in the usual way. The cardiac output may be calculated from the sampling flow rate, the doses of indicator injected into patient and mixing unit, and the areas under the two indicator dilution curves (Emmanuel *et al.* 1966).

Many attempts have been made to sense the changes in indicator concentration non-invasively. Earpiece densitometers have been extensively studied and have proved adequate for monitoring the direction of change in cardiac output but have not proved reliable for absolute measurements. The use of radioactive indicators and external counting over the heart, has also proved disappointing.

Thermal indicator dilution

This technique is now used routinely in the intensive care situation where pulmonary artery catheterization is frequently required for the monitoring of left-sided filling pressures. The principle of the method is similar to other indicator dilution methods but the injection and sampling are performed on the right side of the heart. Typically a slug of 10 ml normal saline or 5% dextrose solution at room temperature is injected into the right atrium and the temperature change is recorded by a thermistor in the pulmonary artery. The dilution curve which results is similar in shape to a dye dilution curve but there is no recirculation. The calculation is also similar but must naturally be worked out in terms of the 'heat dose'. Thus the numerator is the product of the difference in temperature between the injectate and blood multiplied by the density, specific heat and volume of the injectate. The denominator is the area under the temperature–time graph multiplied by the density and specific heat of blood.

---

* A planimeter is an instrument for manual measurement of the area of a curve. One end of the instrument is fixed whilst the small wheel on the other end is moved round the area to be measured. The instrument mechanically integrates the movements of the wheel in the x- and y-axes and so gives a direct reading of the area of the curve.

Thermal dilution methods have a number of advantages (Weisel *et al.* 1975; Buchbinder & Ganz, 1976). The indicator is cheap, non-toxic and repeated measurements may be made without much alteration in the baseline. (With dyes or isotopes the background level builds up progressively so limiting the number of estimations which can be performed.) Arterial puncture and blood withdrawal is not necessary and the absence of a recirculation curve greatly facilitates measurement of the area under the curve, particularly in low output, high central blood volume states where the recirculation curve may make dye dilution estimates of output grossly inaccurate. There are, however, a number of disadvantages to the thermal dilution technique. Firstly, it requires the passage and correct placement of a special catheter with a thermistor probe which is carefully matched to the processor. Such probes are expensive, particularly if combined with triple lumen catheters which permit injection of indicator and the recording of pulmonary artery and wedge pressures. A second disadvantage is that the bolus is large and mixing with the venous blood may be incomplete. The third disadvantage is that pulmonary arterial flow varies much more with intermittent positive pressure ventilation than does systemic flow; furthermore there are respiratory fluctuations in temperature in the pulmonary artery. Injection during inspiration may thus give very different results from those obtained with injection during expiration (Jansen *et al.* 1981). Finally, there is always the problem of correcting for the change of temperature of the injectate as it passes along the catheter.

Both dye- and thermal-dilution methods may now be used in association with minicomputers. With the dye technique the initial part of the down-slope is sampled automatically by the computer and all the computations are then carried out in a similar manner to those already described. The computer rejects the curve if the section sampled is not exponential or if the quality of the curve is unsatisfactory for some other reason. The dye calibration is also incorporated in the processing so that a direct digital or printed display is available within a few seconds of the curve being inscribed.

The thermal-dilution computer similarly utilizes the volume and temperature of the injectate, the patient's blood temperature and the dilution curve to produce the result. The use of such on-line techniques has greatly improved the understanding of acute circulatory problems.

For comprehensive reviews of indicator dilution techniques for cardiac output measurement see Chamberlain (1982) and Hillis *et al.* (1985).

INDICATOR TECHNIQUES FOR ESTIMATION OF CARDIAC OUTPUT AND STROKE VOLUME

Although much progress has been made in the development of non-invasive methods for the measurement of cardiac output, none has proved to be as accurate as the Fick or indicator dilution techniques. However, the non-invasive techniques provide beat-by-beat measurements and so are useful in following rapid changes in stroke output.

Doppler ultrasonography

When ultrasound with a frequency of 1–10 MHz is directed along the long axis of the ascending aorta from a transducer in the suprasternal notch, the sound is reflected back with a frequency shift which is proportional to the velocity of blood flow (Chapter 9). The velocity (V) can then be calculated from the equation:

$$V = \frac{\Delta f C}{2 f_t \cos \theta}$$

where Δf is the Doppler frequency shift, f_t is the known frequency of the transmitted ultrasound, C is the speed of sound in tissue and θ is the angle between the direction of blood flow and the ultrasound beam. If the latter is less than 30° the error from lack of alignment is small. The blood flow velocity curve is integrated to give the average velocity over time and the stroke volume then calculated by multiplying the average velocity during each heartbeat by the cross-sectional area of the aorta. Multiplication of stroke volume by heart rate yields cardiac output.

Both continuous and pulsed Doppler systems are in use. The continuous system can measure high velocities but averages the frequency shifts along the whole length of the ascending aorta so that the exact point at which the velocity is measured is unknown. It is therefore difficult to know where to measure the aortic diameter. The pulsed Doppler again uses the same transducer to generate and receive the ultrasound but this produces short pulses instead of a continuous stream of ultrasound. The great advantage of the system is that the beam can be focussed so that the operator knows the precise depth at which the measurement is being made. However, there is a limit to the velocity of blood flow which can be measured since high velocities lead to a large Doppler shift. If the sampling rate is inadequate, it may prove impossible to measure the velocity. Increasing the pulse repetition frequency extends the range of velocity measurement, but decreases the possible depth of the measurement since the signals must have time to return to the transducer before the next pulse is emitted.

There are three major problems with Doppler measurements of cardiac output. First, the aortic diameter must be measured accurately since the cross-sectional area is πr^2. It has been shown that aortic diameter can be measured reasonably accurately by echocardiography, but errors also arise because the aorta is not completely circular and it expands by up to 12% during systole. Furthermore, the site of diameter measurement may not correspond to the position where velocity is measured.

The second problem is the shape of the velocity profile. This is flat at the orifice of the aortic valve, but may change shape as the blood passes into the larger diameter of the aorta. Although the central core probably has a velocity close to that in the aortic valve opening, lower velocities may be recorded if the beam is not aligned exactly along the aortic axis.

The third problem, the direction of the ultrasound beam relative to the axis, does not usually cause large errors for if θ is 20°, the error in cardiac output will only be about 6%.

There are now a number of studies demonstrating a good correlation between Doppler cardiac output measurement and simultaneous measurements made by the Fick and thermodilution techniques (Dobb & Donovan, 1987). In critically ill patients, pulsed Doppler measurements were approximately $0.5 \, L \cdot min^{-1}$ lower than thermodilution measurements but the standard deviation of the difference between the two measurements exceeded $1.6 \, L \cdot min^{-1}$. This suggests that the accuracy of the method is not adequate for clinical purposes (Donovan et al. 1987). However, it should be remembered that the thermal dilution technique is, in itself, subject to many sources of error.

The measurement of output via the suprasternal notch is only suitable for intermittent measurements. During anaesthesia better results can be obtained by using a transducer on an oesophageal probe. This is positioned so that it views the descending aorta. Three steps are required (Mark et al. 1986). First, the internal diameter of the aorta just above the sinuses of Valsalva must be measured using pulsed A-mode echocardiography. It is assumed that the aorta is circular at this point so that the cross-sectional area can be computed from the diameter. The measurement takes 5–30 min depending on the skill of the operator but in some commercial systems this measurement is derived from a nomogram. The oesophageal Doppler probe is inserted after the patient has been anaesthetized and is then positioned to yield the maximal signal. This can usually be accomplished in 5–10 min. The third step is to calibrate the measurement derived from the oesophageal probe against the cardiac output calculated from the velocity of blood flow in the ascending aorta (measured by a separate transducer placed in the suprasternal notch) and the cross-sectional area of the aorta (Fig. 16.14). This calibration assumes that the proportion of the ascending aortic flow distributed to the upper part of the body remains constant throughout the period of measurement. Whilst the absolute comparison with the thermal dilution is poor, the method provides a useful indication of trends.

Thoracic electrical bioimpedance

Since the electrical impedance of a block of tissue fluctuates according to the blood volume contained

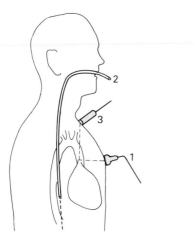

Fig. 16.14. The three steps required in the measurement of cardiac output using an oesophageal Doppler probe. (1) Measurement of the internal diameter of the ascending aorta. (2) Placement of oesophageal probe. (3) Comparison of oesophageal probe measurement with cardiac output calculated from aortic root diameter and aortic flow velocity measured by a probe in the suprasternal notch.

therein, it follows that a study of thoracic impedance changes should yield a signal from which stroke volume might be derived. Two circumferential electrodes are placed around the neck and two around the upper abdomen. A small (<1 mA), constant, high frequency (>1 kHz) alternating current is passed between the outer electrodes and the resulting potential difference detected by the inner pair. This potential is rectified, smoothed, and 'backed off' to yield a zero value. Changes in impedance due to respiration and cardiac activity are now seen as voltage fluctuations about this zero value. The respiratory signals are appreciably larger than those due to cardiac activity, so that measurements must be made either with the subject breath holding, or by utilizing an averaging technique. This is accomplished by using the ECG R-wave as a synchronizing signal and averaging the impedance cardiogram over several cardiac cycles, so that the respiratory artefact, being asynchronous, is eliminated. The signal thus obtained represents changes in thoracic blood volume, and clearly resembles the pulse waveform.

Continued modification of the original technique has now resulted in an instrument which produces results which are in closer agreement with other invasive methods. The new instrument uses a modified formula for its calculations, enables measurements to be made during spontaneous or mechanical ventilation and generates results which are closer to indicator dilution results than previous models (Porter & Swain, 1987; Mattar, 1988). The device underestimates cardiac output in septic shock and aortic regurgitation and is inaccurate when there are intracardiac shunts or dysrhythmias. Nevertheless, it is proving valuable in the study of rapid changes of output which could not be followed by other more invasive techniques.

LIVER BLOOD FLOW

The investigation of liver blood flow is rendered difficult by the inaccessibility of the liver circulation and by the dual nature of the hepatic blood supply. Most measurements yield values of total liver blood flow in $ml \cdot min^{-1}$, but other techniques produce measures of tissue perfusion in $ml \cdot min^{-1} \cdot g^{-1}$ of liver tissue.

Total liver blood flow may be measured by electromagnetic flow probes in animals and by indicator dilution or clearance techniques in humans.

The clearance techniques may be divided into those which measure hepatocyte clearance, reticuloendothelial clearance or hepatic drug extraction. Early measurements utilized bromosulphthalein (BSP) which was removed by the hepatocytes and excreted into the bile. The dye was infused at a rate which maintained a constant arterial level and by measuring both the infusion rate and arterio-venous difference, liver blood flow could be calculated by the Fick principle. In recent years, reticulocyte clearance has been measured using colloidal gold or sulphur whilst hepatic drug extraction has been measured with lignocaine or propranolol.

Total liver blood flow has also been measured by indicator dilution, the indicator (labelled red cells or serum albumin) being injected into the hepatic artery or portal vein and the dilution curve being obtained by hepatic venous blood sampling or external monitoring of hepatic radioactivity (Mathie, 1982).

KIDNEY: EFFECTIVE RENAL PLASMA FLOW

This was originally measured with *p*-aminohippuric acid (PAH) but most workers now use *o*-iodohippuric acid (hippuran) labelled with ^{121}I or ^{131}I.

In the constant infusion methods, urine and plasma samples are taken at a time when the rate of excretion equals the rate of infusion so that clearance (C)

$$C = \frac{UV}{PT}$$

where V is the volume of urine produced during time T, and U and P are the measured concentrations of activity in urine and plasma respectively.

Other techniques using single injections or external monitoring are described by Testa *et al.* (1982).

References

Bellhouse, B.J., Schultz, D.L., Karatzas, N.B. & Lee, G. de J. (1968) A catheter-tip method for the measurement of pulsatile blood flow velocity in arteries. In Bain, W.H. & Harper, A.M. (eds), *Blood flow through organs and tissues.* Churchill Livingstone, Edinburgh.

Buchbinder, N. & Ganz, W. (1976) Hemodynamic monitoring: invasive techniques. *Anesthesiology* **45**, 145–155.

Chamberlain, J.H. (1982) Cardiac output measurement by indicator dilution. In Mathie, R.T. (ed.), *Blood flow measurement in man*, chapter 4. Castle House Publications, Tunbridge Wells, Kent.

Dobb, G.J. and Donovan, K.D. (1987) Non-invasive methods of measuring cardiac output. *Intensive Care Medicine* **13**, 304–309.

Donovan, K.D., Dobb, G.J., Newman, M.A., Hockings, B.E.S. & Ireland, M. (1987) Comparison of pulsed Doppler and thermodilution methods for measuring cardiac output in critically ill patients. *Critical Care Medicine* **15**, 853–857.

Emmanuel, R., Hamer, J., Ching, B. Norman, J. & Manders, J. (1966) A dynamic method for the calibration of dye dilution curves in a physiological system. *British Heart Journal* **28**, 143–146.

Geddes, L.A. & Baker, L.E. (1975) *Principles of applied biomedical instrumentation*, 2nd edn. John Wiley and Sons, New York.

Greenfield, A.D.M., Whitney, R.J. & Mowbray, J.F. (1963) Methods for the investigation of peripheral blood flow. *British Medical Bulletin* **19**, 101–109.

Hillis, L.D., Firth, B.G. & Winniford, M.D. (1985) Analysis of factors affecting the variability of Fick versus indicator dilution measurements of cardiac output. *American Journal of Cardiology* **56**, 764–768.

Jansen, J.R.C., Schreuder, J.J., Bogaard, J.M., Van Rooyen, W. and Versprille, A. (1981) Thermodilution technique for measurement of cardiac output during artificial ventilation. *Journal of Applied Physiology* **50**, 584–591.

Kety, S.S. and Schmidt, C.F. (1945) Determination of cerebral blood flow in man by use of nitrous oxide in low concentrations. *American Journal of Physiology* **143**, 53–56.

Mark, J.B., Steinbrook, R.A., Gugino, L.D., Maddie, R., Hartwell, B., Shemin, R., DiSesa, V. & Rida, W.N. (1986) Continuous non-invasive monitoring of cardiac output with esophageal Doppler ultrasound during cardiac surgery. *Anesthesia and Analgesia* **65**, 1013–1020.

Mathie R.T. (1982) Measurement of liver blood flow in man. In Mathie, R.T. (ed.), *Blood flow measurement in man*, Chapter 13. Castle House Publications, Tunbridge Wells, Kent.

Mattar, J.A. (1988) Non-invasive cardiac output determination by thoracic electrical bioimpedance. *Intensive and Critical Care Digest* **7**, 14–17.

McDowall, D.G. (1969) Regional blood flow measurement in clinical practice. *British Journal of Anaesthesia* **41**, 761–777.

McDowall, D.G. (1976) Monitoring the brain. *Anesthesiology* **45**, 117–134.

Mills, C.J. (1968) A catheter tip electromagnetic velocity probe for use in man. In Bain, W.H., & Harper, A.M. (eds), *Blood flow through organs and tissues*, p. 38. Churchill Livingstone, Edinburgh.

Porter, J.M. & Swain, I.D. (1987) Measurement of cardiac output by electrical impedance plethysmography. *Journal of Biomedical Engineering* **9**, 222–231.

Rowan, J.D. & Harper A.M. (1982) Measurement of cerebral blood flow in man. In Mathie, R.T. (ed.), *Blood flow measurement in man*, Chapter 10. Castle House Publications, Tunbridge Wells, Kent.

Testa, H.J., Lupton, E.W. & Shields, R.A. (1982) Renal blood flow measurement. In Mathie, R.J. (ed.), *Blood flow measurement in man*, Chapter 19. Castle House Publications, Tunbridge Wells, Kent.

Visscher, M.B. & Johnson, J.A. (1953) The Fick principle: analysis of potential errors in its conventional application. *Journal of Applied Physiology* **5**, 635–638.

Weisel, R.D., Berger, R.L. & Hechtman, H.B. (1975) Current concepts: measurement of cardiac output by thermodilution. *New England Journal of Medicine* **292,** 682–684.

Whitney, R.J. (1953) The measurement of volume changes in human limbs. *Journal of Physiology (London)* **121**, 1–27.

Wesseling, K.H., Smith, K.T., Nichols, W.W., Weber, H., De Wit, B. & Beneken J.E.W. (1974) Beat to beat cardiac output from the arterial pressure contour. In Feldman, S.A., Leigh J. & Spierdijk (eds.), *Measurement in anaesthesia.* University Press, London.

Further reading

Mathie, R.T. (ed.) (1982) *Blood flow measurement in man.* Castle House Publications, Tunbridge Wells, Kent.

Prys-Roberts, C. (1980) Measurement of cardiac output and regional blood flow. In Prys-Roberts, C. (ed.), *The circulation in anaesthesia*, p. 536. Blackwell Scientific Publications, Oxford.

Smith, N.T. (1980) Non-invasive assessment of the cardiovascular system. In Prys-Roberts, C. (ed.), *The circulation in anaesthesia*, p. 561. Blackwell Scientific Publications, Oxford.

17: Gas and Vapour Analysis

There are four main applications of gas and vapour analysis to clinical practice. They are:

1 To establish the identity and concentrations of gases and vapours delivered to the patient by an anaesthetic circuit, incubator, oxygen tent or pipeline installation.

2 To detect the presence of atmospheric pollution.

3 To assess metabolic or cardiorespiratory function either by the analysis of the respired gases (O_2, CO_2 and N_2) or by the use of inert tracer gases such as He, CO or Ar.

4 To detect the presence of traces of hydrogen, methane or pentane in respired air as indices of abnormal bacterial colonization of the gut or oxygen free radical damage to the tissues.

Chemical methods

Chemical methods of gas analysis are most commonly used for the estimation of oxygen and carbon dioxide. They involve the removal of fractional volumes from the gas phase by the production of nongaseous compounds, the fractional concentration being determined by the reduction in volume which occurs.

CARBON DIOXIDE

The concentration of CO_2 in gas mixtures can be determined by measuring the reduction in volume after absorption of the gas in 10–20% potassium hydroxide solution. This method cannot be used without modification if another gas soluble in potassium hydroxide (e.g. N_2O) is present. The difficulty can be overcome by using saturated sodium hydroxide, in which N_2O is relatively insoluble, to absorb the CO_2. However, this is difficult since the solution is extremely viscous and

forms a precipitate of sodium carbonate which obscures the meniscus. A better method is to saturate the absorbent solution with N_2O before use (Owen-Thomas & Meade, 1975). Many types of apparatus have been described for carrying out this analysis, the best known being the Haldane, Lloyd–Haldane (Lloyd, 1958) and the Scholander (Scholander, 1974). A simple modification of the Haldane apparatus described by Campbell (1960) illustrates the principle of the method.

This apparatus consists of a burette, absorption chamber and reservoir for the absorbent solution (Fig. 17.1). The burette has a volume of 10 ml and the stem is graduated from 8.5 to 10 ml in 0.1 ml increments. A mercury column driven by a syringe is used to transfer gas from one chamber to another.

Before starting the analysis the absorption chamber is opened to atmosphere and the height of the absorbent reservoir is adjusted until the meniscus is aligned with the hair line. This ensures that the volumes of absorbent in the reservoir and absorption chamber are exactly balanced when at atmospheric pressure. The gas sample to be analysed is attached to the side limb of tap A. A preliminary sample is aspirated into the burette by raising the syringe plunger, and discharged to atmosphere through tap B. Another sample is then aspirated into the burette and the excess gas is discharged through tap B, approximately 10 ml being retained in the burette for analysis. (The 10-ml volume shown on the scale of this apparatus includes the volume in the tube joining taps A and B.) The burette and absorption chamber are then interconnected by the appropriate adjustment of taps A and B and the gas is driven to and fro between the gas burette and the absorption chamber between ten and fifteen times. The absorbent meniscus is again

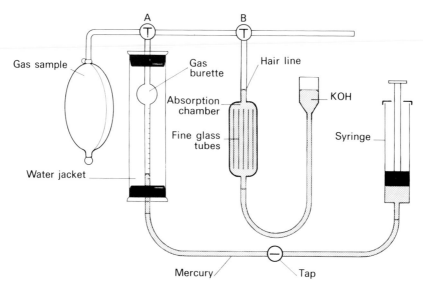

Fig. 17.1. Simplified CO_2 analyser. (Campbell, 1960.)

adjusted to the level of the hair line by manipulating the syringe plunger, and the reduction in volume of the gas in the burette is read from the level of the mercury meniscus in the stem of the burette. The absorption process is repeated and the gas volume checked to ensure that absorption is complete. Thus:

$$\text{fractional concentration of } CO_2 = \frac{\text{reduction in gas volume}}{\text{original volume}}.$$

If the original volume is adjusted exactly to 10 ml the concentration may be read directly from a second scale on the opposite side of the burette.

Care should be taken to ensure that the taps are well lubricated and that the apparatus is free from leaks. The burette must be kept acidified with a few drops of dilute sulphuric acid and the tube between the taps must be cleaned with a pipe-cleaner soaked in dilute H_2SO_4 if the KOH is accidentally drawn into it. The KOH should be replaced whenever absorption takes longer than 12–15 swings. After a little practice operators should be able to achieve duplicates within $\pm 0.1\%$ CO_2 (approximately 1 mmHg).

OXYGEN

The concentration of oxygen in a gas mixture can be determined by absorbing the gas in alkaline pyrogallol or sodium anthraquinone. Since these solutions also absorb CO_2, the CO_2 analysis must be completed first. A standard Haldane apparatus with two absorption chambers is necessary (Haldane & Graham, 1935). This apparatus has an additional burette which automatically compensates for changes in temperature during the analysis. The accuracy is therefore somewhat greater than the simplified apparatus ($CO_2 \pm 0.05\%$; $O_2 \pm 0.1\%$).

Physical methods

The main advantage of the physical methods of gas analysis is their speed. Indeed, they can usually be adapted for continuous operation.

When a machine is designed to follow rapid changes in gas concentration it is essential to know the speed of response of the complete system. This may be divided into two components — the time required for the sample to flow along the sampling

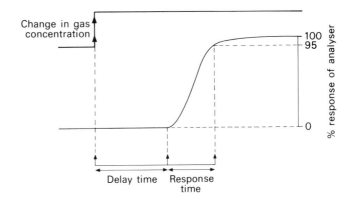

Fig. 17.2. Transit (or delay) time and rise (or response) time after square wave change in sampled gas concentration.

catheter, and the time required for the instrument to react to the change in gas concentration (Fig. 17.2). The former is often called the transit, or delay, time, whilst the latter is usually called the response, or rise, time.

The transit time usually accounts for the greater part of the total delay. It is reduced by using a narrow and short sampling catheter with a rapid sampling flow rate. The response time of the instrument is chiefly a function of the time required to wash out the analysis cell, but additional delays may be imposed by the mechanism used to detect the change in gas concentration. Commonly, the instrumental response to a square wave change in gas concentration is sigmoid in shape. It is therefore usual to express the instrumental response time as the time required to obtain a 90 or 95% response to the change in gas concentration.

A square wave change in gas concentration can be produced in several ways. One of the simplest is to move the tip of the sampling catheter rapidly in or out of a small hole in the wall of a tube which is transmitting a rapid flow of the gas to be analysed. Another, is to burst a small balloon of the gas within a small tube containing the sampling catheter. For regular testing, it is best to utilize a solenoid valve system connected to two high pressure gas sources. The electrical signal used to activate the valves can then be used to measure the transit time down the catheter as well as the rise time of the instrument (Fig. 17.3).

Most gas analysers are subject to zero drift and variations in gain and, therefore, have to be

calibrated frequently. The initial calibration should check the linearity of the instrument over the potential range of use, and this should be repeated at reasonable intervals thereafter. For routine use it is usually sufficient to check the zero with the analyser exposed to the background gas only and then to check the gain with a known input signal. In some analysers the signal is generated electrically, whilst in others it may be generated by interposing a special filter between the light source and analysis cell. However, for most purposes it is preferable to use a known gas mixture. With some gas analysers the calibration gases are readily available: for example, an anaesthetic machine O_2 analyser can be calibrated with N_2O and O_2 and then exposed to air to check the linearity. However, with other instruments it is necessary to generate special gas mixtures. Appropriate mixtures with a certificate of analysis can be purchased commercially and are then delivered in pink cylinders. For some applications, standard gas mixtures, such as 5% CO_2 in O_2, can be used, but these must be subjected to chemical analysis since their composition may differ from the nominal value. More complicated mixtures can be generated by decanting from larger cylinders using calculated pressures to obtain the desired proportion and then subjecting them to chemical analysis (Hill, 1961). However, this should *never* be attempted by those without special training and the mixture should always be made in special cylinders. Yet another technique is to mix the appropriate gases at atmospheric pressure using volumetric mixing

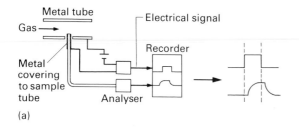

(a)

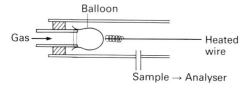

(b)

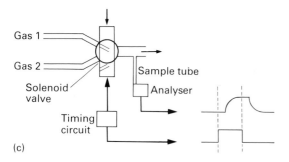

(c)

Fig. 17.3 Methods of producing a square wave change in gas concentration to measure the delay and response times of a rapid gas analyser. (a) Tube moved rapidly in and out of moving stream of gas. Electrical contacts can be used to mark the beginning or end of the square wave. (b) Bursting a balloon of gas in a tube. (c) Use of solenoid valve to switch between two pressurized gas sources.

pumps to produce a constant flow of mixed gas. With the appropriate pump (e.g. the Wosthoff) a very high degree of accuracy may be achieved ($\pm 0.1\%$ v/v). However, this technique is not suitable for the production of mixtures containing volatile anaesthetic agents since these dissolve in the pump oil.

Known concentrations of a vapour may be prepared by using a highly-accurate vaporizer such as the Dräger 'Vapor' (Hill, 1963), by preparing

saturated vapours at a known temperature and the then diluting them (Herchl, 1970; Nunn, et al. 1970), or by vaporizing known weights of a liquid in known volumes of a diluent gas. For example 1 gram-molecule of halothane vapour (molecular weight 197 g) occupies 22.4 L at standard temperature and pressure (STPD.) Therefore, 1 L of halothane vapour weighs 197/22.4 = 8.8 g. To make a 2% v/v concentration 8.8 g of halothane must be vaporized in 50 L of air at 101.3 kPa and 0°C.

Physical methods of analysis may be classified into specific and non-specific methods according to the property of the gas which is to be analysed.

Non-specific methods

These methods use a property of the gas which is common to all gases but possessed by each gas to a differing degree. Examples of the properties used are density, viscosity, thermal conductivity, refractive index, velocity of sound in the gas and magnetic susceptibility (Table 17.1). Non-specific methods are most useful when the particular physical property of the gas to be analysed differs markedly from the background gas. Normally, non-specific methods are only suitable for use with binary gas mixtures but they can be used for the analysis of more complex mixtures if the background gas mixture is constant (e.g. CO_2 in air), or if the relevant physical properties of the gas to be analysed differ widely from the background gases whilst the properties of the background gases differ little from each other.

Specific methods

By using some property of the gas which is unique to that gas, it can be identified in a gas mixture. Such methods may therefore be used when there are a number of background gases whose identity and concentration are unknown. Examples of the specific properties used are the absorption and emission of radiation of a particular wavelength, the detection of atomic nuclear properties or the conduction of electricity in response to an applied voltage (polarography).

Table 17.1. Physical properties of some common gases and vapours

	Refractive index*[†] (Sodium D line) STP	Relative magnetic susceptibility (change in zero reading with 100% gas)[‡]	Thermal conductivity* $(mW \cdot m^{-1} \cdot K^{-1})$	Velocity of sound* $(m \cdot s^{-1} \, STP)$	Viscosity* $(Pa \cdot s)$	Density* $(kg \cdot m^{-3} \, STP)$
Air	1.000 29	—	24.283	331	17.1	1.29
Argon	1.002 81	– 0.22	16.621	319	21.0	1.78
Carbon dioxide	1.000 45	– 0.27	14.235	259	13.9	1.98
Carbon monoxide	1.000 33	+ 0.01	23.404	338	16.7	1.25
Chloroform	1.001 45	NS	12.099 (16°C)	171	9.9	5.34[§]
Diethylether	1.001 55	NS	137.452 (30°C)	206	7.2	3.31[§]
Enflurane	1.001 44	NS	—	—	—	8.25[§]
Halothane	1.001 58	NS	—	—	—	8.78[§]
Helium	1.000 04	+ 0.30	147.375	965	18.9	0.18
Hydrogen	1.000 14	+ 0.24	174.170	1284	8.5	0.09
Krypton	1.000 43	– 0.51	8.876	—	23.3	3.71
Methane	1.000 44	– 0.20	30.186	430	10.3	0.72
Methoxyflurane	1.000 47[§]	NS	—	—	—	7.36[§]
Nitrogen	1.000 30	0.00	24.283	334	16.7	1.25
Nitric oxide	1.000 30	+ 43.00	23.864	324	18.8	1.34
Nitrous oxide	1.000 52	– 0.2	15.407	263	13.5	1.98
Oxygen	1.000 27	100.00	24.492	316	19.5	1.43
Trichloroethylene	1.001 78	NS	116.184 (20°C)	—	—	5.86[§]
Xenon	—	– 0.95	5.191	—	21.0	5.85

NS = no significant effect with concentrations used in clinical practice.
* Data from *Handbook of physiology* (1964). [†] Data from *Handbook of chemistry and physics* (1974).
[‡] Data from Taylor Instrument Analytics Ltd. Instrument calibrated with N_2 = 0%, and O_2 = 100%.
[§] Data from Lowe (1972).

NON-SPECIFIC METHODS

Density

This is one of the oldest methods and was employed by Waller (1908) in his chloroform balance. The principle of the balance is shown in Fig. 17.4.

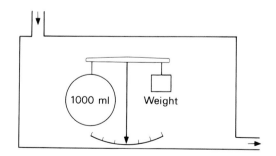

Fig. 17.4. Waller's chloroform balance.

A sealed glass bulb filled with air and of about 1000 ml capacity is exactly counterbalanced by a small weight within a gas-tight chamber. When a heavier than air vapour is admitted to the chamber there is an apparent decrease in weight of the glass bulb due to the difference in density between the vapour/air mixture and the air which it displaces. One thousand millilitres of air weighs 1.3 g and 1000 ml of chloroform vapour weighs 5.3 g at STP. Hence the apparent reduction in weight when pure chloroform vapour is passed through the chamber is 5.3 – 1.3 = 4.0 g. If the reduction in weight is 0.04 g the vapour concentration must be 1%.

Viscosity

Viscosity is an important determinant of flow along a parallel-sided tube when flow is laminar.

Use has been made of a pneumatic 'Wheatsone bridge' to measure the difference in pressure across a capillary tube but the method has not found wide application because of the relatively small differences in viscosity between the common gases.

Thermal conductivity

A gas with a high thermal conductivity conducts heat more readily than one with a low conductivity. This property is utilized in instruments known as katharometers. In these instruments the gas is passed over a heated wire. The degree of cooling of the wire depends on the temperature of the gas, the rate of gas flow and the thermal conductivity of the gas. The reduction in temperature of the wire reduces its resistance, and so provides a signal which can be related to the concentration. The change in resistance is detected with a Wheatstone bridge circuit and the output displayed on a meter (Fig. 17.5).

Katharometers can be made to detect changes in helium concentration of $\pm 0.1\%$ and, by situating the resistors out of the main gas stream, they can be made relatively insensitive to changes of sample flow rate. The response time is then slow. If flow rate is rigidly controlled and the gas samples are passed through small analysis chambers at a very low pressure a katharometer can be made to respond quickly to changes in gas concentration. In one instrument the response was sufficiently rapid to permit breath-by-breath analysis of CO_2.

The use of this type of instrument is obviously dependent on the difference in thermal conductivity between analysis and background gas (Table 17.1). For example the thermal conductivities of N_2 and O_2 are very similar and therefore analysis for one of these gases in the presence of the other is difficult. Helium, however, has a high thermal conductivity. Since a complete change of background gas from N_2 to O_2 would only produce a small change in indicated helium concentration, the apparatus can easily be used for the analysis of helium in nitrogen/oxygen mixtures. In clinical practice katharometers are usually used for the measurement of CO_2 and He; they are also used as detectors in gas chromatography systems (see p. 244 *et seq.*).

Refractive index

Light travels at a speed of about $3 \times 10^8 \, \text{m} \cdot \text{s}^{-1}$ (186 282 miles per second) through a vacuum but at a slower speed through transparent materials. The relationship between the velocity of light through a vacuum and the velocity through a transparent substance determines the refractive index of that substance. Thus the speed of light through water is approximately $2.3 \times 10^8 \, \text{m} \cdot \text{s}^{-1}$ (143 000 miles per second) and the refractive index of water is therefore $3.0 \div 2.3 = 1.3$ approximately. The delay caused by the passage of light through a gas is less than that produced by an equal length of water so that the refractive indices of gases are smaller than the refractive index of water (Table 17.1). Since the delay depends on the number of gas molecules present, the refractive index varies with both the pressure and the temperature of the gas.

The only practicable way of measuring the extremely small delay resulting from the passage of light through a gas is to measure the phase lag by the principle of interference. This is illustrated in Fig. 17.6. Light consists of transverse waves, the colour being determined by the wavelength and the brightness by the amplitude of the wave. When light waves from a common source (and hence in

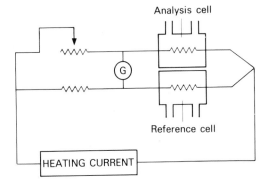

Fig. 17.5. Wheatstone bridge circuit used in a thermal conductivity analyser (katharometer). The cell resistances are heated by passing an electric current through them and the imbalance of the bridge produced by the analysis gas is shown by the galvanometer (G).

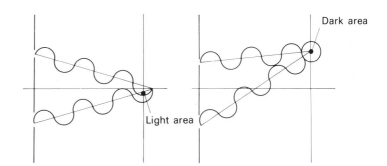

Fig. 17.6. Formation of interference bands. Left: light waves arriving in phase augment each other producing bright areas. Right: light waves arriving 180° out of phase cancel each other producing dark bands.

Dark area

Light area

the same phase) are passed through two linear slits in an opaque sheet and focussed onto a screen an interference pattern is produced. Waves which reach the screen at a point equidistant from the two slits will be in phase and so will reinforce each other and produce a central bright area. On each side there will be two dark bands. These are situated at a point where one light path is exactly half a wavelength longer than the other so that the waves reaching the screen are out of phase and thus cancel each other. Outside the dark bands, where the waves arriving at the screen are exactly in phase because one light path is exactly one wavelength longer than the other, there are two light bands, and outside these there will be two more dark bands and so on. The pattern is only observed when the light source is monochromatic, i.e. emits light of only one wavelength. In many commercial interferometers white light is used; this consists of a mixture of wavelengths each of which produces an interference band at a different distance from the axis. In such instruments only the two innermost dark bands are clearly defined, the remainder of the field tailing off into spectral colours.

When a gas is introduced into one light path it delays the transmission of the light waves. Since the frequency of the waves is unchanged this must lead to a reduction in the wavelength and an alteration in the position of the dark bands. If the refractive index of the gas is known, the change in position can be related to the number of gas molecules in the light path and hence to the partial pressure of the gas.

Two types of refractometers are in common use. The Rayleigh refractometer is a large instrument (about 2 m long) which is used in the laboratory.

Small and robust portable instruments, originally developed for the measurement of methane gas concentrations in mines, are used in clinical surroundings.

Rayleigh refractometer. Light from a tungsten bulb is focused into a parallel beam and passed through two vertical slits and then through two chambers closed at each end with optically flat glass plates (Fig. 17.7a). One chamber (A) contains the gas to be analysed whilst the other (B) contains the background gas. The two beams of light then pass through two glass plates (X, Y) which are inclined at an angle to the optical axis. Plate X is fixed but plate Y can be rotated so that the length of the light path through the glass can be varied. Both light paths are then focused onto a lens at the eye-piece of the instrument which magnifies the image in the horizontal plane. When the two tubes are filled with the same gas and X and Y are inclined at the same angle to the optical path an interference pattern is produced. This appears at the eyepiece as a spectrum with a series of dark bands at its centre (Fig. 17.7b). If the gas in tube A is changed, the position of the interference bands is shifted. However, the shift can be counteracted by varying the thickness of glass in the light path by rotating Y so that the interference bands once again appear in their original position. The degree of rotation of plate Y can be measured with a Vernier scale and calibrated to indicate the gas concentration in tube A.

In order to ensure that the interference pattern is correctly returned to the original position a duplicate pattern is reproduced below this movable

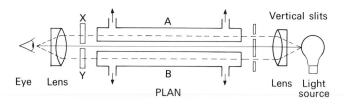

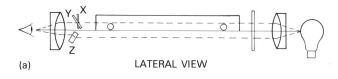

(a)   LATERAL VIEW

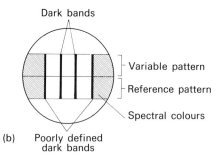

(b)   Poorly defined
        dark bands

Fig. 17.7. (a) Plan and lateral view of the Rayleigh refractometer. (b) The interference pattern viewed at the eye-piece. For description see text.

pattern (Fig. 17.7b). This duplicate pattern is produced by the bottom half of the two beams of light issuing from the vertical slits. These beams pass beneath the two tubes and are diverted by the prism Z, so that their interference pattern appears immediately below the other.

Portable interference refractometers. The detailed arrangement of the optical pathways varies with the instrument but the basic principle is illustrated in Fig. 17.8. Light from a common source is split into two beams, one of which travels through a cell containing the gas to be analysed whilst the other forms the reference pathway. The beams form an interference pattern on a translucent scale which is viewed through the eyepiece. The zero is initially set with the background gas in both the analysis and reference cells and the gas to be analysed is then aspirated through the analysis cell. The dark bands are shifted across the scale and the concen-

tration is read directly from a previously prepared calibration graph (Hulands & Nunn, 1970).

Both types of refractometer are usually calibrated by passing known concentrations of the gas or vapour through the instrument and plotting these against the reading on the instrument. The calibration lines are linear and once the calibration has been performed it remains stable. Although it is possible to encompass a range of sensitivities by adjusting the cell length, most instruments do not incorporate this facility. The main use of this method of analysis is in checking the output from anaesthetic machines and vaporizers, for one analyser can cover a range of gases and vapours, the readings may be made quickly, and the calibration is only likely to change if the machine is damaged.

Although an interferometer is only suitable for the analysis of binary mixtures, it can be used to analyse more complex gas mixtures by analysing the mixture at each stage of the mixing process. For

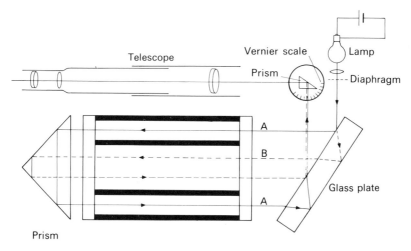

Fig. 17.8. Light path in a portable interference refractometer. A = reference cell. B = analysis cell.

example, Sugg *et al.* (1988) have described how such an analyser may be used to monitor the fresh gas composition on an anaesthetic machine. The interferometer is first used to check that the gas supplies are connected correctly by measuring the refractive index of the gases in the O_2 and N_2O supply lines. The refractive index of the mixture is then determined and the respective concentrations calculated and displayed. The refractive index is again determined after addition of vapour and compared with that of the O_2/N_2O mixture so that the vapour concentration can be measured.

Velocity of sound

This property has been utilized in two ways, both now of only historic interest. In one type of instrument (Faulconer & Ridley, 1950; Stott, 1959), the gas was resonated in a small chamber by an electronic circuit. The frequency of oscillation which caused the gas to resonate depended on the velocity of sound in the gas mixture, and hence on the gas composition. In another instrument (Molyneux & Pask, 1959) a pulse of sound was emitted at the end of a pair of one metre tubes. One tube contained the gas mixture and the other the background gas. The difference in time taken by the sound to travel down the tubes gave a measure of the gas concentration.

Solubility

A number of gases and vapours are soluble in other substances and alter their physical characteristics. An example of an analyser using this principle was the Dräger 'Narkotest' (Fig. 17.9). Four bands of silicone rubber were linked to a pointer and maintained under slight tension by a counterweight. The strips elongated as they absorbed vapour and so moved the pointer across the scale. The length of the strips was also affected by humidity and temperature so that compensation devices had to be included. The 'Narkotest' gave a

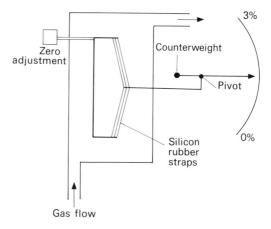

Fig. 17.9. Drager 'Narkotest' halothane analyser.

linear response to cyclopropane, fluroxene, enflurane, diethyl ether, halothane and methoxyflurane
but it was also affected by nitrous oxide, a 70%
mixture of N_2O in O_2 yielding a reading of about
0.3%. When this gas was used with an anaesthetic
vapour the zero had to be adjusted with the
N_2O/O_2 mixture (Lowe & Hagler, 1971; White &
Wardley-Smith, 1972). Normal concentrations of
O_2 had little effect on the instrument.

SPECIFIC METHODS

Magnetic susceptibility

Because of their molecular structure gases may be
influenced by a magnetic field. Most gases are
repelled from the field and are called diamagnetic.
Only two common gases, oxygen and nitric oxide,
are strongly paramagnetic (i.e. attracted into a
magnetic field). However, the paramagnetism displayed by oxygen is so characteristic that methods
based on this property have been incorporated in
this section on specific methods of analysis.

The analyser consists of a cell containing the
pole pieces of a permanent magnet. Suspended
within the non-homogeneous magnetic field are
two small glass spheres connected by a short bridge
to a taut wire suspension. The spheres are filled
with a weakly-diamagnetic gas such as nitrogen and
are free to rotate though the suspension tends to
return the spheres to a position in the strongest
part of the magnetic field. When the molecules of a
paramagnetic gas such as oxygen enter the cell they
are attracted to the centre of the magnetic field and
so displace the glass spheres to a zone where the
magnetic field is weaker. Since the spheres are fixed
by the vertical suspension the only movement open
to them is rotation against the torsion of the
vertical wire. The displacing force exerted by the
oxygen molecules is related to the number of
molecules present so that the new position of the
glass spheres is determined by the concentration of
oxygen present in the cell.

In the simplest instrument, such as that described by Pauling *et al.* (1946), the rotation of the
sensing element is detected by shining a light onto
a small mirror attached to the bridge joining the

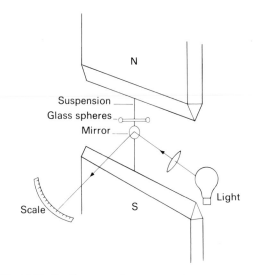

Fig. 17.10. Pauling type of paramagnetic oxygen
analyser.

spheres to the suspension (Fig. 17.10). The resulting light spot is directed onto a translucent scale
calibrated from 0 to 100% O_2. This instrument is
relatively delicate and the accuracy is limited by
the nonlinearities introduced by variations in the
strength of the magnetic field and by the mechanical suspension. More accurate readings are obtained by returning the sensing element to its zero
position by an electrical method. In one instrument
an electrical current from a constant voltage source
is fed into a small coil of wire which is mechanically linked to its sensing element (Fig. 17.11). The
current passing through this coil is gradually increased by a helical potentiometer until the turning
moment produced by the coil in the magnetic field
exactly opposes the turning moment produced by
the gas. The zero position is detected by a beam of
light shining onto a small mirror attached to the
sensing element and reflected onto a translucent
screen with a zero marking. The helipot is calibrated in term of oxygen percentage and can be
read to an accuracy of 0.1% O_2 (Nunn *et al.* 1964).
In a more recent instrument the movement of the
light beam reflected from the mirror is detected by
two photocells (Fig. 17.12). Displacement of the
mirror causes an imbalance between the amount of
light received by the photocells and this alters their

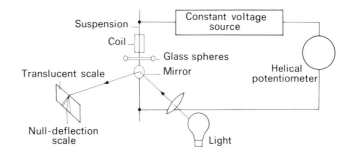

Fig. 17.11. Null-deflection type analyser.

electrical outputs. The difference in output from the two cells is amplified and fed back to the coil, so returning the sensing element to its zero position. The current passing through the coil is directly related to the turning moment produced by the paramagnetic gas and can be displayed on a meter which can be calibrated in terms of oxygen concentration. Two scales are provided: 0–25% O_2 and 0–100% O_2, the discrimination between readings being 0.25% O_2 and 1% O_2, respectively.

In fact, the accuracy of the analyser is much greater than that displayed by the meter and by recording the electrical output on a digital voltmeter it is possible to achieve a degree of accuracy which is probably far in excess of that obtainable on a standard Haldane apparatus (Ellis & Nunn, 1968).

Paramagnetic analysers are affected by the presence of high concentrations of a diamagnetic background gas. For accurate work it is therefore necessary to set the zero point with 100% background gas (e.g. N_2 or N_2O) and then to set the span with 100% O_2. However, small concentrations of a diamagnetic gas (such as carbon dioxide

in expired air) have an insignificant effect on the reading. Another source of error is the presence of water vapour in the gas to be analysed. It has been recommended that all gases should be dried by passage through a tube of silica gel before entering the cell. However, when nitrous oxide is present in the gas mixture it appears to be adsorbed onto the drying medium so that a variable reading is obtained. When working with respired gas it is better to saturate both the calibration gases and the gases to be analysed by passing them over water at room temperature. The cell is then dried by flushing with dry gas when the analyses have been completed.

Conventional paramagnetic analysers have a slow response and are affected by external vibration, excessive flow rate or pressurization of the cell (e.g. by mechanical ventilation). These disadvantages have now been overcome by a new design based on the pneumatic bridge principle (Merilainen, 1988). The device consists of two tubes which are connected by a T-piece to a common suction pump (Fig. 17.13). The sample to be analysed is fed into one tube and the reference gas (air) into the other.

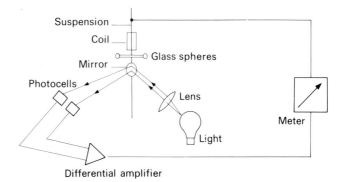

Fig. 17.12. Direct reading type of paramagnetic oxygen analyser utilizing photocells to detect deviations from the zero position of the glass sensing element.

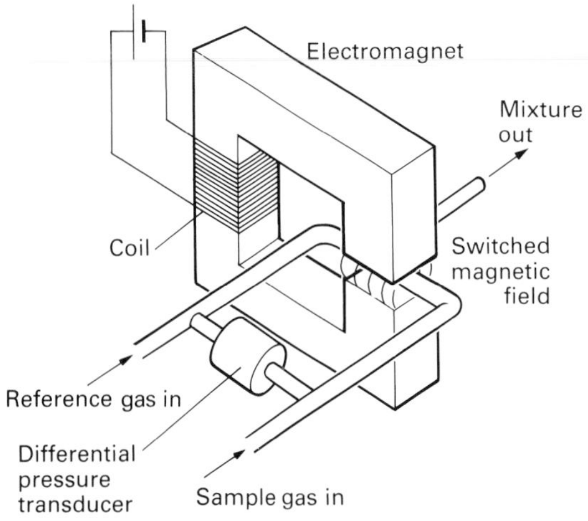
Electromagnet
Mixture out
Coil
Switched magnetic field
Reference gas in
Differential pressure transducer
Sample gas in

Fig. 17.13. Rapid paramagnetic oxygen analyser. The gas to be analysed (sample) and a reference gas (air) are sucked through a T-piece surrounded by an electromagnet. The difference in pressure in the two tubes caused by the attraction of oxygen molecules into the magnetic field is sensed by the differential pressure transducer. (After Merilainen, 1990.)

The T-piece is surrounded by an electromagnet which is switched on and off with a frequency of 110 Hz. When the magnetic field is switched on it creates pressure differences along the two horizontal limbs of the T which are related to the paramagnetic susceptibilities of the sample and reference gases. If the susceptibilities are known, the proportion of oxygen in the sample and reference gases can be determined from the difference in pressure measured at the proximal ends of the two tubes. The difference in pressure is extremely small (about 30 μbar, for a 100% O_2 difference) and is therefore measured with a miniature microphone which is much more sensitive than a conventional pressure transducer. Changes in temperature produce complex effects on the performance of the device so the sensing unit is maintained at a constant temperature. Vibrational effects produced by the magnet and external sources have been overcome by careful mechanical design and construction whilst alternations in pressure due to mechanical ventilation have been minimized by incorporating a pneumatic filter in the sensor. There is a small N_2O effect (equivalent to -1.5% with 100% N_2O), whilst the water vapour effect has been overcome by using sample tubing which is selectively permeable to water vapour and so enables the sampled gas to equilibrate with the humidity of ambient air. The device is linear, very stable and has a response time of less than 150 ms with a sample flow rate of 100 $ml \cdot min^{-1}$. Another device using a variation of the paramagnetic principle is described on p. 240.

Emission of electromagnetic radiation

If suitably excited, all gases will emit electromagnetic radiation in some part of the ultraviolet, visible or infrared portions of the spectrum, the 'neon sign' being a common example of this phenomenon. This principle has been used in a number of gas analysers, but the only instrument available commercially is the nitrogen meter (Daniels *et al.* 1975). This is used in such tests of respiratory function as the single-breath method of measuring anatomical dead space and closing volume, and the nitrogen washout test for assessing the distribution of ventilation.

A powerful suction pump draws the gas sample through a fine needle valve (placed close to the patient) to a gas discharge tube (Fig. 17.14). Two electrodes are sealed into the ends of this tube and a potential of about 1500–2000 V is applied. This ionizes the gas, which glows, the wavelengths of the radiation emitted being characteristic of the gas. A reflector placed behind the tube directs the light through a filter onto a photoelectric cell. This cell produces a current which is proportional to the intensity of the radiation falling on it, and this current is then amplified and displayed on a meter.

The great advantage of the N_2 meter is its specificity and rapid response. The transit time from needle valve to discharge tube and the time required to wash out the tube are minimized by the reduction in pressure in the system and the delay time and response time are accordingly very short, the total delay being in the order of 20–40 ms.

Unfortunately, the light output from the gas discharge tube is not directly proportional to the concentration of the gas and linearizing circuits have to be added. This makes the machine expensive.

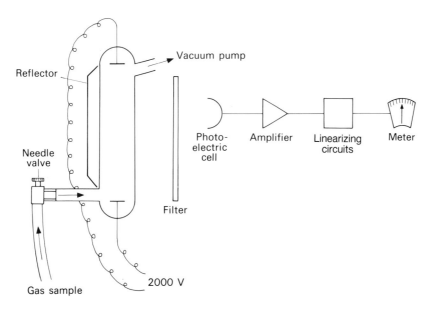

Fig. 17.14. A nitrogen meter.

Absorption of radiation

All gases absorb electromagnetic radiation in either the infrared or ultraviolet regions of the spectrum. The wavelengths are specific for each gas and depend on the molecular configuration (see Chapter 8).

Infrared gas analysers. Infrared radiation in the range 1–15 μm is absorbed by all gases with two or more atoms in the molecule provided these atoms are dissimilar. Thus O_2 does not absorb infrared radiation but CO does.

The instruments utilizing this analytical principle may be classified as *dispersive* or *non-dispersive*.

The infrared spectrophotometer is an example of the dispersive type of analyser. In this instrument radiation from an infrared source passes through a prism or diffraction grating and is so dispersed that the radiations of different wavelengths are arranged in sequence. If now the gas to be analysed is placed in the path of the radiation it will absorb maximally in one or more regions of the spectrum. By scanning the whole spectrum a graph of absorption against wavelength can be plotted. Alternatively, the absorption at a particular wavelength can be studied. This type of instrument is versatile and

can readily be adjusted for measurements on different gases which have different absorption spectra (see Chapter 8).

If interest is centred on only one gas the non-dispersive type of analyser is usually employed (Mogue & Rantala, 1988). In this instrument (Fig. 17.15) light from an infrared source (yielding a wide range of wavelengths) is directed down two tubes whose ends are sealed with a substance which transmits infrared radiation. The gas sample to be analysed is aspirated through the analysis cell, whilst the remainder of the tube on this side, and the reference tube, is flushed with air or other background gas. The gas in the analysis cell absorbs a small proportion of the infrared radiation and the strength of the radiation reaching the detector is therefore less than that impinging on the detector on the reference side.

The Luft type of detector (so-named after the originator) was commonly used. This consisted of two chambers containing the gas or vapour to be analysed. The gas in the chamber also absorbed the infrared radiation, and was therefore heated. This caused the gas to expand. The detector on the reference side received more radiation than that on the analysis side and the difference in pressure in

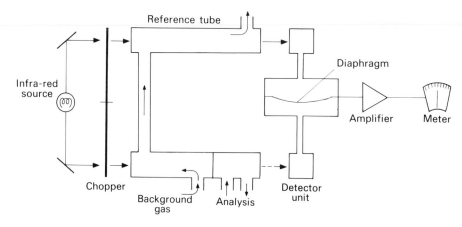

Fig. 17.15. Infrared analyser using Luft-type detector unit.

the two chambers was measured by recording the deflection of the elastic membrane separating them. This part of the detector was therefore a pressure transducer, the capacitance principle being most commonly used. To prevent drift due to slow heating of the detector cells the light from the infrared source was 'chopped' by a rotating shutter so that it cycled on and off at a frequency of 25–100 Hz. This produced an alternating output from the transducer which was then amplified and displayed.

Unfortunately, there are several sources of error with infrared analysis. In the first place there is often some overlap in the absorption wavebands of different gases. For instance, the fundamental absorption bands for carbon dioxide, nitrous oxide, and carbon monoxide are at 4.3, 4.5 and 4.7 μm, respectively. The absorption spectrum of each gas is in fact quite complex, centred about the fundamental wavelength, so that overlap is inevitable. As a result, a CO_2 analyser given a sample containing both CO_2 and N_2O will read high, since the N_2O will absorb some infrared energy *within* the absorption bandwidth for CO_2. This error can be overcome by narrowing the absorption band by special optical filters, or by filling the analyser (except the cuvette) with N_2O, so that no energy within the N_2O absorption band reaches the Luft detector.

A second error arises from the phenomenon of 'collision broadening' (also called 'pressure broad-

ening') in which the absorption spectrum of one gas (i.e. CO_2) is actually *widened* by the physical presence of certain other gases such as N_2, N_2O or C_3H_6, so that absorption is increased. Collision broadening is not altogether prevented by the 'background gas filter' method. Correction factors for different concentrations of N_2O and CO_2 have been published (Kennell *et al.* 1973), but the simplest method of eliminating this error is to calibrate the instrument with gas mixtures which contain the same background gas concentration as that to be analysed.

Since this type of analyser detects the *number* of molecules of absorbent gas in the cuvette, it is really a partial pressure detector, so that changes in atmospheric pressure will alter the reading for a given gas. Frequent calibration checks are therefore necessary to minimize errors from this source. Alternatively, the analyser can be calibrated in partial pressure terms by calculating the P_{CO_2} of the calibrating gas. Errors due to changes in atmospheric pressure will then be minimal. Errors may also be produced by the pressurization of a breathing system by mechanical ventilation or by aspirating the sample through a needle or other orifice with a high resistance. To ensure accuracy it is essential to calibrate the instrument with the intended sampling system in place and then to ensure that the sampling flow rate does not vary.

Modern CO_2 analysers designed for clinical use are very stable but should be subjected to a three-point calibration at regular intervals. It is also important to check the speed of response, for a slow response may result in a failure to reach the true maximum and minimum values at normal breathing frequencies. With the long sample tubes and relatively low sampling rates (less than 500 ml·min^{-1}) used clinically, there will inevitably be a long delay between a square wave change in the composition of the sampled gas and the commencement of the analyser response. However the 90 or 95% rise time should be less than 150 ms to ensure accuracy at normal breathing frequencies. A slower response is usually due to a low sample flow rate caused by blockage in the sampling line due to condensation of water or aspiration of sputum, or to suction pump failure. Most analysers now include a water trap in the sample line and provision is usually made to flush out the cell and sample line if contamination occurs. Some analysers utilize special sampling tubes which are impermeable to gases but permeable to water vapour, so that the humidity of the aspirated gas equilibrates with that of the atmosphere during its passage to the analysis cell.

In modern infrared analysers the infrared radiation is detected by special photocells and the effect of nitrous oxide is minimized by providing an electrical offset operated by a push-button control. The offset provides a reasonable correction when the nitrous oxide is present at the appropriate concentration (usually 70%) but may not be correct at other concentrations. Recently introduced instruments provide a simultaneous breath-by-breath analysis of CO_2, N_2O and the volatile agents, and correct for the problem of interference by using microprocessor technology. Because of differences in the magnitude of absorption two analysis cells are usually used, one for CO_2/N_2O and one for the volatile agents, but since the latter are all analysed at 3.9 μm it is necessary to switch the analyser to the appropriate vapour before use. Most commercial machines are reasonably stable and accurate if warmed up for some minutes before use, but it is a wise precaution to check the calibration at regular intervals using the compressed gas canisters provided by the manufacturers. It should also be remembered that other exhaled vapours, such as ethyl alcohol or cyclopropane, may cause errors with measured vapour concentrations (Foley et al. 1990).

The problem of sampling delay is overcome in some instruments by siting the analysis cell in the airway. Modern 'flow-through cells' have a relatively small dead space, but they are liable to sustain damage by being dropped on the floor.

The accuracy of most analysers is about $\pm 0.1\%$ in the range 0–10% CO_2 although the accuracy of an analyser can be improved tenfold with appropriate modifications (Cormack & Powell, 1972).

Very high resolution analysers are also available for measuring gas concentrations in the parts-per-million (p.p.m.) range required for monitoring gas pollution in operating theatres.

Laser analysers. A number of organic compounds absorb strongly at 3.39 μm which is the wavelength omitted by a helium–neon gas laser. By utilizing the intense, narrow beam generated by the laser it is possible to make the sample cell long and narrow, so that very high sensitivity is easily achieved. A reference beam and the 'sample' beam are chopped alternately by a rotating shutter, and directed onto a photocell so that the intensity of the two beams can be compared. The method has been used for the analysis of trace quantities of ethyl alcohol in expired air and is fast enough to follow breath-by-breath variations in end-tidal CO_2.

Photoacoustic spectroscopy (PAS). This technique, which is based on the absorption of infrared radiation, has only recently been applied to the analysis of anaesthetic gases and vapours.

The gas sample (about 90 ml·min^{-1}) is drawn into a measurement chamber through a flow regulator so that the sample flow is independent of airway pressure. Light from an infrared source is reflected by a mirror and passed through a chopper wheel to a window in the measurement chamber (Fig. 17.16). The chopper wheel contains three concentric bands of windows, each band passing pulses of radiation at a different frequency. Radiation from each band is focused on one of the three optical filters on the front of the measuring

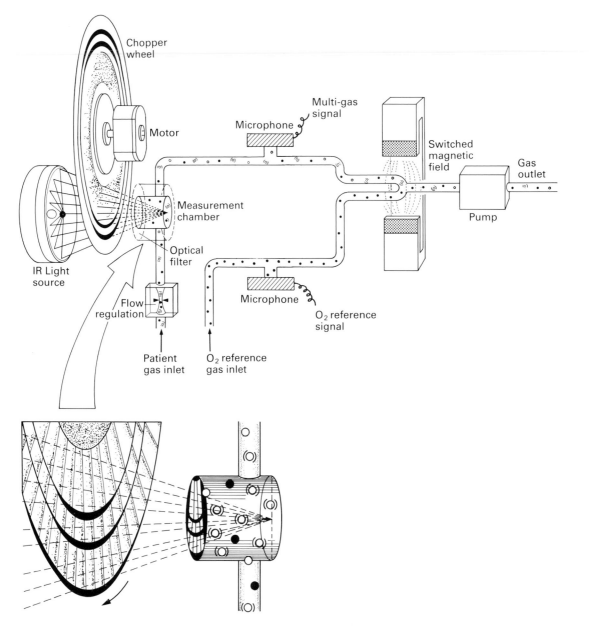

Fig. 17.16. Photoacoustic and magnetoacoustic analyser. Infrared radiation passes through a chopper wheel with three concentric frequency bands to a measuring cell. Radiation from each frequency band is focused onto an appropriate optical filter on the front of the measuring cell, so that the sample to be analysed is exposed to three beams of radiation each having a characteristic wavelength and frequency. The pulses of radiation produce an audio signal due to expansion and contraction of each gas species and the amplitude of each signal is related to the concentration of gas or anaesthetic agent present. The signal is detected by a sensitive microphone which also detects the oxygen signal originating from the pulsed magnetic field. The latter is compared with the signal from the microphone on the reference gas line. (From instruction manual by permission of Brüel & Kjær.)

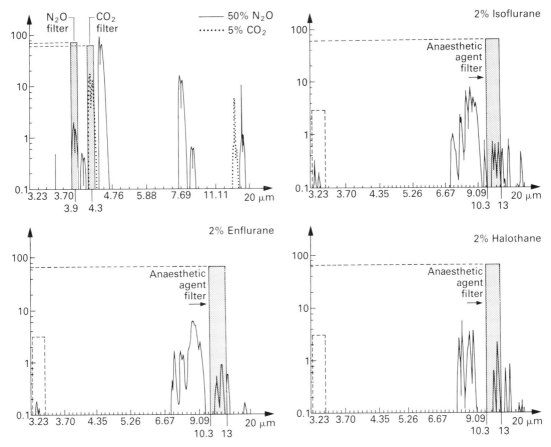

Fig. 17.17. Infra-red absorption spectra for CO_2, N_2O, isoflurane, enflurane and halothane. The identity of the anaesthetic agent must be keyed into the analyser. Note that the filter for the inhalational agent transmits in the range $10.3-13\,\mu m$ where the absorption characteristics of halothane, enflurane and isoflurane are similar. (From instruction manual by permission of Brüel & Kjær.)

chamber so that the gas mixture inside the chamber is exposed to three beams of radiation each with a characteristic frequency and wavelength. The wavelengths selected are $3.9\,\mu m$ for N_2O and $4.3\,\mu m$ for CO_2 whilst the anaesthetic agent filter transmits over a band from 10.3 to $13\,\mu m$ where there is greater absorption than at the shorter wavelengths used in other infrared analysers (Fig. 17.17). The pulses of radiation are absorbed by the components of the mixture to be analysed and create changes of pressure in the measurement cell as they expand and contract. The amplitude of the pressure pulse depends on the concentration of the gas or vapour present whilst the identity of the component can be determined from the frequen-

cies of pulsation assigned to each wavelength. The complex audio signal generated by the expansion and contraction of the gases present is detected by a sensitive microphone, subjected to filtering to identify the signal due to each component of the mixture and then subjected to further processing which fits an 'envelope' over the sine waves to enable the breath-by-breath changes in gas composition to be recorded (Fig. 17.18).

One of the advantages claimed for PAS is that the amount of energy absorbed by the gas is measured directly by measuring the sound energy produced whereas in conventional infrared analysers the absorption is measured indirectly by comparing the light transmitted through the mea-

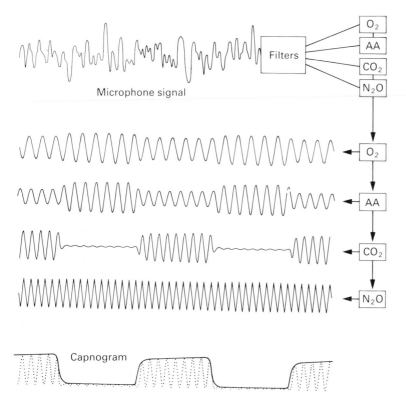

Microphone signal

Capnogram

Fig. 17.18. Photoacoustic analyser. The multi-gas signal from the microphone is subjected to filtering so that the amplitude of the signal resulting from each component can be identified. Further signal processing then superimposes an envelope around the peaks of the sine waves so that real-time traces of concentration are produced. (From instruction manual by permission of Brüel & Kjær.)

suring cell with light transmitted through a cell containing the reference gas. The PAS system thus has greater zero and gain stability, recalibration being required only at 3-monthly intervals. The 10–90% response time is quoted as less than 300 ms for the gas and anaesthetic agents so that the instrument should prove satisfactory for breath-by-breath measurements at adult respiratory frequencies.

Magnetoacoustic spectroscopy (MAS). Since oxygen does not absorb infrared radiation, it cannot be analyzed by the PAS technique. Simultaneous oxygen analysis is therefore performed using a magnetoacoustic technique. This is based on the paramagnetic property of oxygen (i.e. that molecules are attracted into a magnetic field). The gas mixture leaving the measurement cell passes through an electromagnet which is pulsed with an alternating current (a.c.) current at a frequency which differs from that used to identify the other components of the mixture (Fig. 17.16). The

alternating compression and expansion of the gas molecules within the electromagnet generates an audio signal the magnitude of which depends on the concentration of oxygen in the mixture. This signal is detected by the microphone used to detect the other gases and processed in a similar manner. However, to improve tha accuracy of the measurement this signal is continously compared with that from another microphone which measures the changes in pressure in a reference gas (air).

Ultraviolet gas analysers. A number of gases such as hydrogen, oxygen and nitrogen do not absorb in the infrared region of the spectrum but have characteristic absorption patterns in the ultraviolet region. However the greatest use for this method has been in the analysis of halothane which has a useful absorption band in the region of 200 nm. Ultraviolet light from a mercury lamp is filtered and passed through the analysis chamber to a photocell (Fig. 17.19). The output from this cell is compared with a similar reference photocell (to

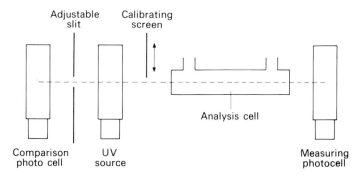

Fig. 17.19. Ultraviolet gas analyser.

minimize errors due to changes in the output from the lamp) and is then amplified and displayed on a meter. The accuracy obtainable is about ±0.2% in the range 0–5% halothane (Robinson *et al.* 1962). Halothane decomposes to a certain extent when exposed to the intense radiation from the mercury lamp so it must not be returned to the circuit. Similar considerations apply to trichloroethylene which can also be analysed by this technique. A rapid response halothane analyser suitable for use with small sample flow rates has also been described (Tatnall *et al.* 1978).

Mass spectrometry

Mass spectrometers are capable of separating the components of complex gas mixtures according to their mass and charge by deflecting the charged ions in a magnetic field. There are basically two types of mass spectrometer, the magnetic sector type and the quadrupole.

Magnetic sector mass spectrometer. The earliest mass spectrometers built for medical purposes were of this type (Fowler & Hugh-Jones, 1957). A gas sample of about 25 ml·min⁻¹ is aspirated continously through the sampling catheter and a small proportion of this sample is drawn into an evacuated ionization chamber through a molecular leak. In this chamber the molecules are bombarded by a transverse beam of electrons. The charged ions then diffuse out of a slit in the chamber wall and are accelerated by a plate to which a negative voltage is applied. The stream of ions passes out through a hole in this plate and comes under the influence of a magnetic field whose lines of force run at right angles to the stream of ions. The magnetic field deflects the ions according to their mass: charge ratio. Since most ions carry a single charge the separation is effectively governed by the mass of the ions, the lightest ions being deflected most and the heaviest least. This results in a fan-like series of beams of ions of different molecular weight (Fig. 17.20).

The position of the deflected beams may be altered by changing the velocity of the ions entering the magnetic field; this is achieved by varying the accelerating voltage on the plate. It is thus possible to direct each beam of ions across the detector unit in turn. The detector measures the rate at which ions impinge on it so that a measure of gas partial pressure is obtained. By relating the detector output on the *y*-axis to the accelerating voltage on the *x*-axis it is possible to display a mass spectrum on an oscilloscope screen (Fig. 17.21). The height of the peaks then represents the concentration of each gas whilst the position of the peak on the *x*-axis identifies the mass number of each peak.

Quadrupole mass spectrometer. The magnetic sector instrument is now being replaced by the quadrupole analyser, which is smaller and lighter. Furthermore, the balance between sensitivity and resolving power (ability to differentiate different masses) can be adjusted easily to suit a particular application.

As in the magnetic sector instrument a beam of ions is accelerated out of an ionization chamber. The ions then pass through the quadrupole mass filter. This consists of four parallel cylindrical rods

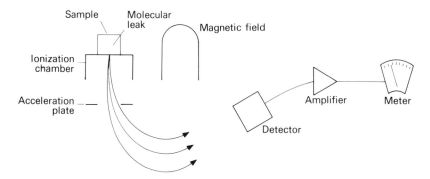

Fig. 17.20. Magnetic sector type of mass spectrometer.

(each about 0.5 cm in diameter and 5 cm long), the opposite pairs being electrically connected. A standing d.c. voltage is applied to the rods and a radio-frequency a.c. component is then applied to the opposite pairs (Fig. 17.22).

By adjusting this frequency it is possible to filter out all the ions except those with a particular mass:charge ratio and these then pass down the filter to the detector at the opposite end of the filter. All the other ions undergo increasing oscillations and eventually hit the rods and lose their charge. By varying the voltage applied to the plate it is possible to scan the mass spectrum and so to determine the proportions of various masses present in the gas mixture.

Mass spectrometers are relatively bulky and expensive, although the introduction of specialized quadrupole machines for particular applications has greatly reduced both their size and cost. They have a very short response time (about 100 ms for

a 95% response) and they require very small sample flow rates (about 20 ml·min^{-1} for normal respiratory work). The sample flow rates can be greatly reduced if a rapid response is not required; indeed the instrument can be used to measure blood gases by sampling the gases which diffuse into the interior of a thin Teflon catheter inserted into a blood vessel. However, there are still many practical problems in the application of this technique. All mass spectrometers operate under conditions of very high vacuum and it takes some time for the various pumping systems to achieve the required working pressures. When these have been achieved the pumps must run continously. Water vapour condensation in the sampling tube is prevented by heating the tube but the response time for water vapour is often longer than that for other gases and vapours. Another problem is that some molecules may lose two electrons without disintegrating and so become doubly charged. They then

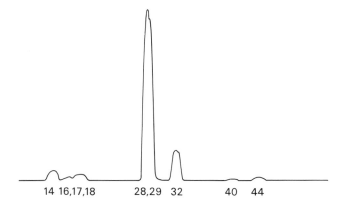

Fig. 17.21. Mass spectrum of room air. Concentration is on the vertical axis and mass/charge ratio along the abcissa. The large N_2 and O_2 peaks occur at 28 and 32. The other peaks are due to doubly- charged O_2 at 16, water vapour at 18. Ar at 40 and CO_2 at 44.

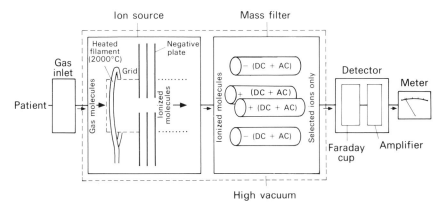

Fig. 17.22. Quadrupole type of mass spectrometer.

behave like ions with half the mass. Some fragmentation of molecules also occurs in the ionization process resulting in the production of a mass spectrum rather than a single peak for each molecule. These secondary peaks can usually be recognized easily and can often be used to advantage. For example in anaesthesia it would be impossible to separate CO_2 from N_2O since the parent peak of each occurs at 44 daltons. However, nitrous oxide produces a strong secondary peak which is about 30% of the parent peak height at 30 daltons and carbon dioxide produces a secondary peak at 12 daltons. Since the ratio of secondary peaks to parent peaks remains reasonably constant these can be used to determine the concentrations of the two gases in a mixture. In most instruments the spectrum is scanned 25 times per second so that it is possible to produce a continuous record of the changing concentration of any gas. Commonly a mass spectrometer can provide a continous record of the changing concentrations of up to eight separate gases. These are selected by tuning the analyser to the appropriate peaks on the mass spectrum and then setting the zero and gain controls of each channel of the recorder to provide the appropriate scale on the recording.

Raman scattering

The Raman effect was first observed in 1928 and was widely used for spectroscopy in the ensuing decade. Its use declined in the 1940s when high speed infrared detectors were developed but there has recently been a renewal of interest in the technique due to the ready availability of cheaper lasers and the need for rapid analysis of multi-gas mixtures.

When light interacts with gas molecules two types of scattering occur. In the first, Rayleigh scattering, the light is scattered without energy loss or alteration of frequency. In the second, Raman scattering, the photon gives up a portion of its energy to the gas molecule and is re-emitted with a longer wavelength, shifted frequency and lower energy. The extent of the frequency shift depends on the vibrational and rotational energy of the gas molecule which is specific to the gas. Thus the frequency components present in scattered light permit identification of the gas species present whilst the amplitude of the peaks in the spectrum provides an approximate indication of the concentrations of each gas or vapour molecule present. Some gases (e.g. N_2O and CO_2) have more than one peak whilst the non-overlapping peaks of halothane, enflurane and isoflurane differ markedly in height, the amplitude of the halothane peak being much larger than those of the other two vapours when equal concentrations are present. The peak for water vapour does not interfere with the other peaks of interest.

The intensity of the scattered light is less than 1 millionth of the incident light so an argon laser is used to provide an intense monochromatic light source. The scattered light passes through a

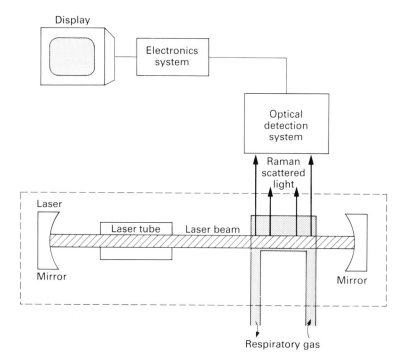

Fig. 17.23. Components of a Raman spectrometer.

number of interference filters to photomultiplier detectors which enable up to eight molecular species to be identified simultaneously (Fig. 17.23). The response time of the instrument is less than 100 ms (so that it can be used to provide accurate breath-by-breath analysis in children) and calibration is automatic. The accuracy appears to be perfectly adequate for clinical purposes and the gases are not altered by passage through the instrument so that they can be returned to the breathing system (Van Wagenen *et al.* 1986). A commercially available instrument is small enough to be used in the operating theatre and the price is somewhat less than that of a mass spectrometer having a similar specification. However, current instruments require a great deal of electrical power (Westenskow *et al.* 1989a,b).

Gas chromatography

This is a contraction for the term gas–liquid chromatography. The use of the word chromatography to describe the process of separating colourless gas or vapour mixtures into their constituents

is derived from the older technique of liquid–liquid chromatography, in which the separated components were identified by their natural colours, or by colours produced by chemical treatment.

The principle used to achieve separation of the components of a mixture is that of partition chromatography: this is based on the fact that molecules of a solute partition between two solvents in a way that reflects the balance of attractive and repulsive forces between solute and solvent. In the gas–liquid chromatograph one solvent is absorbed onto an inert material such as firebrick granules or a diatomaceous earth. This constitutes the stationary phase and is packed into a narrow, stainless steel or glass tube (up to 2 m long) to form the chromatographic column. The second solvent is a stream of gas, such as helium, nitrogen or argon, which flows through the column at a rate of about 50 ml·min^{-1}. The mixture to be analysed is injected as a bolus into this stream of carrier gas and its constituents then partition between the two solvents as the mixture is carried down the column (Fig. 17.24). Components which have a high volatility or low solubility in the stationary phase are

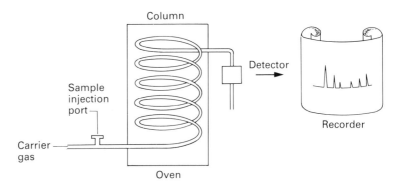

Fig. 17.24. Gas chromatography. The sample is injected into a stream of carrier gas and passes over a column which separates the species in the sample which thus arrive at the detector in sequence. If good separation has been achieved the concentration of each species will be related to the height of the peak.

eluted before the less volatile or more soluble compounds and so are the first to appear at the outlet of the column. The various components of the mixture thus emerge at varying time intervals after the injection and pass to a non-specific detector unit which yields an electronic signal proportional to the quantity of each substance present.

When the substance is a gas or vapour at room temperature it is injected directly into the stream of carrier gas. In order to ensure than an accurately known volume of gas is delivered into the system it is a common practice to use a special gas sampling valve to isolate a known volume of gas before injection. When the substance is a liquid it is necessary to heat part or all of the column to volatilize the components of the mixture. It is also often necessary to heat the column to ensure that the stationary phase is a liquid when the column is in use. For this reason the column is usually enclosed in a thermostatically controlled oven.

Columns are of two main types: the packed columns already mentioned, and open tubular columns in which the liquid phase is deposited on the wall of the tube. The latter have a high resolving power (i.e. produce good separation of the components of the mixture), but the packed columns are cheaper and easier to work with and have a much greater sample capacity, i.e. permit more samples to be analysed before the column has to be changed. The liquid phase is usually a wax or gum with a carbon or silicon base. The column filling must be free from absorptive or catalytic sites and is usually acid-washed and treated with a special blocking agent to prevent such action.

The temperature of the column is of great importance. As the temperature is increased beyond the melting point of the stationary phase, the partition is pushed towards the gaseous phase. This shortens the retention time of the compound (the interval between the injection and the peak of the signal on the detector). It is quite common for two components of a mixture to have widely different retention times, so increasing the duration of each analysis. To overcome this problem most modern instruments have facilities for temperature programming. The temperature is maintained at a constant level for a preset period after injection and then programmed to rise at a finite rate to a maximum value. This method may also be used to separate two substances which have a similar solubility in the liquid phase, but different volatility.

Unfortunately, temperature programming may give rise to the troublesome phenomenon of 'column bleed', in which small amounts of the liquid phase volatilize and pass to the detector. At constant temperature and carrier gas flow rate this effect gives rise to a constant background current which can be offset electronically. However, when the temperature is increased the effect is more pronounced and leads to a constantly shifting baseline.

The first essential, then, is to choose the most appropriate column for the mixture to be analysed and to arrange the temperature programming so that each constituent in the mixture arrives at the end of the column over a narrow time interval which is clearly separated from each of the other constituents. It is then necessary to record the quantity and identity of each component present.

These are the functions of the detector. Many different types of detector are used for this purpose but all are non-specific; that is they produce a signal proportional to the quantity of the substance present but they are incapable of identifying the substance. The choice of detector is governed by the nature of the substances being analysed.

Perhaps the simplest detector is the *thermal conductivity* or katharometer detector (p. 228). The detector consists of a heated resistance wire which forms part of a Wheatstone bridge. When a gas with a thermal conductivity different from that of the carrier gas passes the detector there will be a difference in the amount of heat conducted away from the wire. As a result its temperature will change and so will its resistance. This change in resistance unbalances the bridge and produces a signal which can be amplified and displayed on a chart recorder. This type of detector is chiefly used when inorganic gases such as oxygen, nitrogen, carbon dioxide and nitrous oxide are being analysed. Since the thermal conductivity of helium differs widely from the other inorganic gases (Table 17.1) it is often used as a carrier gas in such situations.

The *flame ionization detector* is commonly employed when trace amounts of organic vapours have to be analysed. The detector contains a small flame produced by hydrogen burning in air and the carrier gas emerging from the column is fed into this flame. The presence of an organic component results in the production of positive ions which are then attracted to a charged collecting electrode. The resulting ionization current is detected and fed to a suitable amplifier and recorder. This type of detector is widely used, gives a linear response over a wide range of concentrations, is very sensitive and has a small background current. The detector responds to all compounds containing carbon and has the added advantage of not being affected by water vapour.

The *electron-capture detector* is used for the selective analysis of organic compounds containing electron-capturing atoms such as a halogen. The detector consists of a small chamber containing a radioisotope which emits beta-radiation, i.e. nega-

tively charged electrons. A small voltage is applied to the collector electrode (anode) and the resulting current (carried by the electron stream) detected and amplified. When electron-capturing molecules pass through the detector, some of the electrons are 'captured', and so fail to reach the anode. The reduction in current can then be recorded. The detector is very sensitive but the output is only linear over a narrow range of concentrations. It is particularly useful when measuring anaesthetic agents in blood, for these are commonly extracted into heptane before being injected into the chromatograph. Heptane tends to produce a wide peak which masks the smaller halothane peak when the flame ionization detector is used, but this problem does not arise with the electron capture detector.

Many other forms of detector have been used for specific purposes but perhaps one of the most powerful analytical tools is provided by a combination of a gas chromatograph with a mass spectrometer. The latter instrument can identify the molecular fragments present in any component eluted from a chromatograph column and so greatly aid identification of an unusual compound.

However, in normal practice it is still necessary to identify the source of the deflection produced by the non-specific detector. When analysing known mixtures identification can usually be performed by determining the retention time for each constituent of the mixture and identifying the peaks on this basis. It is then necessary to quantify the amount of each substance present, for the response of the detector varies with the substance. One way of calibrating the deflection is to inject a known quantity of each of the substances being analysed and to relate these to the deflections produced. However, the injection of small quantities (often in the microlitre range) is not very accurate and it is therefore wise to incorporate an internal standard into each sample. This standard must have characteristics similar to those of the constituents of the sample but must be readily identifiable and must not interfere with the other components of the mixture. The inclusion of such a standard obviates errors due to changes in column conditions, gas flow or amplifier gain and greatly improves the accuracy of the technique. If the column has once been calibrated for this internal standard and the test substance, the concentration of the latter can be derived.

The electrical output of a detector is proportional to the mass of the substance passing through the detector at that instant. If the sample size is fixed, concentrations can be derived. The output appears as a deflection from the baseline, and if this is drawn on paper moving at constant speed, the area between the curve and the base line is proportional to the total mass of that compound in the sample. If the chromatographic separation is good, the deflection has an abrupt onset, short duration, and abrupt termination, and appears as a peak. Under these conditions, the peak bears a close approximation to a triangle, and the area can be found as:

$$\frac{\text{half height}}{\text{base}}$$

or, more commonly, height times width at half height (since the base may be distorted by contaminants). If the base is always the same, then the peak height alone is proportional to area, and is an acceptable simplification. However, where peaks are broad, area must be measured. This can be done mechanically or electronically.

The gas–liquid chromatograph may be used for purposes other than gas analysis. Thus, it can be used to analyse blood samples containing volatile or local anaesthetic agents (Wortley *et al.* 1968; Douglas *et al.* 1970; Jones *et al.* 1972). It is also widely used to measure the concentrations of other drugs such as the anticonvulsants, barbiturates and tranquillizers. For further references to the use of this technique readers are referred to Hill (1973) and Moore & McVittie (1978).

Electrochemical devices

Polarography. If two electrodes are connected by a buffered electrolyte and a potential of about 0.6 V is maintained between them, it is found that the current which flows is proportional to the concentration of oxygen present in the electrolyte. By imprisoning a thin layer of electrolyte under a membrane, the electrode can be made to respond to changes in oxygen concentration in the gas on the other side of the membrane (Adams & Hahn, 1987). This is the basis of the oxygen electrode described in Chapter 18. The technique can also be used to measure N_2O and halothane concentrations (Albery *et al.* 1978).

CO_2 electrodes. The concentration of CO_2 in gas may be measured by determining the change in pH within a thin layer of bicarbonate solution surrounding a pH-sensitive electrode (Chapter 18).

Galvanic cell. Galvanic cells convert energy from an oxidation–reduction chemical process into electrical energy. They are analogous to a primary cell in a battery though they differ from a battery in that the output is dependent on the oxygen concentration present. The chemical reaction uses up the components of the cell so that its life depends on the concentration of oxygen to which it is exposed and on the duration of exposure. Modern galvanic cell analysers for oxygen are compact, not affected by N_2O and reasonably accurate though the response is not fast enough to permit breath-by-breath measurements (Torda & Grant, 1972). Their life depends on the product of oxygen concentration and time and most of the modern cells may be expected to last for 6–12 months, under normal conditions of use.

Radioactive isotopes

Respired gases can be 'labelled' by incorporating radioactive isotopes in the mixture. This enables their fate in the body to be followed with great accuracy. There are many technical difficulties associated with this type of work, but the principle has now been widely used in respiratory physiology and has contributed greatly to our knowledge of the distribution of pulmonary ventilation and blood flow (see Chapter 10).

References

Adams, A.P. & Hahn, C.E.W. (1987) *Principles and practice of blood-gas analysis.* Churchill Livingstone, Edinburgh.

Albery, W.J., Brooks, W.N. Gibson, S.P. & Hahn, C.E.W. (1978) An electrode for P_{N_2O} and P_{O_2} analysis in blood and gas. *Journal of Applied Physiology: Respiratory, Exercise & Environmental Physiology* **45**, 637–643.

Campbell, E.J.M. (1960) Simplification of Haldane's apparatus for measuring CO_2 concentration in respired gases in clinical practice. *British Medical Journal* **i**, 457–464.

Cormack, R.S. & Powell, J.N. (1972) Improving the performance of the infra-red carbon dioxide meter. *British Journal of Anaesthesia* **44**, 131–141.

Daniels, A.U., Couvillon, L.A. & Lebrizzi, J.M. (1975) Evaluation of nitrogen analyzers. *American Review of Respiratory Disease* **712**, 571–575.

Douglas, R., Hill, D.W., & Wood, D.G.L. (1970) Methods for the estimation of blood halothane concentration by gas chromatography. *British Journal of Anaesthesia* **42**, 119–123.

Ellis, F.R., & Nunn, J.F. (1968) The measurement of gaseous oxygen tension utilizing paramagnetism: an evaluation of the 'Servomex' 0A 150 analyser. *British Journal of Anaesthesia* **40**, 569–577.

Faulconer, A. & Ridley, R.W. (1950) Continuous quantitative analysis of mixtures of oxygen, nitrous oxide and ether with or without nitrogen. *Anesthesiology* **11**, 265–278.

Fenn, W.O. & Rahn, H. (eds) (1964) *Handbook of physiology*, Section 3, *Respiration*, Vol. 1, Chapter 3. American Physiology Society, Washington DC.

Foley, M.A., Wood, P.R., Peel, W.J., Jones, G.M. & Lawler, P.G. (1990) The effect of exhaled alcohol on the performance of Datex Capnomac. *Anaesthesia* **45**, 232–234.

Fowler, K.T. & Hugh-Jones, P. (1957) Mass spectrometry applied to clinical practice and research. *British Medical Journal* **i**, 1205–1211.

Haldane, J.S. & Graham, J.I. (1935). *Methods of air analysis*, 4th edn. Griffin, London.

Herchl, R. (1970) The preparation of accurate standard mixtures of inhalation anaesthetic agents *Canadian Anaesthetists' Society Journal* **17**, 624–629.

Hill, D.W. (1961) The production of accurate gas and vapour mixtures. *British Journal of Applied Physics* **12**, 410–413.

Hill, D.W. (1963) Halothane concentrations obtained from a Drager 'Vapor' Vaporizer. *British Journal of Anaesthesia* **35**, 285–289.

Hill, D.W. (1973) *Electronic techniques in anaesthesia and surgery*, 2nd edn. Butterworth, London.

Hulands, G.H. & Nunn, J.F. (1970) Portable interference refractometers in anaesthesia. *British Journal of Anaesthesia* **42**, 1051–1059.

Jones, P.L. Molloy, M.J. & Rosen, M. (1972) A technique for the analysis of methoxyflurane in blood by gas chromatography. *British Journal of Anaesthesia,* **44**, 124–130.

Kennell, E.M., Andrews, R.W. & Wollman, H. (1973) Correction factors for nitrous oxide in the infrared analysis of carbon dioxide. *Anesthesiology* **39**, 441–443.

Lloyd, B.B. (1958) A development of Haldane's gas analysis apparatus. *Journal of Physiology* **143**, 5P.

Lowe, H. (1972) *Dose-regulated penthrane anaesthesia.* Abbott.

Lowe, H.J. & Hagler, K. (1971) Clinical and laboratory evaluation of an expired anesthetic gas monitor (Narko-Test). *Anesthesiology* **34**, 378–382.

Merilainen, P.T. (1988) A fast differential paramagnetic O_2 sensor. *International Journal of Clinical Monitoring and Computing* **5**, 187–195.

Merilainen, P.T. (1990) A differential paramagnetic sensor for breath-by-breath oximetry. *Journal of Clinical Monitoring* **6**, 65–73.

Mogue, L.R. & Rantala, B. (1988) Capnometers. *Journal of Clinical Monitoring* **4**, 115–121.

Molyneux, L. & Pask, E.A. (1959) A sonic analyser for anaesthetic vapours. *Anaesthesia* **14**, 191–195.

Moore, R.A. & McVittie, J.D. (1978) Gas–liquid chromatography. *British Journal of Clinical Equipment* **3**, 25–32.

Nunn, J.F., Bergman, N.A., Coleman, A.J. & Casselle, D.C. (1964) Evaluation of the Servomex paramagnetic oxygen analyser. *British Journal of Anaesthesia* **36**, 666–673.

Nunn, J.F., Gill, D. & Hulands, G.H. (1970) Apparatus for preparing saturated vapour concentrations of liquid anaesthetic agents. *Journal of Physics E* **3**, 331–333.

Owen-Thomas, J.B. & Meade, F. (1975) The estimation of carbon dioxide concentration in the presence of nitrous oxide, using a Lloyd–Haldane apparatus. *British Journal of Anaesthesia* **47**, 22–24.

Pauling, L., Wood, R.E. & Sturdivant, J.H. (1946) An instrument for determining the partial pressure of oxygen in a gas. *Journal of the American Chemical Society* **68**, 795–798.

Robinson, A., Denson, J.S. & Summers, F.W. (1962) Halothane analyzer. *Anesthesiology* **23**, 391–394.

Scholander, P.F. (1947) Analyser for accurate estimation of respiratory gases in one-half cubic centimetre samples. *Journal of Biological Chemistry* **167**, 235–250.

Stott, F.D. (1957) Sonic gas analyzer for measurement of CO_2 in expired air. *Review of Scientific Instruments* **28**, 914–915.

Sugg, B.R., Palayiwa, E., Davies, W.L. Jackson, R., McGraghan, T., Shadbolt, P., Weller, S.J. & Hahn,

C.E.W. (1988) An automated interferometer for the analysis of anaesthetic gas mixtures. *British Journal of Anaesthesia* **61**, 484–491.

Tatnall, M.L., West, P.G. & Morris, P. (1978) A rapid response u.v. halothane meter. *British Journal of Anaesthesia* **50**, 617–622.

Torda, T.A. & Grant, G.C. (1972) Test of a fuel cell oxygen analyzer. *British Journal of Anaesthesia* **44**, 1108–1112.

Van Wagenen, R.A., Westenskow, D.R., Benner, R.E., Gregonis, D.E. & Coleman, D.L. (1986) Dedicated monitoring of anesthetic and respiratory gases by Raman Scattering. *Journal of Clinical Monitoring* **2**, 215–222.

Waller, A.D. (1908) The chloroform balance. A new form of apparatus for the measured delivery of chloroform vapour. *Journal of Physiology* **37**, 6P.

Weast, R.C. (Ed.) (1974) *Handbook of chemistry and physics*. CRC Press, Cleveland, Ohio.

Westenskow, D.R., Smith, K.W., Coleman, D.L., Gregonis, D.E. & Van Wagenen, R.A. (1989a) Clinical evaluation of a Raman scattering multiple gas analyzer for the operating room. *Anesthesiology* **70**, 350–355.

Westenskow, D.R. & Coleman, D.L. (1989b) Can the Raman scattering analyzer compete with mass spectrometers: an affirmative reply. *Journal of Clinical Monitoring* **5**, 34–36.

White, D.C. & Wardley-Smith, B. (1972) The 'Narkotest' anaesthetic gas meter. *British Journal of Anaesthesia* **44**, 1100–1104.

Wortley, D.J., Herbert, P., Thornton, J.A. & Whelpton, D. (1968) The use of gas chromatography in the measurement of anaesthetic agents in gas and blood. *British Journal of Anaesthesia* **40**, 624–628.

18: Acid–base, Blood Gas and Other Analysers used by Clinicians

Clinical diagnosis is often assisted by laboratory investigation and the subsequent management of the patient will rarely be undertaken without analysis of body fluids for a large number of variables. In intensive care, the analysis may need to be repeated frequently and the results obtained quickly if they are to be of value. For this reason blood gas analysers were the first instruments to be placed in the clinical environment. As intensive care developed, rapid analysis of other important variables was demanded. Paper strip tests for blood glucose and for urine testing have been available for many years but recent developments in microprocessor technology have now resulted in a new generation of analytical systems which enable a wide range of measurements to be made at the bedside. At the same time blood gas analysers have recently been given increasing capability and are being complemented by the new generation of 'stat' or clinical-user analysers.

Blood gas analysis

At the time of the severe poliomyelitis epidemic in Copenhagen in 1952, the acid–base status was determined by measuring bicarbonate with the manometric Van Slyke apparatus and pH with a glass electrode, and then calculating P_{CO_2} from the Henderson–Hasselbalch equation. This method was time consuming and the calculated P_{CO_2} relatively inaccurate. The immense laboratory load generated by this epidemic stimulated the chemical pathologist Paoul Astrup to develop a new technique based on the equilibration of the blood sample with two gases of known P_{CO_2}. Astrup noted that there was a linear relationship between pH and log P_{CO_2} and that the slope of this line was governed by the haemoglobin concentration; its position was dependent on the non-respiratory component of acid–base balance. The position of the line was fixed by equilibrating two aliquots of the blood sample with 3 and 7% CO_2, and measuring the pH of each of them. The P_{CO_2} of the blood sample was then determined by interpolating the original blood pH value on the buffer line so plotted (Astrup, 1956). To enable these measurements to be made Astrup and Schroder (1956) developed a thermostatted chamber which enabled the blood pH measurement to be made anaerobically at body temperature and also permitted the blood sample to be equilibrated with the different CO_2 gas mixtures. This technique revolutionized acid–base measurement and led to the development of the micro method which utilized capillary blood samples equilibrated in a vibrating tonometer (Siggaard-Andersen *et al.* 1960).

In 1954, Stow and Randall described the basic principle of a CO_2 electrode using a pH electrode covered by a rubber membrane with a layer of distilled water trapped between the two. Severinghaus and Bradley (1958) modified this by trapping a layer of salt and sodium bicarbonate solution in a cellophane spacer between the pH electrode and the rubber membrane and found that the pH reading was stable and a linear function over a wide range of log P_{CO_2} values. Meanwhile, Clark *et al.* (1953) & Clark (1956) had developed the polarographic oxygen electrode and had described the use of a plastic membrane to prevent the poisoning of the platinum cathode by blood proteins. In 1958 Severinghaus demonstrated a composite blood gas apparatus containing pH, P_{CO_2} and P_{O_2} electrodes at a CIBA symposium in London. This device was the forerunner of today's combined systems which not only provide automatic control of the calibration and washing procedures, but also measure sodium, potassium, ionized calcium or chloride, haematocrit, glucose and urea accompanied by a variety of calculated parameters.

With this increased capability the problems associated with the results from clinical user instruments have also increased proportionately.

pH

The pH unit was defined by Sörensen in 1909 as 'the log to the base 10 of the reciprocal of the hydrogen ion concentration'. pH is used as an indication of acidity or alkalinity, which in turn depends on the concentration of free hydrogen (H^+) ions present in solution. In acid solutions, defined by Brønsted and Lowry as proton donors, there is a predominance of hydrogen ions; the converse is true of basic solutions. The SI unit used to define the acidity or alkalinity of blood is the hydrogen-ion concentration [H^+], expressed in $nmol \cdot L^{-1}$. However, it is not possible to measure [H^+] directly in aqueous solutions and [H^+] is therefore expressed in terms of pH units measured using a glass electrode. Even in those laboratories reporting hydrogen ion concentration, the value is obtained from the measured pH (Table 18.1).

pH can also be calculated using the Henderson–Hasselbalch equation, which assumes that there are only three variables:

$$pH = pK' + \log \frac{[HCO_3^-]}{[H_2CO_3]}.$$

Since the equilibrium of the reaction: $CO_2 + H_2O \Leftrightarrow H_2CO_3$ is well to the left under normal conditions (less than 1% of the CO_2 being in the hydrated form) it is customary to calculate the denominator from the P_{CO_2} and the solubility coefficient (α). This has a value of 0.51 and leads to the production of conversion factors of $0.231 \ mmol \cdot L^{-1} \ kPa^{-1}$ (or $0.0301 \ mmol \cdot L^{-1} \ mmHg^{-1}$) at 37 °C thus:

$$pH = pK + \log \frac{[HCO_3^-]}{\alpha \cdot P_{CO_2}}$$

Table 18.1. Conversions between pH and hydrogen ion activity ($nmol \cdot L^{-1}$)

pH	[H^+] ($nmol \cdot L^{-1}$)
6.80	158.3
6.90	125.7
7.00	100.0
7.10	79.4
7.20	63.1
7.25	56.2
7.30	50.1
7.35	44.6
7.40	39.8
7.45	35.5
7.50	31.6
7.55	28.2
7.60	25.1
7.70	20.0

Example 1
Convert pH = 7.40 to $nmol \cdot L^{-1}$

$$pH = -\log [H^+]$$

$$-\log [H^+] = pH$$

which is

$$\log [H^+] = -pH$$

$$\log [H^+] = -7.40$$

which may be written as

$$\log [H^+] = +0.6 - 8.0$$

$$[H^+] = antilog\ 0.6 - antilog\ 8.0$$

$$= 3.98 \times 10^{-8}$$

or, as $nmol \cdot L^{-1}$ are the preferred units, 39.8×10^{-9} or $39.8 \ nmol \cdot L^{-1}$.

Example 2
Convert 50.1 $nmol \cdot L^{-1}$ to pH:

$$[H] = 50.1 \ nmol \cdot L^{-1}$$

$$= 50.1 \times 10^{-9} \ mol \cdot L^{-1}$$

$$pH = -\log [H^+]$$

$$= -[(\log 50.1) + (\log 10^{-9})]$$

$$= -[(1.70) + (-9)]$$

$$= -[-7.30]$$

$$pH = 7.30.$$

or

$$pH = pK + \log \frac{[CO_2] - \alpha \cdot P_{CO_2}}{\alpha \cdot P_{CO_2}}$$

where $[CO_2]$ is the total CO_2 content measured by vacuum extraction (e.g. in the Van Slyke technique). Unfortunately, pK′ (normally 6.1) varies with pH and temperature and α also varies with temperature so that calculation of pH is relatively inaccurate (Severinghaus *et al.* 1956). Thus blood pH is now always measured with glass electrodes.

Glass pH electrode

The first practical apparatus for measuring blood pH anaerobically was described by McInnes and Belcher (1933). This has since been modified substantially in order to produce a stable, sensitive measurement with progressively smaller quantities of blood. The pH measurement electrode, the first ion-selective electrode, utilizes a glass membrane which is selectively permeable to hydrogen ions. In reality, no single electrode will respond exclusively to an individual anion, cation, atom or molecule and the 'membrane' has to be tailored to allow the electrode to be maximally selective to the ion to be measured.

In the case of pH measurement the composition of the glass will determine the stability and response of the electrode system. The pH measurement system, shown diagrammatically in Fig. 18.1, consists of the two electrodes Ag : AgCl and Hg:Hg$_2$Cl$_2$ (calomel) each of which maintains a constant potential. It can be seen that each electrode consists of two conductors, a metal component which conducts electrons and the electrolytic component which conducts ions. A potential difference or electromotive force (e.m.f.) exists at the interface between the two conductors, and this is referred to as the electrode potential. The only variable in the circuit, given a constant temperature, is the difference in pH between the inner buffer of the electrode and that of the sample.

The circuit between the sample and calomel electrode is completed using a saturated solution of KCl. Potassium chloride is used as a salt bridge as the relative mobility of potassium and chloride in aqueous solution is the same. This connection is made via a porous plug placed at the end of the measurement pathway, thus minimizing the effect of any KCl diffusion into the sample at the measurement electrodes. A commercial electrode is illustrated in Fig. 18.2. The glass electrode produces an e.m.f. which is approximately 60 mV per pH unit change at 37 °C. Since the internal resistance of the cell is high it is important to minimize the amount of current drawn from the cell to ensure an accurate reading of e.m.f. This is achieved by using a voltmeter with a very high input impedance (in the range 10–100 MΩ at 25 °C).

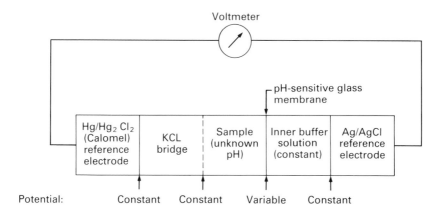

Fig. 18.1. The measurement of pH showing arrangement of reference electrodes, pH sensitive glass and sample reference solutions.

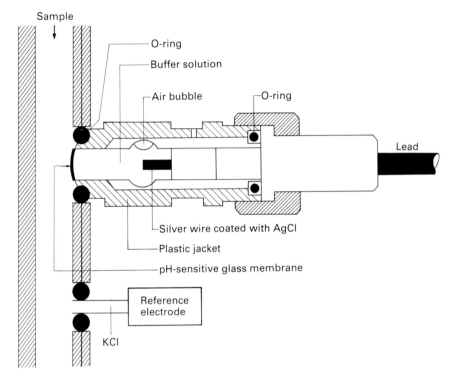

Fig. 18.2. Glass electrode assembly (Radiometer). The electrode is held in a thermostated block (37 °C). The blood is pumped over both the pH sensitive glass membrane and the porous plug of the calomel reference electrode, immersed in KCl (not shown).

Molecular interaction within any ionic species results in a difference between the activity and concentration of a given solution and it is only at infinite dilution that these are equal. The pH electrode, being an ion-selective electrode, responds to the activity and not the concentration of hydrogen ions. The output of the electrode is therefore standardized using buffer solutions, the pH scale being related to these solutions rather than to the absolute concentration of hydrogen ions. The pH unit is defined by the British and US National Bureau of Standards, as 'the difference in the hydrogen ion activity of the two standards which at 25 °C, and using the same standard H_2 electrode (i.e. 1 atmosphere H_2 pressure) and the same reference electrode, gives an e.m.f. difference of 0.05916 V'. The hydrogen electrode is used as it does not produce liquid junction potentials.

Modern blood gas analysers use two buffers of pH 6.841 and 7.383 at 37 °C. The 6.841 buffer has

the same pH as the buffer inside the electrode and therefore is used as an arbitrary system zero. The pH 7.383 buffer is used as a reference against which the blood samples are read.

CARBON DIOXIDE

In conscious patients with normal lungs the P_{CO_2} of the arterial blood is approximately equal to the end-tidal, or alveolar, P_{CO_2}. In anaesthetized patients and in patients with lung disease there is an increase in alveolar dead space which results in an arterial to end-tidal P_{CO_2} difference. In anaesthetized patients with normal lungs the end-tidal P_{CO_2} is approximately 0.7 kPa (5 mmHg) lower than the arterial P_{CO_2}. However, in patients with lung disease this difference can be as much as 2–3 kPa (15–20 mmHg). The end-tidal P_{CO_2} may, therefore, be used to monitor blood P_{CO_2} in normal patients but not those with lung disease. An increase in the arterial to end-tidal P_{CO_2} difference also occurs when cardiac output is markedly reduced, so that end-tidal sampling cannot be used to estimate P_{CO_2} in shock states. Conversely, if ventilation is being controlled at a fixed volume, end-tidal monitoring can be used to detect acute disturbances of the circulation. Under these circumstances a sudden reduction in end-tidal P_{CO_2} indicates an acute reduction of blood flow to the lungs, whilst an end-tidal P_{CO_2} of zero indicates cardiac arrest or a disconnection.

Re-breathing methods have been used in which gas in a reservoir bag is re-breathed resulting in the gas attaining equilibrium with the mixed venous blood. The normal difference between arterial and mixed venous P_{CO_2} is 0.8 kPa (6 mmHg) and this is subtracted from the mixed venous P_{CO_2} in order to obtain a value for arterial P_{CO_2}. This difference is inversely proportional to cardiac output and cannot, therefore, be used unless cardiovascular status is normal (McEvoy *et al.* 1974). Although the method is simple and easy to repeat, it has fallen

out of use with the ready availability of blood–gas analysers (see p. 309).

Calculation of P_{CO_2} from pH and bicarbonate concentrations is subject to the same errors as outlined in the pH calculation above and has also fallen out of use.

Astrup interpolation technique

The indirect method of estimating P_{CO_2} using the Astrup interpolation technique was used extensively until about 1970. This technique was based on the linear relationship between pH and log P_{CO_2} over the physiological range. It relied upon three measurements of blood pH, one before, and two after equilibration with known tensions of carbon dioxide. The pH measurements of the two equilibrated samples were then plotted against the respective P_{CO_2} with pH on the abscissa (x-axis) and P_{CO_2} plotted on a logarithmic scale on the ordinate (y-axis) using a Siggaard–Andersen nomogram (Fig. 18.3).

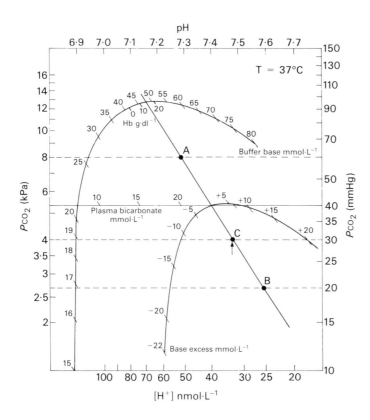

Fig. 18.3. Principle of the Astrup interpolation technique plotted on a Siggaard–Andersen nomogram (1962). Points A and B are obtained by measuring the pH of two samples of the patient's blood which have been equilibrated with two O_2–CO_2 gas mixtures of known P_{CO_2}, in this case 8 kPa (60 mmHg) and 2.7 kPa (20 mmHg). Point C is interpolated from the measured pH of the patient's blood. The P_{CO_2} can then be read off the ordinate. The base excess (zero in the figure) is read from the lower curve. In a non-respiratory alkalosis the buffer line A–B is shifted to the right and in a non-respiratory acidosis it is shifted to the left.

The original pH was then used to read the P_{CO_2} from the y-axis. The standard bicarbonate and base excess were also obtained from the same nomogram. Errors occurred if the equilibration gas was different from the nominal value. Incomplete equilibration also caused errors as the P_{CO_2} in the sample differed from that of the gas.

The slope of the buffer line becomes steeper with increasing haemoglobin concentration (as would be expected from the increased buffering power of the blood) and the position of the line in relation to the ordinate is dependent on the metabolic or non-respiratory component of the sample, being displaced to the left in acidotic and to the right in alkalotic conditions.

The standard bicarbonate and base excess are the two most commonly used indicators of non-respiratory disturbances but actual bicarbonate, total CO_2 and standard base excess are also used. The definitions and methods of calculating these variables are as follows.

The *standard bicarbonate* is the bicarbonate concentration in the plasma of fully oxygenated blood which has been equilibrated with gas having a P_{CO_2} of 5.3 kPa (40 mmHg) at 37 °C. The normal range is 22–26 mmol·L^{-1}.

The *base excess* is the amount of strong acid or base required to titrate 1 L of blood back to a pH of 7.40 at a P_{CO_2} of 5.3 kPa (40 mmHg) and 37 °C. A base deficit is the same as a negative base excess. The normal range is ±2 mmol·L^{-1}.

The *actual bicarbonate* is the amount of (HCO_3^-) present in plasma. This is calculated from the P_{CO_2} and pH measurements on the whole blood sample.

$$[HCO_3^-]\ \text{mmol·L}^{-1} = \alpha \cdot P_{CO_2} \times 10^{(\text{pH} - 6.1)}$$

where α = 0.231 when P_{CO_2} is in kPa and 0.0301* when P_{CO_2} is in mmHg.

Note that the electrodes actually measure plasma P_{CO_2} and pH so that the actual bicarbonate value also refers to plasma. The normal value is 24 mmol·L^{-1}. The *total CO_2* is the sum of the dissolved CO_2 and actual bicarbonate = 1.2 + 24 = 25.4 mmol·L^{-1} in arterial blood.

* The correct value is 0.0301 but all commercial instrument makers use 0.031.

The *buffer base* is the sum of all the buffer anions in the blood (haemoglobin, bicarbonate, protein and phosphate) and the normal value is 44–48 mmol·L^{-1}. Since the value is affected by haemoglobin concentration it has been suggested that the *normal buffer base* is a more useful measure of the non-respiratory component of acid–base balance. The normal buffer base (mmol·L^{-1}) = 41.7 + [0.42 × Hb (g·dl^{-1})].

These measurements refer to *in vitro* conditions. *In vivo* a certain amount of the bicarbonate generated by the addition of CO_2 diffuses into the extracellular fluid. The body as a whole therefore, does not buffer a change in P_{CO_2} as well as blood alone and the *in vivo* buffer line has a slope which approximates to that of a haemoglobin of about 5 g·dl^{-1}. Thus if the blood is sampled when the P_{CO_2} is high and then equilibrated with gas having a normal P_{CO_2} there will appear to be a non-respiratory acidosis (Fig. 18.4). The magnitude of this error will depend on the P_{CO_2} at the time of sampling and the duration of the change in respiratory state, but in most circumstances the error in base excess is less than 3–4 mmol·L^{-1}. To overcome this problem some blood gas analysers calculate a *standard base excess* which assumes a haemoglobin of 5 g·dl^{-1} to relate the measurement more closely to *in vivo* conditions (Siggaard–Andersen, 1966).

The difference between the *in vitro* approach to the interpretation of acid–base disorders (utilized widely in Europe) and the emphasis put on the *in vivo* changes by workers in the US has been well summarized by Severinghaus (1976).

Errors will also occur if the haemoglobin and oxygen saturation are not measured on a sample taken at the same time as that for pH and P_{CO_2}. These variables are included in the calculations but will have to be assumed unless a co-oximeter is interfaced with the blood gas analyser, so that the actual haemoglobin and saturation can be used.

The CO_2 electrode

The electrode consists of a glass pH electrode assembly with the pH-sensitive glass in contact with a thin layer of bicarbonate buffer (Fig. 18.5).

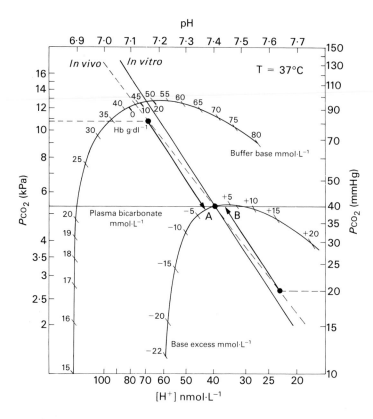

Fig. 18.4. Error in acid–base measurement due to the difference between *in vitro* and *in vivo* equilibration lines. It is assumed that the patient normally has a P_{CO_2} of 5.3 kPa (40 mmHg) and base excess of zero. An acute respiratory acidosis is then induced (*in vivo* curve) and the blood sampled at P_{CO_2} = 10.7 kPa (80 mmHg). When this blood sample is equilibrated *in vitro* the equilibration line will be displaced to the left. The apparent base deficit is indicated by the arrow (A). The opposite effect occurs during a respiratory alkalosis (B). A revised chart incorporating *in vivo* changes has been published by Siggaard–Andersen (1971).

The buffer is trapped in a nylon mesh spacer and separated by a thin Teflon or silicone membrane which is permeable to CO_2 but not to blood cells, plasma or charged ions. The whole unit is maintained at 37 °C. CO_2 diffuses from the blood into the buffer and so changes its pH, a change of about 0.01 pH units being produced by a 0.1 kPa (1.25 mmHg) change in P_{CO_2}.

The electrode is calibrated by equilibrating the buffer with two known CO_2 concentrations to establish the relationship between pH and P_{CO_2}. The calibrating gases may be humidified, warmed and then passed through the electrode cuvette directly or may be dissolved in the buffer solutions which then serve as a composite calibration solution for all of the measurement electrodes. The majority of blood gas analysers use humidified gases for calibration but those produced by Radiometer use two buffers equilibrated with different CO_2 concentrations from an inbuilt gas mixer (Holbeck, 1989). The advantage of this is that the

'blood gas factor' of the O_2 electrode is eliminated: the disadvantage is the time taken to equilibrate the buffers fully after any disruption in gas supply, as in humidifier maintenance. In operation, the CO_2 from a small cylinder is mixed with room air to provide CO_2 concentrations of 5.61 and 11.22%. These concentrations differ slightly between any two instruments, but each gas mixer is accurately calibrated to two decimal places. The analyser then calculates the partial pressure of CO_2 from:

$$P_{CO_2} = \frac{CO_2 \text{ concentration}}{100} \times (BP - WVP)$$

where BP is the barometric pressure and WVP is the water vapour pressure at 37 °C.

Other blood gas analysers use either an inbuilt gas mixer, or pre-mixed gases, which are certified by the suppliers. Again, the P_{CO_2} is calculated from the CO_2 concentration each time calibration occurs. The CO_2 electrode output from the two

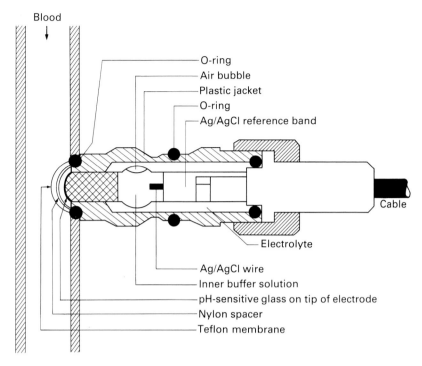

Fig. 18.5. The CO_2 electrode.

calibration gases is used by the analyser to construct a reference line to which the electrode output of the blood sample is referred. The response time taken for a CO_2 electrode to reach a stable reading will be directly related to the difference between the calibration or conditioning gas and the CO_2 of the sample (Smith & Hahn, 1975). Modern electrode technology allows a reading to be made in less than 1 min.

OXYGEN

Oxygenation may be assessed by measuring the tension, saturation or content of oxygen, the relationship between these three measurements being determined by the shape and position of the oxygen dissociation curve (Fig. 18.6). Since there are many causes of variations in both the shape and position of the curve it is usually necessary to measure the variable of interest directly. However, if content is required, it is usual to measure those variables which allow it to be calculated (see below). Thus tension measurements are required for most respiratory problems, though saturation or content may be required if the percentage shunt is to be calculated. Saturation and tension are necessary to define the dissociation curve whilst content measurements are required when O_2 transport is being considered.

Although there was a brief period when Po_2 was determined directly by the analysis of a gas bubble equilibrated with the blood sample (Riley *et al.* 1957), this technique was soon superceded by the use of the oxygen electrode. Saturation is determined by photometric techniques involving the transmission or reflection of light at certain wavelengths, or from measurements of oxygen content and capacity. Oxygen content is measured by vacuum extraction and chemical absorption, by driving the O_2 into solution and measuring the increase in Po_2, or by a galvanic cell analyser. O_2

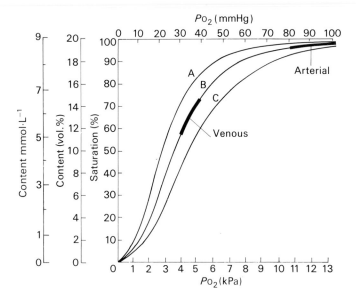

Fig. 18.6. The oxygen dissociation curves for (A) P_{CO_2} = 2.7 kPa (20 mmHg); (B) P_{CO_2} = 5.3 kPa (40 mmHg); (C) P_{CO_2} = 8 kPa (60 mmHg). The normal arterial and mixed venous ranges are shown.

capacity is determined by measuring the O_2 content of the blood sample after it has been fully saturated with oxygen. Then:

$$\% \text{ saturation} = \frac{O_2 \text{ content}}{O_2 \text{ capacity}} \times 100.$$

Since measured content and capacity include dissolved oxygen, this must be subtracted before calculating saturation.

The oxygen electrode

The oxygen electrode (Clark, 1956) consists of a platinum wire, nominally 20 Å (2 nm) in diameter, which is embedded in a rough surfaced glass rod. This is immersed in a phosphate buffer which is stabilized with KCl and contained in an outer jacket (Fig. 18.7). At the end of the outer jacket is a membrane which is usually polyethylene or polypropylene, each being permeable to oxygen. The polyethylene membrane will allow faster diffusion of oxygen than the polypropylene, making the system more sensitive but less stable. A polarizing voltage of between 600 mV and 800 mV is applied to the platinum wire and as oxygen diffuses through the membrane electro-oxidoreduction occurs at the cathode:

$$O_2 + 4e^- \rightarrow 2O_2$$
$$2O_2 + 2H_2O \rightarrow 4OH^-.$$

Corresponding oxidation occurs at the Ag:AgCl anode:

$$4Ag \rightarrow 4Ag^+ + 4e^-$$
$$4Ag^+ + 4Cl^- \rightarrow 4AgCl.$$

Thus a half cell is set up and a current generated. The current is of the order of 10^{-11} A·mmHg^{-1}, and therefore cannot be measured using an ammeter. The resistance in the circuit is mathematically adjusted to unity and from Ohms Law:

$$V = IR. \quad \text{If } R = 1, \text{ then } V = I.$$

The change in current is then measured as a change in voltage using the same potentiometric circuit as the pH and P_{CO_2} measurement systems.

If the polarizing voltage at the cathode is set at − 675 mV with reference to the anode, interference from the reduction of other gases is largely eliminated, although there is still a potential interference from halothane (Norden & Flynn, 1979).

The oxygen electrode in most blood gas analysers is calibrated using two standard gases, one containing no oxygen, the other about 12% O_2. It is not now thought necessary to utilize 'white spot'

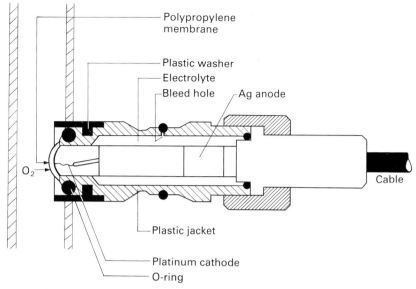

Fig. 18.7. The oxygen electrode.

nitrogen (guaranteed 0% O_2) or solutions of sodium dithionite for the zero point; two manufacturers, AVL and Radiometer, simply 'short out' the electrode producing an electronic zero. The error which this produces is minimal. The linearity of the oxygen electrode will vary depending on the physical circumstances, such as cathode diameter, polarizing voltage and type of membrane used. Generally, the current generated begins to reach a plateau at an output equivalent to a Po_2 of about 19.95 kPa (150 mmHg) and some manufacturers use a curve fitting programme which 'linearizes' the Po_2 measurement above this point. Other sources of error are discussed below.

A 'disposable' electrode has been introduced in the 200 series from Ciba Corning. Replacing the membrane of the Pco_2 and Po_2 electrodes has been eliminated and the electrodes, held together by a spring loaded retainer, are designed to form the flow path for the blood, the gas or the calibration buffer.

Although several authors have described electrodes with a response time which is rapid enough to follow breath-by-breath changes in Po_2, these have not become commercially available.

Intravascular monitoring of oxygen tension

Miniature electrodes have been used for the continuous intravascular monitoring of oxygen tension, but these are subject to a build-up of fibrin which alters the electrode sensitivity. The short response time of the electrode makes the system useful for monitoring acute changes in Po_2 such as those resulting from nursing procedures such as opening an incubator, turning the patient, extubating or temporarily disconnecting the patient from a ventilator. A composite tip containing both Pco_2 and Po_2 electrodes (Parker *et al.* 1978) found limited use but these systems have been largely replaced by non-invasive techniques.

Transcutaneous electrodes

There are advantages in monitoring blood gases non-invasively, particularly when dealing with infants, and transcutaneous electrodes have been extensively used for the monitoring of neonatal blood gas status (Huch *et al.* 1977; Blackburn, 1978; Skeates, 1978).

The electrodes are based on similar principles to those used in blood gas analysers but also incorporate a heating element. The electrode is attached to the skin to form an airtight seal using a contact liquid and the area is heated to 43 °C. At this temperature the blood flow to the skin increases and the capillary oxygen diffuses through the skin allowing measurement of the diffused gases by the attached electrode. A combined electrode (Fig. 18.8) has been produced by Radiometer which will simultaneously measure both the trancutaneous carbon dioxide tension (tcP_{CO_2}) and oxygen tension (tcP_{O_2}) and is claimed to have the same sensitivity as the individual transcutaneous electrodes. The electrodes are calibrated using room air for oxygen and a gas of known CO_2 concentration for carbon dioxide. Changes in barometric pressure are largely ignored in the calibration procedures and errors of only ± 1 mmHg for tcP_{CO_2} and ± 2 mmHg for tcP_{O_2} are claimed.

Problems can occur with surgical diathermy; the heating current circuit provides a return path for the cutting current which can cause the transcutaneous electrode to overheat. At 45.6 °C the Radiometer TCM3 electrode will cease operation and display an error warning, although first, and occasionally second, degree burns do occur (Jennis & Peabody, 1985).

The values obtained from transcutaneous electrodes will generally be lower than those obtained from a simultaneous arterial specimen. As blood in the skin capillaries is heated, the solubility of the dissolved gases decreases as does the haemoglobin oxygen affinity, resulting in an increase in the oxygen tension in the capillary blood. This increase offsets the diffusion gradient and the increased tissue metabolism resulting from the increased temperature. The net effect is a tcP_{O_2} close to

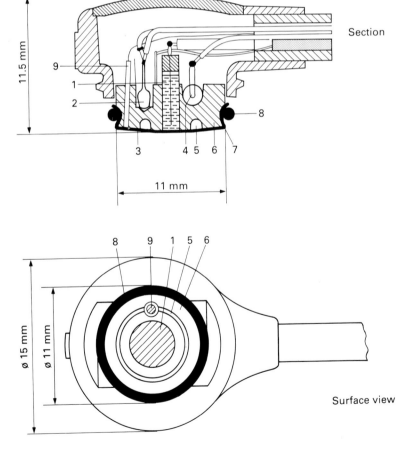

Fig. 18.8. Combined transcutaneous electrode for P_{CO_2} and P_{O_2} measurement.
1 P_{CO_2} electrode.
2 Thermistor.
3 Polypropylene membrane over O_2 electrode.
4 Heating element.
5 Electrolyte.
6 Silver body acting as P_{O_2} electrode anode and P_{CO_2} reference electrode.
7 Teflon membrane over whole electrode (permeable to gas but not [H$^+$]).
8 O-ring.
9 P_{O_2} electrode cathode.

arterial P_{O_2}. It is possible to calibrate transcutaneous electrodes with reference to values obtained from a blood gas analyser. P_{CO_2} and P_{O_2} results from a blood sample are entered into the transcutaneous monitor and a set factor is then applied to the measurements obtained from the transcutaneous electrodes. When this procedure is accomplished the monitor displays 'in vivo cal' in order to differentiate from the alternative calibration procedure.

The electrode reads low with severe hypotension and microcirculatory perfusion failure and it has been claimed that the device is a useful monitor of oxygen transport as well as P_{O_2}. Rome et al. (1984) and Hamilton et al. (1985) found tcP_{O_2} was lower than P_{aO_2} in post-term infants and postulated that this was due to the increasing thickness of the epidermal layer and decreasing density of the underlying capillaries in the skin, which occurs with advancing postnatal age.

Fluorescence-based blood–gas analysis

Gehrich et al. (1986) and Miller et al. (1987) have described a fluorescence based fibre-optic measurement system for the measurement of pH, P_{CO_2} and P_{O_2}. A sensor is incorporated into a probe which is inserted through a 20 standard wire gauge (SWG) radial artery catheter. This is claimed not to affect blood withdrawal or pressure measurement.

The Miller system depends upon light from a pulsed xenon lamp being selectively filtered at 410, 460 and 385 nm for the respective measurements of pH, P_{CO_2} and P_{O_2}. A fluorescent weak acid, bonded to a hydrophilic matrix, is attached directly to the end of the sensor fibre. The dissociated and undissociated forms of the acid are selectively excited by light at 410 and 460 nm, and both emit at 520 nm. The ratio of the intensity of light at 520 nm is related to the pH at the tip of the sensor.

The P_{CO_2} sensor uses the same principle as the pH, but measures the ratio of output from a buffer encapsulated in silicone which is at equilibrium with the CO_2 tension of the blood.

The P_{O_2} measurement utilizes an oxygen-quenchable dye dissolved in silicone. The dye is excited with light at 385 nm, and the *decrease* in light emitted at 515 nm is directly proportional to the oxygen tension. The system is calibrated before insertion of the sensor using two gases of known concentration sequentially bubbled into a calibration device. Subsequent calibration is possible if an arterial blood specimen is analysed using a blood gas analyser and the system adjusted accordingly. The fluorescence based system is available commercially from Cardiovascular Devices Inc. as the 'CDI System 1000'. The sensor is coated in covalently bonded heparin (Heparon[TH]) which is said to make it bio-compatible (non-toxic, non-haemolytic and non-thrombogenic), for single use up to 72 h. There was no interference from a variety of antibiotics, morphine, succinylcholine or thiopentone, but there was a small increase in P_{O_2} measured in the presence of nitrous oxide and a greater increase with halothane. Miller et al. (1987) claimed a coefficient of correlation (r) of more than 0.98 for all three sensors against simultaneous blood gas measurements on withdrawn samples.

Ion-selective electrodes

The pH electrode utilizes a glass membrane, the composition of which is tailored selectively to allow hydrogen ions to pass through, thus producing an e.m.f. Eisenman et al. (1957) varied the composition to produce a triple glass system containing $Na_2O–Al_2O_3–SiO_3$ which is selectively permeable to sodium ions.

Since then, many electrode systems have been devised which are selective for either cations or anions. The most commonly used are those which are selective for sodium, potassium and calcium, but lithium and particularly chloride electrodes are being incorporated into more instruments. Many others are available for research purposes (e.g. fluoride).

There are three basic types of membrane in addition to the original glass membrane:

1 Solid state (e.g. lanthanum fluoride for F^- ions).
2 Liquid ion exchange (e.g. calcium di-*n*-decyl phosphate for Ca^{++} ions).
3 Neutral carrier (e.g. valinomycin for K^+ ions).

The membranes, although different, all produce an electrical response when in contact with salt solution containing the particular ion to which the electrode is sensitive. The magnitude of the e.m.f. produced is based on the Nernst equation.

Unfortunately, when the solution contains another ion there is an interference since no electrode is perfectly selective. However, as long as the selectivity is much greater than the relative concentrations in the solution being measured this is not a major problem. For example, the Na^+ electrode has a selectivity for Na^+ versus K^+ of approximately 200 to 1. Given the physiological ratio of Na^+/K^+ in plasma of 30 to 1, it can be seen that interference with the sodium reading from potassium will be minimal.

Systems incorporating ion-selective electrodes have the advantage that they can measure the relevant substances directly without the need for pretreatment or even centrifuging. Minimal technical ability is required and they are virtually hazard free. In the case of sodium measurement, the ion-selective electrode will produce a 'true' sodium value without the problems which lead to falsely low values in emission flame photometry. The measurement of calcium using ion-selective electrode technology produces a value for 'ionized calcium' as opposed to total calcium and as such provides a value for that portion which is physiologically active.

Oxygen saturation and oxygen content

The standard method of determining the percentage oxygen saturation (Sao_2) is to measure the oxygen content of the blood sample and then to relate this to the oxygen capacity. This is the oxygen content of the same blood sample after it has been equilibrated with air to achieve full saturation of the red cells. Since the equation:

$$Sao_2\% = \frac{oxygen\ content\ (ml \cdot dl^{-1})}{oxygen\ capacity\ (ml \cdot dl^{-1})} \times 100$$

refers to the quantities of oxygen in the red cells it is necessary to subtract the dissolved O_2 from the measured values before inserting these in the equation (van Slyke & Neill, 1924). In this definition the two forms of haemoglobin which do not

bind with oxygen (COHb and MetHb) are not included. However, oximeters using four or more wavelengths are capable of measuring COHb and MetHb and report their results as fractional haemoglobin saturation or O_2Hb:

$$O_2Hb\% = \frac{O_2Hb}{O_2Hb + Hb + COHb + MetHb} \times 100.$$

Most pulse oximeters measure the absorption of red light at around 660 nm and infrared at around 940 nm. In the red region the absorption produced by COHb is close to that produced by O_2Hb whilst MetHb produces similar absorption to that of Hb. However, at 940 nm COHb absorption is close to zero whilst the absorption of MetHb and Hb differ markedly. It follows that the reading of a pulse oximeter ($Spo_2\%$) will differ from $Sao_2\%$ and $O_2Hb\%$ when either of these haemoglobins are present (Barker & Tremper, 1987; Tremper & Barker, 1989).

Oxygen content and capacity. Various methods have been used to measure content and capacity. In 1924, van Slyke introduced a volumetric method whereby the gases dissolved in a blood sample were liberated using lactic acid and vacuum extraction and the volume measured at a fixed (atmospheric) pressure. This was later superceded by a manometric method (Fig. 18.9) in which the pressure of the liberated gases was measured at a fixed volume. The CO_2 liberated was absorbed in KOH and the pressure measured. An O_2 absorbent was then added and the pressure measured again. This method is technically difficult and time consuming and is now rarely used.

Another method of measuring O_2 content is to add a small sample of blood (50–500 μl) to a large volume (e.g. 50 ml) of potassium ferricyanide solution. The latter haemolyses the red cells and drives the oxygen into solution. By measuring the Po_2 of the solution before and after adding the blood and knowing the solubility of oxygen in the solution it is possible to calculate the O_2 content of the original sample. Modifications to the original techniques have been suggested by Horabin and Farhi (1978).

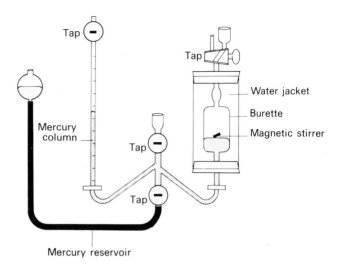

Fig. 18.9. The manometric apparatus of van Slyke.

A direct reading galvanic cell system of oxygen content measurement, the Lex-O-Con was introduced in 1974 (Fig. 18.10). Here a carrier gas consisting of 1% carbon monoxide, 2% hydrogen and 97% nitrogen is passed over a palladium catalyst (to ensure that it contains no O_2) and bubbled through a haemolysed sample of blood. The liberated oxygen is reduced at a carbon cathode which gives rise to four electrons per molecule of oxygen. The current generated is proportional to the amount of oxygen in the sample. This system was evaluated by Selman *et al.* (1975). It is unaffected by the presence of volatile anaesthetic agents but is, however, not widely used.

A colorimetric method of oxygen content measurement was introduced by Zander *et al.* (1977). In this, a 10 μl sample of whole blood is injected anaerobically into a sealed cuvette containing an alkaline catachol solution and the change in absorbance at 511 nm is measured. From this a blank representing fully reduced haemoglobin has to be subtracted and this is obtained by injecting a similar volume of sample into an identical cuvette containing a solution of 0.1 M NaOH. A commercial application of this system called 'Oxystat' is available in Germany but has not been introduced to the UK.

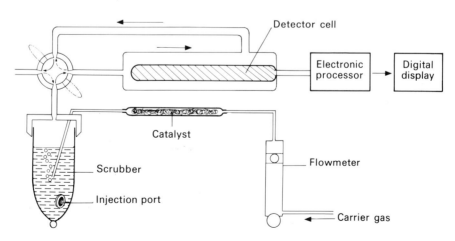

Fig. 18.10. The Lex-O-Con galvanic cell analyser for O_2 content.

Oxygen saturation: oximetry. This technique utilizes the difference between the characteristic absorption spectra of haemoglobin and oxyhaemoglobin to quantify the relative concentrations of the two forms in the sample. The instruments may use reflected or transmitted light and measurements may be made *in vitro* or *in vivo*. In the past *in vitro* measurement was chiefly used for calculating the degree of right to left shunt at cardiac catheterization. In recent years intravascular measurements have been made with catheters passed into the pulmonary artery. Now the non-invasive *in vivo* technique of pulse oximetry is finding a wide application in anaesthesia, intensive care and many other clinical situations.

Reflection oximetry

One of the earliest *in vitro* instruments was the Kipp haemoreflector. This measured the intensity of reflected light from a layer of blood at two wavelengths, the ratio of the logarithms of the reflected light intensity being a linear function of the oxygen saturation (Brinkman & Zijlstra, 1949). A similar technique was developed for use in patients and utilized a sensor placed on the forehead — the so-called Cyclops oximeter (Brinkman *et al.* 1952).

The next development was an *in vivo* reflectance oximeter which utilized flexible optical fibres to transmit the radiation along a catheter which could be inserted into the heart or major vessels (Polanyi & Hehir, 1962). In the early models the catheters were very stiff, light transmission was impaired by breakage of the optical fibres and aberrant signals were produced by the proximity of the catheter tip to the vessel wall or deposition of fibrin on the fibre-optic window at the end of the catheter. Changes in haematocrit also affected the results.

In modern *in vivo* oximeters many of these problems have been minimized by microprocessor technology. Currently, one system uses two wavelengths whilst the other uses three wavelengths. In the latter, three light-emitting diodes (LEDs) send alternating pulses of radiation of three different wavelengths down one fibre-optic channel at a frequency of approximately 4 Hz. The radiation is absorbed and refracted by the haemoglobin and reflected back up the second fibre-optic channel. The oxygen saturation is then computed over a 5 s interval and updated each second. Fibrin deposition is minimized by a continuous flush of heparinized lactated Ringer's solution and fibrin deposition sensed by an absence of a pulsatile response from the sensing channel. The system is calibrated before insertion by a standard reference, but can also be calibrated *in situ* by a standardized optical device which is contained in each catheter pack. The three wavelength system has proved to be reasonably accurate in use (Baele *et al.* 1982; Divertie & McMichan, 1984; Gettinger *et al.* 1987) and measurements are not affected by changes in body temperature, haematocrit or cardiac output. The catheter incorporates a balloon to assist placement in the pulmonary artery, injection and sampling ports, and a thermistor for thermal dilution cardiac output measurement.

Transmission oximetry

Spectrophotometric analysis of haemoglobin has been carried out using a variety of combinations of wavelengths. The method is based on the fact that if a mixture of oxyhaemoglobin and deoxyhaemoglobin is read at two wavelengths, one at which there is a significant difference between oxy- and deoxyhaemoglobin, the other at the isobestic point of oxy- and deoxyhaemoglobin, the percentage saturation can be obtained.

The difference in absorbance between oxygenated and deoxygenated haemoglobin is greatest at 625 nm: 805 nm is the isobestic point of oxyhaemoglobin and deoxyhaemoglobin (Fig. 18.11). Spectrophotometric analysis with automatic calculation was introduced in 1970 with the IL 182 co-oximeter (Instrumentation Laboratory, England), which measured the absorbance at three different wavelengths (548.5, 568.6 and 578.7 nm). The system used an analogue computer to solve three simultaneous equations, producing values not only for oxy- and deoxyhaemoglobin, but also carboxy- and total haemoglobin (Fallon, 1973).

The third generation co-oximeters utilize the absorption spectra of the different haemoglobin

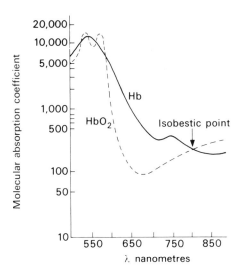

Fig. 18.11. Optical absorption spectra of oxygenated and reduced haemoglobin.

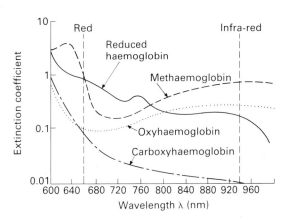

Fig. 18.12. Optical absorption spectra of various haemoglobins. The vertical broken lines show the absorption at the two wavelengths customarily used in pulse oximeters (660 and 940 nm). (After Tremper and Barker, 1989.)

derivatives (Fig. 18.12) to determine their concentrations and from the sum of these derivatives produce a total haemoglobin (Dennis & Valeri, 1980). The absorbance is measured at four (Il 482), six (Radiometer OSM 3) and seven (Ciba-Corning 2500) different wavelengths. In addition to those parameters previously mentioned, values for methaemoglobin, oxygen content and oxygen capacity are produced. Blood is injected or aspirated into the co-oximeters and haemolysed, either ultrasonically (Ciba-Corning, Radiometer) or chemically (Instrumentation Laboratory). The concentrations of the haemoglobin derivatives are calculated by solving a series of simultaneous equations using the absorptions at the different wavelengths.

Oxygen content of whole blood is calculated from the formula:

$$\text{oxygen content} = (SO_2/100 \times Hb \times Hf) + \alpha Po_2$$

where Hb is the total haemoglobin, Hf is the Hufner factor (1.39 ml·g^{-1}) and α is the solubility coefficient of oxygen (0.0031 ml·mmHg^{-1} at 37 °C).

Oxygen capacity is the oxygen content when all the reduced haemoglobin is converted to oxyhaemoglobin.

Carboxyhaemoglobin will normally be present as a result of haem metabolism at concentrations of less than 2%, but in heavy smokers, concentrations of 10–12% may be found. Increases are also found if there is exposure to fumes from car exhausts or fires.

Methaemoglobin is formed when the ferrous (Fe^{++}) atom in the haemoglobin molecule is oxidized to ferric (Fe^{+++}). This can be caused by the inhalation of agricultural chemicals, chlorates or nitrates (Harris *et al.* 1979) or as a side effect of the administration of prilocaine (Atkinson *et al.* 1987).

Fetal haemoglobin has an absorption spectrum which is fairly similar to adult haemoglobin but reads as carboxyhaemoglobin in modern co-oximeters which use more measurement wavelengths (Cornelissen *et al.* 1983). The OSM 3 has a correction factor.

The relationship between saturation and oxygen tension

The co-oximeters now available measure saturation quickly, easily and reliably. They can be interfaced with blood gas analysers, the results being printed out with other blood gas variables. The combination can then be used to provide additional parameters that can assist in the management of patients with respiratory disorders. The relationship between saturation and oxygen tension

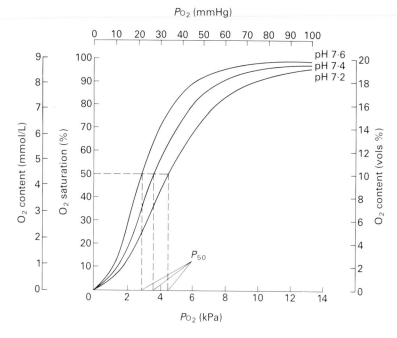

Fig. 18.13. A normal oxyhaemoglobin dissociation curve and normal P_{50} and curves showing a left and a right shift.

Table 18.2. Factors affecting haemoglobin oxygen affinity

Left shift	Right shift
Decreased temperature	Increased temperature
Decreased [H$^+$]	Increased [H$^+$]
Decreased P_{CO_2}	Increased P_{CO_2}
Decreased 2,3-DPG	Increased 2,3-DPG
Decreased [Hb]	Increased [Hb]
Decreased cation concentration	Increased cation concentration
Abnormal haemoglobin	Abnormal haemoglobin
Carboxyhaemoglobin	Cortisol
Methaemoglobin	Aldosterone
	Methylprednisolone

Table 18.3. Factors influencing the production of 2,3-DPG

Decreased 2,3-DPG	Increased 2,3-DPG
Increased [H$^+$]	Decreased [H$^+$]
Decreased thyroid hormone	Thyroid enzyme deficiency
Erythrocyte enzyme deficiency (hexokinase)	Erythrocyte enzyme deficiency (pyruvate kinase)
Cell age (old)	Cell age (new)
Decreased organic phosphate	Increased organic phospate
	Inosine
	Increased sulphate

is described by the sigmoid-shaped oxygen dissociation curve (ODC, see Fig. 18.13). The position of the curve will depend on the affinity of the haemoglobin for oxygen and the type or mixture of haemoglobins present in the red blood cells. The affinity changes both naturally and in sickness and is influenced by a number of factors (Table 18.2). These usually affect the affinity by either stabilizing or destabilizing deoxyhaemoglobin.

The decrease in pH as arterial blood loses oxygen and gains CO_2 causes a decrease in the haemoglobin affinity and this results in a right shift in the

ODC. The normal differences between pH and P_{CO_2} in arterial and venous blood are 0.04 and 0.8 kPa (6 mmHg) respectively. This is the Bohr effect and the decrease in affinity shifts the ODC approximately 5% to the right.

Phosphates, in particular 2,3-diphosphoglycerate (2,3-DPG), have a major influence on affinity. 2,3-DPG sits in a pocket in the quaternary structure of deoxyhaemoglobin formed by the $\alpha_1\beta_2$ linkages thus stabilizing that form and decreasing the affinity with a resulting right shift. The factors influencing the production of 2,3-DPG are given in Table 18.3.

Determination of the position and shape of the ODC

A number of methods have been used to locate the position of ODC. These are usually based on simultaneous, sequential or multiple measurements of haemoglobin saturation and oxygen tension. Commercial systems were introduced in the early 1970s from Radiometer (Dissociation Curve Analyser, DCA1) and Instrumentation Laboratory. Neither are now available.

The 'Hem-Ox-Analyser' (TCS Medical Products Co., USA) will plot the complete ODC (or oxygen association curve, OAC) automatically in approximately 10 min, using 5–50 μl of whole blood. The system is based on the simultaneous measurement of oxygen tension and saturation in a cuvette to which an increasing or decreasing oxygen concentration is applied. The saturation is calculated from two wavelengths and therefore only oxy- and deoxyhaemoglobin are measured.

Willis *et al.* (1987) introduced a system which uses saturation, measured with a co-oximeter (Ciba-Corning M 2500), and oxygen tension to compute an *in vivo* ODC. An iterative procedure which alters the constants given in the Kelman and Nunn (1966) and Thomas (1972) algorithms allows the normal ODC to be modified to fit the *in vivo* ODC. This system, which is now available commercially (Ciba-Corning ODC analyser), has the advantage of producing a calculated *in vivo* curve as quickly as a normal blood gas analysis. The curve will not be computed if:

1 significant levels of carboxy- or methaemoglobin are present;

2 the oxygen tension is outside the levels at which the curve can be accurately computed;

3 the measurement limitations of the instruments are exceeded.

The computed *in vivo* curve is then used to calculate additional variables:

1 effective oxygen tension ($Paeo_2$): (measured tension adjusted for ODC shift.)

2 P_{50} *in vivo*, oxygen tension at 50% saturation.

3 P_{95}, oxygen tension at 95% saturation.

4 $C(a - x)O_2$ the conditional oxygen extraction; [three values, where x is the mixed venous oxygen content at a Pvo_2 assumed to be 2.66 kPa (20 mmHg) 3.99 kPa (30 mmHg) and 5.32 kPa (40 mmHg)].

These values are all calculated at the actual pH and CO_2 tension of the patient and not corrected to standard values of temperature and CO_2. Thus they can be used in conjunction with a measurement (or reasonable assumption) of cardiac ouput and the patient's oxygen requirements, when inspired oxygen levels are being adjusted or when decisions regarding mechanical ventilation are to be made (Willis *et al.* 1987).

The expression normally used to determine the position of ihe ODC is a standard P_{50} ($P_{50\,std}$) whereby the P_{50} is calculated at a Pco_2 of 5.32 kPa (40 mmHg) and a pH of 7.4. Unfortunately, those patients in whom information regarding the position of the ODC is most likely to be required may well have abnormal CO_2 tensions which will significantly alter the P_{50} and potentially mislead the clinician about the position of the ODC.

Pulse oximetry

Although devices for measuring arterial saturation *in vivo* have been available since the late 1930s there were always difficulties in calibration due to the variable tissue absorption of the transmitted or reflected light and the need to vasodilate the earlobe to produce arterialization of the capillary bed. These problems were not solved until the 1970s when an eight-wavelength earpiece oximeter was introduced and shown to produce reasonably accurate measurements of saturation without the need for calibration against arterial samples (Flick & Block, 1976). However, the apparatus was expensive and the earpiece was bulky and it was therefore not used widely in clinical practice.

In 1974, Aoyagi *et al.* described the technique of pulse oximetry which overcame the problem of variable tissue absorption by analysing the pulsatile variations in light absorbance. The original design used filtered light sources (similar to Millikan's original oximeter) and was not a commercial success. Present instruments owe their success to two modifications of the original technique, namely the use of LEDs as light sources and

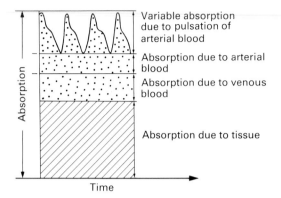

Variable absorption
due to pulsation of
arterial blood

Absorption due to arterial
blood

Absorption due to venous
blood

Absorption due to tissue

Fig. 18.14. a.c. and d.c. signals received by the pulse oximeter.

microprocessor technology to analyse the data (Wukitsch *et al.* 1988).

The sensor may be placed on the finger, earlobe, nasal septum or toe and often works well on the hand or foot in the neonate. It contains two LEDs which emit in the red ($\approx$660 nm) and infrared ($\approx$940 nm) regions of the spectrum, and a photo-diode which measures the intensity of the radiation from both LEDs after it has passed through the tissue. In order to be able to identify the absorption at each wavelength the LEDs are activated sequentially followed by a period when both are off. This sequence is repeated about 30 times a second so that the absorption at both wavelengths can be sampled many times during each pulse beat. The result is a steady (d.c.) signal which depends on the strength of the light source, absorption by the tissues and by the arterial, venous and capillary blood. On this is superimposed a pulsatile signal due to absorbance associated with the greater volume of blood in the light path with each pulse wave (Fig. 18.14). The raw signals are then subjected to very complex processing. First, the a.c. level is divided by the d.c. level to give a 'scaled' a.c. level that is no longer a function of the incident light intensity (Fig. 18.15(a)). The resulting ratio of the amplitude of the red/infrared pulsatile signals can then be related to the arterial saturation (Fig. 18.15(b)).

In clinical practice, movement artefacts and other sources of interference add 'noise' to the signal. The high frequency of sampling is therefore used to enable running averages of saturation to be calculated many times a second, so minimizing the influence of aberrant readings due to 'noise'. Some manufacturers use 'weighting' techniques to give more emphasis to readings obtained during the upstroke of the pulse wave, whilst others allow a choice of averaging times, long averaging times (e.g. 10–15 s) giving a more reliable value but a longer response time. Other algorithms are incorporated to detect errors due to inadequate pulsation or probe misplacement and most machines have both high and low adjustable alarm limits.

Sources of error. The a.c. signal sensed by a pulse oximeter is usually about 1–5% of the d.c. signal when the pulse volume is normal, so it is not surprising that pulse oximeters become inaccurate when the patient is vasoconstricted from cold or hypovolaemia. Signals may also be inadequate in elderly patients with arterial disease. All pulse oximeters should provide an analogue signal of the pulse waveform so that the user can ensure that a satisfactory signal is being obtained. Bargraph displays of pulse amplitude and some analogue displays are misleading because they are subject to an automatic gain control and so do not reveal a decrease in pulse volume. A useful check on the adequacy of the signal is obtained by comparing the pulse oximeter heart rate reading with that derived from the electrocardiograph (ECG). Whilst many pulse oximeters give warning of an inadequate signal, others continue to display an apparent normal reading.

A second problem is that there may be an error in the saturation displayed. Since the relationship of red/infrared absorption to saturation is a non-linear empirical function, pulse oximeters are usually calibrated by comparing their readings with directly determined arterial saturations in volunteers breathing mixtures containing low concentrations of oxygen. Most of the calibration points are therefore in the range of 80–100%. Values below 80% are usually extrapolated from the higher readings. Although there have now been several studies showing significant errors at saturations of 70% or below, it is difficult to ascertain the true

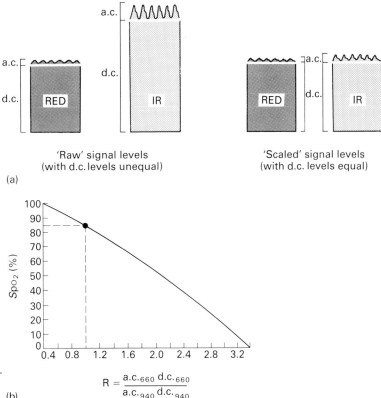

Fig. 18.15. (a) Scaling of a.c. signal. (b) Relationship of red/infrared to Sp_{O_2}.

$$R = \frac{a.c._{660} \quad d.c._{660}}{a.c._{940} \quad d.c._{940}}$$

performance of an individual machine since manufacturers tend to change the software in an attempt to improve performance when gross errors have been detected (Severinghaus & Naifeh, 1987). Since most machines read 95–97% on normal patients there is a tendency to believe that their accuracy is within the manufacturers specification of ±3% saturation. However, as Severinghaus et al. (1989) have shown, mean error varied from 0 to +13%, and precision (the standard deviation of the differences between arterial saturation and Sp_{O_2}) varied from +3.5 to ±16% between instruments tested.

The third source of error is a delay in response. This is due to instrumental delay and circulatory delay. Severinghaus and Naifeh, (1987) showed that with some instruments there was a delay of 10–15 s between a step reduction in alveolar gas concentration and the pulse oximeter response with an ear-probe but that the delay frequently exceeded 60 s when a finger probe was used. Wilkins et al. (1989) showed that cold-induced vasoconstriction and venous engorgement could increase the normal response time two or three-fold.

The fourth problem is interference from intravenous dyes such as methylene blue, bilirubin or dark coloured nail varnish (Cote et al. 1988; Gorman & Schnider, 1988). The problem of MetHb and COHb have already been discussed (p. 265). Fetal haemoglobin has very similar absorption characteristics to adult haemoglobin and should not therefore cause gross errors (Harris et al. 1988). Other sources of interference are large venous pulsations (e.g. in tricuspid incompetence), ambient light or infrared heaters and surgical diathermy. For a critical analysis of pulse oximeter errors see Tremper and Barker (1989).

Interpretation problems. When interpreting the results obtained from pulse oximeters the relationship between saturation and oxygen tension must be considered. This relationship will depend upon the affinity of the haemoglobin for oxygen.

If saturation is monitored using a pulse oximeter, any increase in saturation tends to be interpreted favourably and conversely a decrease unfavourably. Undoubtedly, increasing arterial oxygen saturation will positively reflect the adequacy of pulmonary function, but this must be interpreted in relation to the oxygen tension level. If, for a given Pa_{O_2} of 9.31 kPa (70 mmHg) the saturation increases from 94 to 98% the oxygen content of the arterial blood will increase; however, if this is because the haemoglobin affinity has increased due to changes in some other factor such as hypophosphataemia, the resultant left shift in the oxygen dissociation curve will also provide a relatively higher mixed venous saturation for a given $P\bar{v}_{O_2}$. The net result of the changes is a decrease in the arterio-venous oxygen content difference ($Ca-\bar{v}_{O_2}$) and therefore a decrease in oxygen delivery to the tissues if cardiac output is unchanged. The converse will apply if a decrease in Sa_{O_2} occurs for a fixed Pa_{O_2} giving a greater value for ($Ca-\bar{v}_{O_2}$). In practice, unexpected right shifts are far more common in the intensive care unit than left shifts. In such cases oxygen delivery will be better than the clinician expects.

Pulse oximetry as a monitor of pulmonary function is useful when large changes occur, but the results obtained must be used in conjunction with those from blood gas analysis when small changes occur at high saturations, as these may otherwise be interpreted as advantageous when the converse could well be true.

ERRORS ASSOCIATED WITH BLOOD GAS ANALYSIS

The degree of accuracy obtained when measuring any variable depends on a number of factors. The acceptability of the accuracy which is achieved will depend on the effect that subsequent adjustment will have, and the speed of the patient's response to the change in treatment. Blood gas analysis clearly falls in the class of measurement in which high accuracy is needed. The factors affecting the mea-

surements and calculations fall into five main categories (Adams *et al.* 1967, 1968).

Electrode problems

One of the problems of O_2 electrodes calibrated with gases is that they tend to read low when measuring the P_{O_2} of a liquid which has been equilibrated with gas of a known composition. This blood–gas difference usually varies between 2 and 6% of the reading and is due to the consumption of O_2 by the electrode. In the early electrodes with large diameter cathodes and a relatively high O_2 consumption it was necessary to stir the blood vigorously during the measurement. However, in modern electrodes the effect is minimized by using cathodes of very small diameter. For accurate work the blood gas factor should be determined by the use of tonometered blood samples. However, when buffers equilibrated with known gases have been used for calibration, the blood–gas difference is largely eliminated.

Systematic errors

These are specifically concerned with the performance of the electrodes and the validity of the calibration. Errors also occur if there is lack of membrane integrity. State of the art instruments now produce error codes if systems are not functioning within specified limits. Results can, however, be printed out and could therefore be acted upon.

Quality control solutions

The materials available differ from manufacturer to manufacturer. There are different types of carrier which may be an aqueous buffer, perfluorocarbons or may contain haemoglobin. It is important to select at least one control which has a different type of buffer from that used to calibrate the pH electrode. The different thermal coefficient will highlight a temperature change in the system in the unlikely, but possible occurrence of a malfunction in both the thermostatic control and temperature warning system.

Calculations

Errors associated with the calculation of metabolic variables have been described above (p. 255). These are particularly influenced by increased lipid content of the blood. All modern blood gas analysers calculate haemoglobin saturation; corrections are made for temperature and the Bohr effect before the oxygen tension is applied to the equation, but as none of the other factors are taken into account, the calculated saturation will only be an approximation. Bellingham *et al.* (1971) introduced a correction factor for 2,3-DPG, but the analysis is too time consuming to enable the factor to be incorporated into the equation at the time of blood gas analysis.

Integrity of specimens

It is essential that the specimen analysed contains blood which is unchanged from that in the vessel sampled. Errors will be caused by:

1 incorrect procedure when taking the specimen;
2 undue delay in analysing the specimen.

Sampling. Errors will occur if too much suction is applied when aspirating the sample, if too much heparin is left in the syringe or if there is insufficient discard of the heparinized saline used to maintain the patency of arterial lines. Excess heparin will not only dilute the specimen but will cause haemolysis and any simultaneous measurement of potassium will be falsely elevated. The effect of dilution with heparinized saline on potassium levels will be directly proportional to the dilution factor. Errors in such P_{CO_2} and P_{O_2} results will depend on the actual blood level, the tensions in the heparinized saline and the amount of dilution. The P_{CO_2} measurement will show the largest error as the level of CO_2 in saline is zero. The buffering effect of blood will minimize the change in pH, but calculated parameters based on pH and P_{CO_2} will be incorrect. The amount of heparinized saline which has to be flushed and discarded before an undiluted blood specimen will

be obtained is approximately twice the internal volume of the cannula and lines (Clapham *et al.* 1987).

Before transferring the sample to the blood gas analyzer it should be thoroughly mixed by rotating the syringe in both directions between the palms of the hands. Any gas bubbles present should be expelled and the blood in the nozzle of the syringe discarded before injecting the appropriate volume of sample into the analyser. For samples used to measure content it is advisable to use a mechanical device to ensure that mixing is complete before analysis.

The samples used in blood gas analysis may be arterial, capillary or venous. Venous samples should not be taken with a tourniquet, as stasis markedly influences the pH. Arterialized venous samples taken from the veins on the back of the hand after 10–15 min warming can provide satisfactory pH and P_{CO_2} measurements, though P_{O_2} will usually be lower than arterial. Capillary specimens may be taken, particularly from neonates, where arterial specimens are impractical. They are usually taken from the heel although other sites such as toe, earlobe or thumb may be used. The results obtained, however, will differ from arterial, particularly for P_{O_2}. Arterial blood may be sampled by intermittent puncture using a standard no. 1 (SWG 21) needle or from an indwelling catheter. Catheters may be of the disposable type inserted over a needle or may be inserted by the Seldinger (1953) technique. To minimize complications, catheters should be made of Teflon and should have parallel sides, the diameter being no greater than 20 SWG (Bedford & Wollman, 1973; Bedford, 1975). Catheters may be left in the radial or brachial arteries for 24–48 h provided they are inserted carefully and are flushed with small quantities (0.5–1.0 ml) of heparinized saline (10 $IU \cdot ml^{-1}$) at intervals of 0.5–1.0 hr or are connected to a continuous flush apparatus (e.g. Intraflo, Sorensen; USA).

Storage. Errors due to storage of blood specimens at 4 °C will depend on the following factors:
1 The material from which the syringe is made.

2 The white blood cell count.

3 The anticipated time between collection and analysis.

4 The actual tensions of the gases, particularly oxygen.

Glass does not allow diffusion of gases, but if there are any cracks in the barrel or the plunger does not fit, equilibration of gases with the atmosphere will occur far more quickly than with a plastic syringe. The diffusion of oxygen will be in the direction of the tension gradient (Scott *et al.* 1971a,b). Blood in polypropylene (clear) or polyethylene (opaque) syringes will tend to equilibrate with room air (P_{O_2} = 20 kPa, 150 mmHg) and if the blood P_{O_2} is lower, it will increase. The converse will occur for higher levels of oxygen tension. However, the errors are small with 30 min of storage.

A high white blood cell count (WBC) will increase aerobic respiration with a resultant decrease in oxygen tension and content (Shohat *et al.* 1988). Unless the WBC is very high, refrigeration to reduce such respiration is not necessary if the analysis is to be carried out less than 20 min after the specimen has been taken.

If any bubbles are present, the increased solubility at 4 °C will result in oxygen from the bubbles dissolving in the blood. Air bubbles in the specimen will produce a greater error if the bubble is injected or aspirated undetected onto the face of a measuring electrode.

False assumptions

It is common teaching that an oxygen tension in excess of 9.31 kPa (70 mmHg) will provide a sufficient supply of oxygen to the tissues. This assumption will only be valid if the ODC is normal. In fact, only 10% of patients with an acid–base imbalance will have a normal ODC (Willis & Clapham, 1985). Thus assumptions regarding oxygen delivery made without reference to oxygen saturation and the position of the ODC may well be false.

There is a direct relationship between the oxygen carried in the arterial blood and the haemoglobin concentration and the concurrent measurement of total haemoglobin is essential if decisions on oxygen therapy are to be taken. Haemoglobin concentration will also serve as an indicator of the integrity of the sample taken. Other variables measured during blood gas analysis can change quickly but haemoglobin concentrations will normally change slowly. Thus marked changes in haemoglobin are either indicative of a large blood loss or, more often, of dilution of one or more specimens due to insufficient flushing and discard.

Temperature corrections

Blood gas analysers are thermostatically controlled to measure blood gases at 37 °C. If the patient's temperature differs from this, correction factors must be applied. Hypothermia will decrease the P_{O_2} and P_{CO_2} but as the pH is the reciprocal of the $[H^+]$, this will increase. The converse applies if the patient is pyrexic.

The correction factor which is used for pH is that suggested by Rosenthal (1948):

$$pH_{(temp)} = pH_{(37\,°C)} - 0.0147\,(T\,°C - 37)$$

For P_{O_2} and P_{CO_2} the factors of Kelman (1966) and Kelman and Nunn (1966) are usually used. The equations for correction are as follows:

$$P_{CO_2\,(temp)} = P_{CO_2\,(37\,°C)} \times 10^{0.019\,(T\,°C - 37)}$$

$$P_{O_2\,(temp)} = P_{O_2\,(37\,°C)} \times 10^{A\,(T\,°C - 37)}$$

where

$$A = 0.0052 + 0.027[1 - 10^{-0.13\,(100 - Sat)}].$$

The saturation included in the P_{O_2} correction formula has to be calculated from the measured oxygen tension assuming a normal dissociation curve. If the *measured* saturation is used in the above equation, the results will differ if high oxygen tensions are corrected to low body temperatures, since the correction factor (above) incorporates a saturation figure. At high oxygen tensions the actual saturation will be lower than the saturation calculated from the oxygen tension.

The non-respiratory component of acid–base balance is measured at 37 °C as the significance of pH measurement at low temperatures is not clear.

'Stat' instruments

Until the early 1980s clinical user instruments for pathology investigations were limited to reflectance meters associated with the glucose strip test. Recently a number of 'Stat' instruments for clinical use have been developed with a wide and ever increasing range of tests being offered. They are transportable, bench-top instruments, ideal for small laboratories or for use in clinics, and which give quick and accurate results for a large number of analyses. Recently, large high capacity versions of one type have been developed for use in main laboratories. The clinical instruments are designed to be used by non-technical personnel and are microprocessor controlled with results being obtained from algorithms incorporated into the ROM (read only memory) of the system. They offer speed, acceptable accuracy, flexibility and the ability to produce high quality results with only simple training. The instruments are divided into two main categories; those using liquid reagents held in plastic cassettes which mix the specimen and reagents by a variety of means, usually inversion or centrifugation, with resultant colour reactions being measured spectrophotometrically; and those using solid phase technology and reflection spectroscopy. The theoretical aspect of spectrophotometry has been discussed in Chapter 8. The techniques of solid phase technology are worth further consideration.

SOLID PHASE TECHNOLOGY

Two of the systems using solid phase chemistry are the Ames Seralyser (Miles Laboratories, England) and the Kodak Ektachem (Kodak, England). The principles, although similar, differ sufficiently for both to be described.

Ames Seralyser

A plastic strip, supporting a cellulose matrix is placed into the system on a thermostatted specimen table. The cellulose matrix consists of layers of analytical reagents which have been dried sequentially. The choice of solvent allows layers to be superimposed so that reactive components are separated by inert ones. The strips are stored at room temperature and are usable for at least 60 days after a pack is opened. The reagents dissolve when the pad is rehydrated by the application of a diluted serum sample.

The appropriate reagent strip is placed on a thermostated table and $30\,\mu l$ of a diluted serum specimen is pipetted onto the surface of the strip which is pushed into the instrument. Bar codes on the strip are read and a microprocessor selects the necessary conditions for the test, such as wavelength and algorithm. The conditions under which each test is performed are contained in an interchangeable ROM cartridge.

Light from a xenon flash tube illuminates a surrounding sphere with a series of flashes. The light has a usable spectrum of 340–700 nm and is pulsed for $60\,\mu s$. The internal surface of the sphere is coated with several layers of barium sulphate which diffuse the light and allow it to strike the upper surface of the reagent pad from all angles. The intensity of the light at the specific wavelength, reflected from the pad, is compared to the total light available to illuminate the pad. The comparison of reflected and incident light is used to calculate the concentration of the specific analyte. Calibration for any given test is at two points before each individual analysis or batch of analyses. A series of error codes will highlight errors both procedural and systematic.

A number of investigations are already possible, including enzyme activities, glucose, urea, creatinine and all the common electrolytes; the number will undoubtedly increase. Evaluations of the Seralyser system as a whole have been undertaken by a number of authors (Ito & Niwa, 1982; Karmen & Lent, 1982; Thomas *et al.* 1982). Evaluations of the specific tests offered have been carried out by many authors as each new analyte becomes available. To date there have been in excess of 50 publications.

Kodak Ektachem

Another type of system based on reflectance spectrophotometry has been introduced by Kodak

(Kodak Ektachem DT60 Analyser). This can be complemented by additional modules, one of which will measure electrolytes whilst the other will measure rate reactions to determine the activity of enzymes or measure concentrations of drugs. The reagents are incorporated into a slide on a clear polyester support base. The slides differ from the strips used in the Seralyser in that the reagents are layered in a matrix which contains some water molecules and so storage at 4 °C is required.

The slides are produced with differing numbers of layers, including semi-permeable, with a variety of reagents, depending on the analytes to be measured (Fig. 18.16a). There are two basic types of slide (Fig. 18.16b).

1 Colorimetric, in which reflected light is measured.

2 Potentiometric, in which electrolyte concentra-

tion is measured as a function of the potential difference produced between a sample and a reference solution in a half cell.

Colorimetric. The slide is inserted into the instrument where it is held in a thermostatted block at 37 °C. A bar code is read as the slide is inserted and the relevant information regarding the test is displayed. The $10\,\mu l$ sample is placed, using a specifically designed automatic pipette, onto a spreading layer (barium sulphate or titanium dioxide). This has the dual purpose of spreading the sample and providing a white background to aid reflectance. The spreading layer also contains reagents which will initiate chemical reactions when analytes with large molecules such as cholesterol and triglycerides are to be measured. The reagent layer can contain enzymes, buffers and catalysts, and if several different reactions are to occur, several layers are incorporated into the slide. Macromolecules can be excluded by incorporating a semi-permeable membrane. When, for instance, urea is to be measured, the spreading layer and a semi-permeable membrane allows ammonia to diffuse through to the indicator layer. A solid state fibreoptic system consisting of four separate fibre-optic bundles, carries light from three light emitting diodes at 555, 605 and 660 nm to the slide, while the fourth transmits the reflected light from the colour reaction, through the clear polyester base, to the photodetector.

The microprocessor selects the appropriate LED for the test and the portion of incident light not absorbed by the coloured complex is reflected by the spreading layer and measured by the photodetector. The analogue output from the photodetector is digitized and compared to that obtained from a reference 'white spot', which theoretically reflects all the incident light, and a 'black spot' which is a zero offset for instrument noise. These values are related to three reference values from calibration materials and a value for the sample can then be obtained.

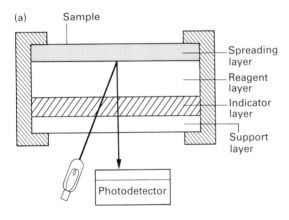

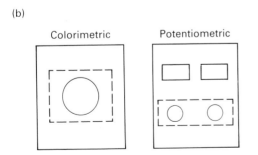

Fig. 18.16. (a) Structure of an Ektachem slide. (b) The two types of cell arrangement (colorimetric and potentiometric).

Potentiometric. The system can measure sodium, potassium, chloride and bicarbonate. When potassium is to be measured, $10\,\mu l$ of the sample and reference fluid are pipetted onto the 'drop holes' in the slide (Fig. 18.17). The two solutions diffuse towards each other on the paper bridge and form an electrochemical junction; the valinomycin is selectively permeable to K^+ ions and a small quantity of water from each solution penetrates to the KCl internal reference layer. The Ag : AgCl layer provides a reference potential and the resulting e.m.f. produced is proportional to the relative concentration of the K^+ ion in the sample and the reference solutions. Again, a number of analytes can be measured including ammonia. Calibration is recommended at 3 monthly intervals for a given batch of slides, and quality control at one level, daily, when the instrument is in use.

The Ektachem system was evaluated by Ayers *et al.* (1987) for the estimation of sodium, potassium, glucose and urea. He found the system gave results comparable in terms of bias and precision, with current methods. O'Leary *et al.* (1988) reported that a lipaemic specimen with a very high triglyceride produced a low value; serial dilution of the specimen confirmed a cut off-point at high levels, resulting in a default low level being produced. Glick and Ryder (1987) found that systems incorporating physical barriers or protein separation steps, such as the Ektachem, were less affected

than other systems by interfering substances such as bilirubin and lipids.

References

Adams A.P., Morgan-Hughes, J.O. & Sykes, M.K. (1967) pH and blood-gas analysis. Methods of measurement and sources of error using electrode systems, Part 1. *Anaesthesia* **22**, 575–597.

Adams, A.P., Morgan-Hughes, J.O. & Sykes, M.K. (1968) pH and blood-gas analysis. Method of measurement and sources of error using electrode systems. Part 2. *Anaesthesia* **23**, 47–64.

Aoyagi, T., Kishi, M., Yamaguchi, K. & Watanabe, S. (1974) Improvement of an earpiece oximeter. *Abstracts of the 13th annual meeting of the Japanese Society for Medical and Electronics and Biological Engineering*, pp. 90–91.

Astrup, P. (1956) A simple electrometric technique for the determination of carbon dioxide tension in blood and plasma, total content of carbon dioxide in plasma, and bicarbonate content in 'separated' plasma at a fixed carbon dioxide tension. *Scandinavian Journal of Clinical and Laboratory Investigation* **8**, 33–43.

Astrup, P. & Schroder, S. (1956) Apparatus for anaerobic determination of pH in blood. *Scandinavian Journal of Clinical and Laboratory Investigation* **8**, 30–32.

Astrup, P. (1961) A New approach to acid–base metabolism. *Clinical Chemistry* **7**, 1–15.

Atkinson, R.S., Rushman, G.B. & Lee, J.A. (1987) *A synopsis of anaesthesia*, 10th edn., pp 395 and 603. Wright, Bristol.

Ayers, G., Rumjen, C.S.S., Woods, I.F. & Burnett, D. (1987) Evaluation of the Kodak Ektachem DT60 analyser for sodium, potassium, glucose and urea. *Journal of Clinical Laboratory Automation* **9**, 119–124.

Baele, P.L., McMichan, J.C., Marsh, H.M., Sill, J.C. & Southorn, P.A. (1982) Continuous monitoring of mixed venous oxygen saturation in critically ill patients. *Anesthesia and Analgesia* **61**, 513–517.

Barker, S.T. & Tremper, K.K. (1987) The effect of carbon monoxide inhalation on pulse oximeter signal detection. *Anesthesiology* **67**, 599–603.

Bedford, R.F. (1975) Percutaneous radial-artery cannulation—increased safety using Teflon catheters. *Anesthesiology* **42**, 219–222.

Bedford, R.F. & Wollman, H, (1973) Complications of percutaneous radial artery cannulation. *Anesthesiology* **38**, 228–236.

Bellingham, A.J., Delter, J.C. & Lenfant, C. (1971) Regulatory mechanisms of haemoglobin affinity in acidosis and alkosis. *Journal of Clinical Investigation* **50**, 700–706.

Blackburn, J.P. (1978) What is new in blood gas analysis? *British Journal of Anaesthesia* **50**, 51–62.

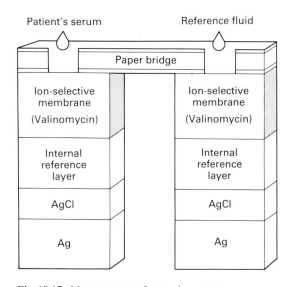

Fig. 18.17. Measurement of potassium on a potentiometric slide.

Brinkman, R. & Zijlstra, W.G. (1949) Determination and continuous registration of the percentage oxygen saturation in small amounts of blood. *Archivium Chirurgicum Neerlandicum* **1**, 177–183.

Brinkman, R.M., Zijlstra, W.G. & Koopmans, R.K. (1952) A method for continuous observation of percentage oxygen saturation in patients. *Archivium Chirurgicum Neerlandicum* **1**, 333–334.

Clapham, M.C.C., Willis, N. & Mapleson, W.W. (1987) Minimum volume of discard for valid blood sampling from indwelling arterial cannulae. *British Journal of Anaesthesia* **59**, 232–235.

Clark, L.C. (1956) Monitor and control of blood and tissue oxygen tension. *Transactions of the Society for Artificial Internal Organs* **2**, 41–48.

Clark, L.C., Wolf, R., Granger, D. & Taylor, Z. (1953) Continuous recording of blood oxygen tensions by polarography. *Journal of Applied Physiology* **6**, 189–193.

Cornelissen, P.J.H., van Woensel, C.L.M., van Del, W.C. & de Jong, P.A. (1983) Correction factors for hemoglobin derivatives in foetal blood, as measured with the IL 282 co-oximeter. *Clinical Chemistry* **29**, 1555–1556.

Cote, C.J., Goldstein, E.A., Fuchsman, W.M. & Hoaglin, D.C. (1988) The effect of nail polish on pulse oximetry. *Anesthesia and Analgesia* **67**, 683–686.

Dennis, R.C. & Valeri, C.R. (1980) Measuring percent oxygen saturation of hemoglobin, percent carboxyhemoglobin and methemoglobin, and concentrations of total hemoglobin in man, dog and baboon. *Clinical Chemistry* **26**, 1304–8.

Divertie, M.B. & McMichan J.C. (1984) Continuous monitoring of mixed venous oxygen saturation. *Chest* **85**, 423–428.

Eisenman, G., Rudin, D.O. & Casby, J.V. (1957) Glass electrode for measuring sodium ion. *Science* **126**, 831–834.

Fallon, K.D., Melenfgant, A.L., Weisel, R.D. & Heachteman, H.B. (1973) Oxygen transport to the tissues. Instrumentation, methods and physiology. *Advances in experimental medicine and biology*, pp. 93–97. Plenum Press, New York.

Flick, M.R. & Block, A.J. (1978) Continuous *in vivo* arterial oxygen saturation measurements by oximetry. *Heart, Lung* **6**, 990–993.

Gehrich, J.L., Lübbers D.W., Opitz, N., Hansmann, D.R., Miller, W.W., Tusa, J.K. & Yafuso, M. (1986) Optical fluorescence and its application to an intravascular blood gas monitoring system. *IEEE Transactions on Biomedical Engineering* BME-33, 117–132.

Gettinger, A., DeTraglia, M.C. & Glass, D.D. (1987) In-vivo comparison of two mixed venous saturation catheters. *Anesthesiology* **66**, 373–375.

Glick, M.R. & Ryder, K.W. (1987) Analytical Systems ranked by freedom from interferences. *Clinical Chemistry* **33**, 1435–1458.

Gorman, E.S. & Schneider, M.R. (1988) Effect of methylene blue on the absorbance of solutions of hemoglobin. *British Journal of Anaesthesia* **60**, 439–44.

Gregory, I.C., Hulands, G.H. & Millar, R.A. (1971) The *in vivo* oxygen capacity of hemoglobin in man. *Journal of Physiology* **219**, 31P.

Hamilton, P.A., Whitehead, M.D. & Reynolds, E.O.R. (1985) Underestimation of arterial oxygen tension by transcutaneous electrodes with increasing age in infants. *Archives of the Diseases in Childhood* **60**, 1162–1165.

Harris, J.C., Rumack, B.H., Peterson, R.G. & McGuire, B.M. (1979) Methemoglobinaemia resulting from absorption of nitrates. *Journal of the American Medical Association* **242**, 2869–2871.

Harris, A.P., Sevdak, M.J., Donham, R.T., Thomas, M. & Duncan, D. (1988) Absorption characteristics of human fetal haemoglobin at wavelengths used in pulse oximetry. *Journal of Clinical Monitoring* **4**, 175–177.

Horabin, A.L. & Farhi (1978) Measurement of blood O_2 and CO_2 concentrations using Po_2 and Pco_2 electrodes. *Journal of Applied Physiology* **44**, 818–820.

Holbeck, C.C. (1989) The radiometer ABL 300 Blood gas analyzer. *Journal of Clinical Monitoring* **5**, 4–16.

Huch, A., Huch, R., Schneider, H. & Rooth, G. (1977) Continuous transcutaneous monitoring of fetal oxygen tension during labour. *British Journal of Obstetrics and Gynaecology* **84**, Suppl. 1, 1–39.

Ito, K. & Niwa, M. (1982) A new clinical chemical analysis device using dry chemistry; an experiment on the Seralyser system. *Journal of Clinical Instruments* **5**, 11–17.

Jennis, M.S. & Peabody, J.L. (1985) No burns, no gradient — pulse oximetry, an alternative to transcutaneous Po_2. *Clinical Research* **33**, 139A.

Karmen, A. & Lent, R. (1982) Clinical chemistry testing with the Ames Seralyser dry reagent system. *Journal of Clinical Laboratory Automation* **2**, 284–296.

Kelman, G.R. (1966) Digital computer subroutine for the conversion of oxygen tension into saturation. *Journal of Applied Physiology* **21**, 1375–1376.

Kelman, G.R. & Nunn, J.F. (1966) Nomograms for correction of blood Po_2, Pco_2, pH and base excess for time and temperature. *Journal of Applied Physiology* **21**, 1484–1490.

McEvoy, D.S., Jones, N.L. & Campbell, E.J.M. (1974) Mixed venous and arterial Pco_2. *British Medical Journal* **iv**, 687–690.

McInnes, D.A. & Belcher, D. (1933) A durable glass electrode. *Industrial and Engineering Chemistry: Analytical Edition* **5**, 199–200.

Miller, W.W., Masao, Y., Cheng, F.Y., Henry, K.H. & Arick, S. (1987) Performance of an *in vivo*, continuous blood–gas monitor with disposable probe. *Clinical Chemistry* **33**, 1538–1542.

Norden, A.G.W. & Flynn, F.V. (1979) Halothane interference with Po_2 measurements and a method of inhibiting its effect. *Clinica Chimica Acta* **99**, 229–234.

O'Leary, T.D., Taylor, T.W. & Langton, S.R. (1988) Spurious triglyceride results with the Kodak Ectachem 700. *Clinical Chemistry* **34**, 744–775.

Parker, D., Delphy, D. & Lewis, M. (1978) Catheter tip electrode for continuous measurement of Po_2 and Pco_2. *Medical Biology Engineering and Computing* **16**, 599–600.

Polanyi, M.L. & Hehir, R.M. (1962) *In vivo* oximeter with fast dynamic response. *Review of Scientific Instruments* **33**, 1050–1054.

Riley, R.L., Campbell, E.J.M. & Shepard, R.H. (1957) A bubble method for estimation of Pco_2 and Po_2 in whole blood. *Journal of Applied Physiology* **11**, 245–249.

Rome, E.S., Stork, E.K., Carlo, W.A. *et al.* (1984) Limitations of transcutaneous Po_2 and Pco_2 monitoring in infants with bronchopulmonary dysplasia. *Pediatrics* **74**, 217–220.

Rosenthal, T.B. (1948) The effect of temperature on the pH of blood and plasma *in vitro*. *Journal of Biological Chemistry* **173**, 25–30.

Scott, P.V., Horton, J.N. & Mapleson, W.W. (1971a) Mechanism and magnitude of leakage of oxygen from blood and water samples stored in plastic syringes. *British Journal of Anaesthesia* **43**, 717–718.

Scott, P.V., Horton, J.N. & Mapleson, W.W. (1971b) Leakage of oxygen from blood and water samples stored in plastic and glass syringes. *British Medical Journal* **iii**, 512–516.

Selman, B.J., White, Y.S. & Tait, A.R. (1975) An evaluation of the Lex-O_2-Con oxygen content analyser. *Anaesthesia* **30**, 206–211.

Seldinger, S.I. (1953) Catheter replacement of the needle in percutaneous arteriography. *Acta Radiologica (Stockholm)* **39**, 368–376.

Severinghaus, J.W. (1976) Acid–base nomogram. A Boston–Copenhagen detente. *Anesthesiology* **45**, 539–541.

Severinghaus, J.W. & Bradley, A.F. (1958) Electrodes for Po_2 and Pco_2 determination. *Journal of Applied Physiology* **13**, 515–520.

Severinghaus, J.W. & Naifeh, K.H. (1987) Accuracy of response of six pulse oximeters to profound hypoxia. *Anesthesiology* **67**, 551–558.

Severinghaus, J.W., Stupfel, M. & Bradley, A.F. (1956) Variations of serum carbonic acid pK′ with pH and temperature. *Journal of Applied Physiology* **9**, 197–200.

Severinghaus, J.W., Naifeh, K.H. & Koh, S.O. (1989) Errors in 14 pulse oximeters during profound hypoxia. *Journal of Clinical Monitoring* **5**, 72–81.

Shohat, M., Schonfeld, T., Zaizoz, R., Cohen, I.J. & Nitzan, M. (1988) Determination of blood gases in children with extreme leucocytosis. *Critical Care Medicine* **16**, 787–788.

Siggaard-Andersen, O., (1962) The pH/log Pco_2 blood acid–base nomogram revised. *Scandinavian Journal of Clinical and Laboratory Investigation* **14**, 598–604.

Siggaard-Andersen, O. (1966) Titratable acid or base of body fluids. *Annals of the New York Academy of Science* **133**, 41–58.

Siggaard-Andersen, O. (1971) An acid–base chart for normal and pathophysiological reference areas. *Scandinavian Journal of Clinical and Laboratory Investigation* **27**, 239–245.

Siggaard-Andersen, O., Engel, K., Jorgensen, K. & Astrup, P. (1960) A micro method for determination of pH, carbon dioxide tension, base excess and standard bicarbonate in capillary blood. *Scandinavian Journal of Clinical and Laboratory Investigation* **12**, 172–176.

Skeates, S.J. (1978) The non-invasive measurement of arterial oxygen. *British Journal of Clinical Equipment* **3**, 63–70.

van Slyke, D.D. & Neill, J.M. (1924) The determination of gases in blood and other solutions by vacuum extraction and manometric measurement. *Journal of Biological Chemistry* **61**, 523–573.

Smith, A.C. & Hahn, C.E.W. (1975) Studies with the Severinghaus Pco_2 electrode. 1: Electrode stability, memory and S plots. *British Journal of Anaesthesia* **47**, 553–588.

Stow, R.W. & Randall, B.F. (1954) Electrical measurement of the Pco_2 of blood. *American Journal of Physiology* **179**, 678.

Thomas, Jr., L.J. (1972) Algorithms for selected blood acid–base and blood gas calculations. *Journal of Applied Physiology* **33**, 154–158.

Thomas, L., Plischke, W. & Stork, G. (1982) Evaluation of a quantitative solid phase reagent system for determination of blood analytes. *Annals of Clinical Biochemistry* **19**, 214–223.

Tremper, K.K. & Barker, S.J. (1989) Pulse oximetry. *Anesthesiology* **70**, 98–108.

Wilkins, C.J., Moores, M. & Hanning, C.D. (1989) Comparison of pulse oximeters: effects of vasoconstriction and venous engorgement. *British Journal of Anaesthesia* **62**, 439–444.

Willis, N. & Clapham, M.C.C. (1985) The validity of oxygen content calculations. *Clinica Chimica Acta* **150**, 213–220.

Willis, N., Clapham, M.C.C. & Mapleson, W.W. (1987) Additional blood gas variables for the rational control of oxygen therapy. *British Journal of Anaesthesia* **59**, 1160–1170.

Wukitsch, M.W., Petterson, M.T., Tobler, D. & Polge, G. (1988) Pulse oximetry: analysis of theory, technology and practice. *Journal of Clinical Monitoring* **4**, 290–301.

Zander, R., Lang, W. & Wolf, H.U. (1977) Oxygen cuvette: a simple approach to the oxygen concentration measurement in blood. *Pflugers Archives* **368**, R16.

19: Thermometry, Thermography and Humidity Measurement

Thermometry

Spontaneous and controlled changes in body temperature are now so commonly encountered in clinical practice that temperature monitoring has become routine in the operating theatre and intensive care unit. Thermometry is also used to monitor the function of therapeutic devices such as humidifiers and extracorporeal circulation equipment, and ancillary equipment such as autoclaves, refrigerators and laboratory apparatus.

TEMPERATURE SCALES AND CALIBRATION

In 1714 the German physicist Fahrenheit developed the first thermometer using mercury in a closed tube. There is some doubt about the fixed points on his scale of temperature but it is believed that he set the zero point with a mixture of sodium chloride and ice and assumed that body temperature was 100 °F. The temperature of melting ice then read 32 °F and that of boiling water 212 °F. In 1742 the Swedish astronomer Anders Celsius adopted a different scale which, in its final form, utilized the temperature of melting ice and boiling water as the two fixed points on the scale. This scale was divided into a 100 steps and so became known by the Latin equivalent 'centigrade'. However, in 1948 the scale was renamed the Celsius scale (°C) in honour of its inventor. The conver-

sions between the two scales are given by:

$$°F = (°C \times 9/5) + 32$$

and

$$°C = (°F - 32) \times 5/9.$$

Normal body temperature is customarily said to be 37 °C or 98.4 °F, although in fact many in the population have a normal oral temperature some 0.2–0.4 °C less than this.

When dealing with gas law equations it is necessary to employ yet another scale of temperature, the Absolute or Kelvin temperature scale. On this scale the zero is the absolute zero, which is the lowest temperature it is theoretically possible to attain. This is – 273.16 °C. The unit of the Kelvin scale used to be called the degree Kelvin but in the SI system is now simply called the kelvin (K). It is defined as 1/273.16 of the thermodynamic temperature of the triple point of water (the point where the solid, liquid and vapour forms of water co-exist). Thus 0 °C is equivalent to 273 K and 100 °C to 373 K. Since each degree Celsius is equal to a kelvin, K = °C + 273 (Fig. 19.1).

The fixed points on most thermometers can be set with melting ice and boiling water. However, the accuracy of intermediate points can only be ensured by checking that the scale is linear. Furthermore some thermometers have a limited scale

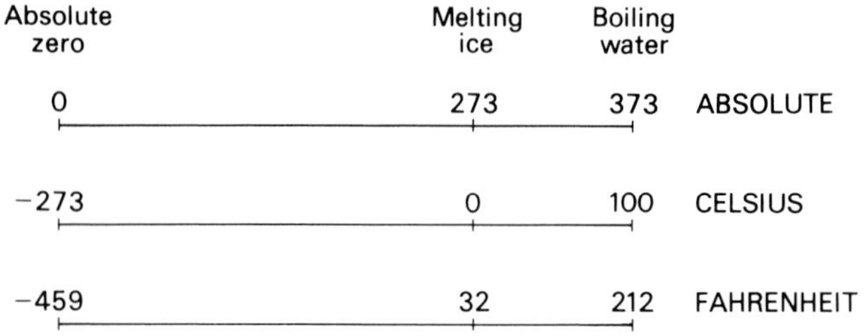

Absolute zero		Melting ice	Boiling water	
0		273	373	ABSOLUTE
−273		0	100	CELSIUS
−459		32	212	FAHRENHEIT

Fig. 19.1. Absolute, Celsius and Fahrenheit temperature scales.

length so that the 0 °C and 100 °C points cannot be established. Thermometers are therefore calibrated by reference to a thermometer whose accuracy has been certified by the National Laboratory at Teddington.

Types of thermometers

DIRECT READING INSTRUMENTS

Liquid expansion thermometers

These are the simplest and most reliable devices for measuring temperature. The instrument consists of a glass bulb, connected to an evacuated, closed capillary tube. The bulb is filled with a liquid (generally alcohol or mercury) and the temperature is indicated by the position of the meniscus in the capillary tube. If the cross-sectional area of the capillary is uniform throughout its length a linear calibration can be achieved.

The coefficient of expansion of mercury is relatively small (about 1.8% of its volume between 0 and 100 °C) so that the clinical thermometer requires a large bulb and a very narrow capillary to increase sensitivity. The narrow capillary is rendered more easily visible by shaping the thermometer so that the glass forms a lens and by incorporating a strip of white glass behind the capillary (Fig. 19.2). A constriction in the capillary tube permits the mercury to expand but hinders its return to the bulb so that the reading is preserved until the mercury is shaken down into the bulb.

This type of thermometer has several disadvantages. It is fragile, has a large thermal capacity and so is slow to respond, is difficult to read and to re-set, is unsuitable for insertion into body cavities and cannot be used for remote reading or recording. Most clinical thermometers also have a limited scale length so that special low-recording thermometers must be used when hypothermia is suspected.

Dial thermometers

It is possible to separate the display from the site of temperature measurement by using liquid or gas expansion thermometers in which the expansion is detected by a pressure measuring device such as a Bourdon gauge. The temperature sensing bulb is connected to the pressure gauge by a narrow metal tube and the cavity is filled either with a liquid or with a volatile liquid and its saturated vapour. The change in pressure produced by the alteration in temperature is sensed by the gauge and displayed on the dial. The volume of the bulb must be large compared with the volume of the connecting tube and gauge (to minimize the effects of changes in ambient temperature on the reading) and the connecting tube must not be bent or narrowed after calibration has been performed. This type of thermometer is relatively cheap and robust but not very accurate. It is therefore generally employed to measure fairly large temperature changes, e.g. in humidifiers, water baths or autoclaves.

Bimetallic thermometers

If strips of two metals with different coefficients of expansion are fastened together throughout their length, the combined strip will bend when heated. In thermometers based on this principle the bimetallic strip is usually bent into a spiral or coil and one end is fixed whilst the other end is attached to a pointer lying in front of a dial. A change in temperature causes the coil to wind or unwind so moving the pointer across the dial. This principle is used in cheap, but not very accurate thermometers for measuring air temperature. A bimetallic strip is also used in a number of anaesthetic vaporizers to compensate for changes in the temperature of the liquid being vaporized. The strip opens and closes an orifice which varies the proportion of gases passing through the bypass

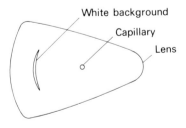

White background

Capillary

Lens

Fig. 19.2. Cross-section through a clinical thermometer.

tube and vaporizing chamber. It thus maintains a constant output concentration of vapour despite changes in vapour pressure due to changes in temperature of the volatile agent.

Chemical thermometers

One clinical instrument consists of an aluminium strip with a transparent cover. The strip contains several rows of small cells along its length. Each cell is filled with a unique mixture of chemicals which melts at a particular temperature, the number of cells being chosen to suit the desired accuracy and temperature range. The chemicals melt within about 30 s and, in doing so, release a dye. The temperature is indicated by the number of cells which have changed colour. By incorporating 50 such cells in one strip it is possible to cover the range 35.5–40.4 °C with an acccuracy of ±0.1 °C. The method is somewhat expensive because a fresh thermometer is required for each temperature reading; however, the use of disposable thermometers eliminates the danger of cross-infection.

Reversible chemical thermometers are also available. These contain a number of cells filled with liquid crystals (long chain polymers), each cell having a slightly different composition from the next. At a critical temperature the optical properties change due to a re-alignment of the molecules, causing reflection instead of absorption of incident light. By selecting suitable materials, temperature intervals of about 0.5 °C can be differentiated (Lees *et al.* 1968).

REMOTE READING INSTRUMENTS

Resistance-wire thermometers

These are based on the principle that the resistance of certain metal wires increases as their temperature increases. The metal most commonly used for this purpose is platinum, since it resists corrosion and has a large temperature coefficient of resistance. Over the range 0–100 °C the change in resistance is linearly related to the change in temperature and is about $0.4 \, \Omega \cdot °C^{-1}$ for a $100 \, \Omega$

resistance element. Copper and nickel are also used. The 'Craftemp' utilizes a piece of copper foil, 5 mm × 1.5 mm, with a thickness of only 50 μm, encased in food quality polyethylene, fabricated as a single-use probe. This need only be placed in the mouth for 10 s or the axilla for 40 s. The resistance change is then measured by a battery operated handpiece which grips the two terminals at the distal end of the probe. An accuracy of ±0.1 °C is claimed. Platinum resistance thermometers can be made to sense very small differences in temperature (±0.0001 °C) but the instrument then becomes somewhat fragile and slow to respond.

Thermistor thermometers

Thermistors are semiconductors made from the fused oxides of heavy metals such as cobalt, manganese and nickel, and can be made to have positive or negative temperature coefficients. Their resistance varies markedly with temperature (about 4% per °C) over the range of body temperature, but the change is non-linear. However, this can be corrected over a limited temperature range by simple electronic circuitry. Thermistors have several other potential disadvantages. First, the resistance of individual thermistors in a batch tends to vary. Second, thermistors tend to 'age' or show a change in resistance with time. Third, they tend to exhibit hysteresis so that the value of a given temperature recorded during a heating cycle is less than the value recorded at the same temperature during a cooling cycle. These disadvantages can be minimized by purchasing matched, pre-aged thermistors which display a much smaller hysteresis effect.

Because the temperature coefficient of a thermistor is much greater than that of a resistance wire element, thermistors can be used to detect very small temperature changes. Furthermore the beads are extremely small (about the size of a pinhead) so that they respond very quickly. They are therefore ideally suited for detecting the change in temperature of pulmonary arterial blood in the thermal dilution method of cardiac output measurement. They have also been used to detect changes in temperature between inspired and expired gas in respiration monitoring and have been incorporated into endoradiosondes or 'radio pills' which are swallowed and then transmit the deep body temperature of mobile patients.

Thermocouple thermometers

If two dissimilar metals are joined to create an electrical circuit and the junctions are at different temperatures, a current will flow from one metal to the other, the electromotive force (e.m.f.) generated being a function of the temperature difference between the two junctions (Fig. 19.3). This phenomenon was first described in 1923 and is known as the Seebeck effect. Common combinations of metals used to make thermocouples are copper–constantan (constantan is 60% copper and 40% nickel) or platinum–rhodium. It is essential to maintain the cold junction at a constant temperature (e.g. ice water) or to include some electronic compensating device which will correct for changes in ambient temperature.

The output from a copper–constantan junction is relatively small (about $40\,\mu V$ per °C temperature difference between the junctions) but can be sensed with sufficient accuracy by a galvanometer or digital voltmeter. The supreme advantage of the thermocouple is that all junctions made from the same materials behave identically, and are very inexpensive, so that multichannel thermometers can be constructed economically.

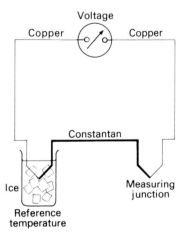

Fig. 19.3. Principle of a thermocouple thermometer.

Wire and thin film thermometers

These are usually made of platinum which makes them more expensive than thermistors, but have a much lower temperature coefficient. However, fine wire and thin film elements can have very fast response times which enable them to sense rapidly changing air or blood velocity.

Transistor detectors

If a current is passed across diodes or transistor junctions, the voltage developed is temperature dependent and is about 50 times greater than that of a copper–contantan thermocouple. The error, drift and variability between sensors are all extremely low.

Crystal Resonators

The resonant frequency of a quartz crystal is temperature dependent and at 28 MHz the variation is about $1\,KHz\cdot°C^{-1}$. Being able to have temperature measurements as a frequency output is advantageous for digital signal processing.

Site of body temperature measurement

Small gradients of temperature exist between different parts of the body in normal subjects but these gradients are often accentuated in disease and when the body is rapidly cooled or heated by external means (Cooper & Kenyon, 1957).

The highest temperature is normally recorded in the rectum. This is usually assumed to represent 'core' temperature but may prove unreliable if faeces are present. The oesophageal temperature is mainly dominated by the temperature of the blood in the heart and is usually 0.5 °C lower than rectal temperature. However, if the probe is situated in the upper oesophagus and the patient is vigorously hyperventilated through a tracheostomy or an endotracheal tube oesophageal temperature may be several degrees below rectal (Whitby & Dunkin, 1968, 1969, 1970). Oesophageal probes should therefore lie about 25 cm below the laryngeal orifice. Tympanic membrane temperature reflects

brain temperature and is usually close to oesophageal (Dickey *et al.* 1970; Holdcroft & Hall, 1978).
However, there is a risk of bleeding and damage to
the tympanic membrane (Webb, 1973). To prevent
such damage, Keatinge and Sloan (1975) recom-
mend that the probe should be placed on the
anterior wall of the aural canal with a servocon-
trolled heating device on the outer ear to prevent
local cooling. Nasopharyngeal temperature can be
used to monitor brain temperature providing that
the probe is maintained in apposition to the
mucosa. However it frequently becomes displaced
and the method is unreliable in practice (Whitby &
Dunkin, 1971).

Skin temperature varies widely and is markedly
affected by skin blood flow. It thus provides a
useful measure of tissue blood flow, the toe–core
temperature difference often being used as a monitor of the adequacy of the circulation in shock or
other low output states (Matthews *et al.* 1974a,b).
In the neonate the abdominal skin temperature
decreases rapidly as the infant cools, thus providing a more sensitive index of body cooling than
rectal temperature. This fact has been utilized in a
number of servo-controlled heaters for neonates
which control their heat output on the basis of the
abdominal skin temperature.

Rapid changes in blood temperature produced,
for example, by extracorporeal circulation, are
reflected immediately by changes in oesophageal
temperature. Temperature changes in the organs
receiving a high proportion of the cardiac output
(brain, heart, kidney) lag slightly behind the
changes in blood temperature whilst changes in
muscle and rectal temperature may be considerably
delayed. When rewarming by the bloodstream
route it is therefore important to continue warming
until full equilibrium between oesophageal and
tissue temperature has been achieved to prevent a
fall in oesophageal temperature when the extracorporeal circulation is discontinued. When skin
cooling is used the gradient is reversed; with this
technique cooling must be terminated at an oesophageal temperature 2–3 °C higher than the final
desired oesphageal temperature to allow for the redistribution of the colder blood from the superficial
tissues.

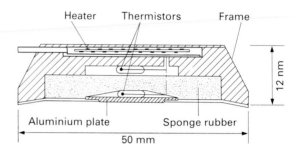

Fig. 19.4. Cross-sectional view of transcutaneous probe
for deep tissue temperature using zero heat flow
method. The sponge rubber acts as the insulating layer.
Heat is applied to the upper surface of the insulator
until the temperature on each side is the same. When
this has been achieved there is no heat loss from the
skin so that there is an equilibrium between skin and
deep tissue temperature.

ZERO HEAT FLOW METHODS

Heat generated in the body core is transported to
the surface by convection and conduction. The
surface loses the heat and so maintains the gradient. If the heat flow across the skin is reduced to
zero, skin surface temperature must be equal to
deep tissue temperature. This provides a means of
measuring the latter at the surface.

The arrangement is shown in Fig. 19.4. Thermistors on either side of a thermal insulator are
used to control a heater which abolishes any
gradient across the insulating layer. When this is
achieved the skin is in equilibrium with the
underlying deep tissues. The probes originally used
were flat pads having a surface are of 30–40 cm^2
but smaller discs 5 cm in diameter have been used
successfully. Results with the method have shown a
correlation with a variety of measures of deep
temperature from sternum (Singer & Lipton,
1975), forehead (Muravchick, 1983; Leeds *et al.*
1980) and occiput (Togwa *et al.* 1976).

Thermography

The human skin behaves almost like a black-body
radiator. This means that it emits infrared radiation with a predictable spectrum. The peak is at
about 9.7 μm and 90% of the radiation energy is
emitted in the range 4–30 μm. The emitted energy
at all wavelengths increases as the temperature

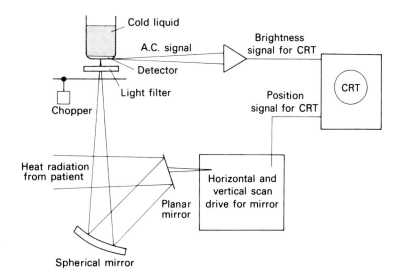

Fig. 19.5. Principle of thermographic unit

rises and if a narrow range of frequencies can be detected, the amount of radiant emission is proportional to the fourth power of the temperature.

Detectors are of two basic kinds: temperature-sensitive devices, such as thermistors and thermocouples, or photon-sensitive devices. The former have a high sensitivity and can discriminate 0.1 °C over the range 0–50 °C: using a spot size of a few millimetres in diameter, the response time can be as low as 1 s. They are thus suitable for measuring the temperature of a small but uniform area whose temperature is not changing quickly but are unsuitable for use in scanning cameras.

For heat scans the most versatile photon-sensitive material is indium antimonide, which is a photoconductive material which produces a small current when infrared radiation between 1 and 6 μm impinges on it. The detector has to be kept very cold in liquid nitrogen to eliminate thermal noise arising in the detector itself. Filters are used to minimize the effects of other wavelengths, such as reflected sunlight, and the elements are shielded from ambient temperatures.

The field is scanned, rather like a television picture, successively, both vertically and horizontally (Fig. 19.5). The speed of response is such that as many as a hundred individual points in a frame can be scanned four times a second. The information can be displayed on a cathode-ray oscilloscope, intensity modulated, so that hotter areas appear brighter.

The main fields of application of thermographic scanning have been in the diagnosis of breast tumours, the location of deep perforating varicose veins of the leg, the site of vascular occlusions, and the location of the placenta. No direct applications to anaesthesia have yet been reported, but the measurement of changes in blood flow in the intensive care unit is an obvious possible future application.

Measurement of humidity

There are several situations in clinical practice in which the control of humidity is of importance. One is when a patient breathes through an endotracheal or tracheostomy tube and extra humidity must be provided to prevent crusting of secretions and to maintain ciliary activity. It has also been customary to maintain a high relative humidity in the operating theatre to decrease the risk of static sparks. This, however, is of lesser importance in theatres in which anaesthetists have given up the use of inflammable anaesthetics, although some humidity is necessary for personal comfort. Relative humidity is an important determinant of body heat loss so that careful control is also required when the patient is kept in a special environment,

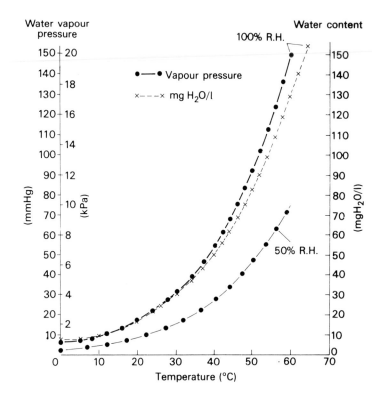

Fig. 19.6. Water vapour pressure and absolute humidity (mg H$_2$O/l) curves for gas which is fully saturated (RH = 100%) and gas which is half saturated (RH = 50%).

e.g. in a plastic isolator or in the treatment of widespread burns.

Two measures of humidity are in common use. *Absolute* humidity is the actual amount of water vapour contained in a given volume of gas at a given temperature and pressure. It is expressed in grams of water vapour per cubic metre of gas. *Relative* humidity is the actual amount of water vapour present in the gas expressed as a percentage of the amount that the same volume of gas would contain at the same temperature and pressure if it were fully saturated. The amount of water vapour required to saturate a given volume of air increases with temperature (Fig. 19.6). Consequently, air which is fully saturated at 20 °C will be only about 40% saturated when warmed to 37 °C. Normally, the additional moisture required to saturate the inspired air is added during its passage through the nose, mouth and trachea.

Measurements of humidity are made by instruments termed hygrometers.

REGNAULT'S HYGROMETER (DEW-POINT HYGROMETER)

A silver tube is cooled gradually by the evaporation of liquid ether. When the tube cools to the dew-point of the surrounding air (i.e. the point at which the air becomes fully saturated), small droplets of water will condense on the outside of the silver tube. If the temperature of the ether is now measured the absolute humidity can be read from the graph (Fig. 19.6) or from tables.

HAIR HYGROMETER

A human hair increases in length as the humidity of the surrounding air increases. If one end of the hair is fixed and the other is attached to a light lever system which magnifies the change in length, the scale can be suitably calibrated and a direct reading of relative humidity obtained. The range is limited to 15–85% relative humidity and the accuracy is not high. However, it is adequate for monitoring the humidity in operating rooms.

WET AND DRY BULB THERMOMETER

Two mercury-in-glass thermometers are mounted side-by-side. The bulb of one is exposed to the air whilst the bulb of the other is surrounded by a small wick which dips into a water reservoir. The temperature of the wet bulb depends on the rate of evaporation, and hence on the humidity of the surrounding air, and is therefore lower than the temperature of the dry bulb. There must, of course, be a minimum airflow over the wet bulb. When humidity is high the rate of evaporation is less and the temperature difference between the two bulbs is, therefore, also less. The relative humidity is determined from tables which relate the dry and wet bulb temperatures to the humidity.

The *whirling hygrometer* works on an identical principle, but is actively 'whirled' in the air in which humidity is to be measured before a reading is made. The tables for this forced-draught device are different from the still-air hygrometer, as evaporation from the wet bulb is greater. The device is insensitive to room-air movements and therefore marginally superior.

HUMIDITY TRANSDUCERS

These utilize the change in electrical characteristics which occurs in a substance when it absorbs water. The substance is usually incorporated into an electronic circuit as a resistor or as the dielectric portion of a capacitor, and the change in resistance or capacitance is detected. Such an instrument can be made extremely sensitive and can be used as part of a servo-system to control humidity in air-conditioning systems. The transducers tend to display hysteresis and this feature makes them unsuitable for critical applications but they can now be made to respond very rapidly.

WEIGHING

When water droplets are present in the air the absolute humidity may exceed the value for saturated air at that temperature. The measurement of humidity can then only be accomplished by either warming the air so that all the droplets are evaporated or by condensing the water vapour and weighing the quantity of water in a known volume of air. Allowance must then be made for the water vapour still present in the saturated vapour over the condensed water. An alternative technique is to absorb the water vapour in concentrated sulphuric acid, silica gel or anhydrous calcium chloride and again to determine the quantity present by weighing. If these methods are used the air must be passed through a number of chambers arranged in series, so that the completeness of absorption can be checked. (There should be no weight gain in the terminal chamber.)

MASS SPECTROMETER

This instrument (see p. 241) can be used to measure the water vapour pressure (Hayes & Robinson, 1967) and is sufficiently rapid to follow breath-by-breath changes. However, the expense of such an instrument precludes its general use for this purpose.

References

Cooper, K.E. & Kenyon, J.R.. (1957) A comparison of temperatures measured in the rectum, oesophagus and on the surface of the aorta during hypothermia in man. *British Journal of Surgery* **44**, 616–619.

Dickey, W.T., Ahlgren, E.W. & Stephen, C.R. (1970) Body temperature monitoring via the tympanic membrane. *Surgery* **67**, 981–984.

Hayes, B. & Robinson, J.S. (1970) An assessment of methods of humidification of inspired gas. *British Journal of Anaesthesia* **42**, 94–104.

Holdcroft, A. & Hall, G.M. (1978) Heat loss during anaesthesia. *British Journal of Anaesthesia* **50**, 157–164.

Keatinge, W.R. & Sloan, R.E.G. (1975) Deep body temperature from aural canal with servo-controlled heating to outer ear. *Journal of Applied Physiology* **38**, 919–921.

Leeds, D.E., Kim, Y.D. & MacNamara, T.E. (1980) Noninvasive determination of core temperature during anesthesia. *Southern Medical Journal (Birmingham, Al)* **73**, 1322–1324.

Lees, D.E., Schuette, W., Bull, J.M., Whang-peng, J., Atkinson, E.R. & MacNamara, T.E. (1968) An evaluation of liquid-crystal thermometry as a screening device for intra-operative hyperthermia. *Anesthesia and Analgesia* **57**, 669–674.

Matthews, H.R., Meade, J.B. & Evans, C.C. (1974a) Peripheral vasoconstriction after open-heart surgery. *Thorax* **29**, 338–342.

Matthews, H.R, Meade, J.B. & Evans, C.C. (1974b) Signficance of prolonged peripheral vasoconstriction after open-heart surgery. *Thorax* **29**, 343–348.

Muravchick, S. (1983) Deep body thermometry during general anesthesia. *Anesthesiology* **58**, 271–275.

Singer, B. & Lipton, B. (1975) Monitoring of core temperature through the skin: a comparison with esophageal and tympanic temperatures. *Bulletin of the New York Academy of Medicine* **51**, 947–952.

Togwa, T., Nemoto, T., Yamazaki, T. & Kobayashi, T. (1976) A modified internal temperature measurement device. *Medical Biological Engineering* **14**, 361–364.

Webb, G.E. (1973) Comparison of esophageal and tympanic temperature monitoring during cardiopulmonary bypass. *Anesthesia and Analgesia* **52**, 729–733.

Whitby, J.D. & Dunkin, L.J. (1968) Temperature differences in the oesophagus: preliminary study. *British Journal of Anaesthesia* **40**, 991–995.

Whitby, J.D. & Dunkin, L.J. (1969) Temperature differences in the oesophagus. The effects of intubation and ventilation. *British Journal of Anaesthesia* **41**, 615–618.

Whitby, J.D. & Dunkin, L.J. (1970) Oesophageal temperature differences in children. *British Journal of Anaesthesia* **42**, 1013–1015.

Whitby, J.D. & Dunkin, L.J. (1971) Cerebral, oesophageal and nasopharyngeal temperatures. *British Journal of Anaesthesia* **43**, 673–676.

Further reading

Benzinger, T.H. (1969) Heat regulation: homeostasis of central temperature in man. *Physiological Reviews* **49**, 671–759.

Hall, G.M. (1978) Body temperature and anaesthesia. *British Journal of Anaesthesia* **50**, 39–44.

Togawa, T. (1985) Body temperature measurement. *Clinical Physics and Physiological Measurement* **6**, 83–108.

Part 3
Principles of Monitoring in Anaesthesia and Intensive Care

20: The Design of a Monitoring System: Alarms

This chapter, and those following, are concerned with the clinical application of the principles and techniques discussed earlier. A number of the techniques outlined in Part 2 were included to illustrate the principles underlying a particular measurement and would not be used in clinical practice. When deciding which instruments are suitable for clinical use it is important to consider not only their size, shape, robustness and accuracy, but also how they may be integrated into a comprehensive monitoring system. The following chapters consider the problems of using monitors to enhance patient safety during anaesthesia, recovery and intensive care. In these circumstances there is a need to monitor not only the patient's condition but also the functioning of the therapeutic apparatus applied to the patient. It will become apparent that the indiscriminate use of a number of separate monitors does not guarantee safety. What is required is an integrated approach which gives early warning of apparatus malfunction or a change in the patient's condition.

Design of the system

A monitoring system is designed to alert the attendant to an alteration in machine function or patient's condition which, if continued, would hazard the patient's safety. The most important factor to be considered when designing any monitoring system is therefore the time interval between the event and the onset of irreversible damage. For example, the patient will lose consciousness and stop breathing within a few seconds of a cardiac arrest whilst irreversible damage will develop over the ensuing 3–4 min. However, severe arterial hypotension may be tolerated for much longer periods without clinical evidence of cerebral dam-

age. It is, therefore, more important to have a continuous monitor of the presence of a pulse than it is to have intermittent measurements of arterial pressure. Again, a sudden oxygen supply failure resulting in continued ventilation of the lungs with a hypoxic gas mixture will produce severe arterial desaturation within 20–40 s if a nonrebreathing system is being used, whereas disconnection of the patient from a ventilator may not result in desaturation until several minutes have elapsed if the patient has been ventilated with an oxygen-enriched gas mixture. This indicates that there should be an immediate warning of oxygen supply failure with a simultaneous N_2O cut off, whilst a disconnection alarm could be delayed for 15–20 s to minimize the incidence of false alarms, e.g. during endotracheal suction. Thus the designer must always take into account, not only the inevitable delays associated with the development and recognition of the fault, or change in patient's condition, but also the time taken to diagnose the problem, correct it and finally restore normal conditions in the patient.

The second problem with monitoring devices is that they may not provide an accurate measurement of the variable being measured. Such errors may result from zero or gain instability, non-linearity or lack of specificity. For example, a polarographic O_2 analyser may be calibrated with N_2 and 100% O_2 but may read 5% v/v O_2 too high in the mid-range of concentrations due to non-linearity. Again, it is not infrequent for this type of analyser to develop a sensitivity to N_2O. For example, one electrode calibrated on N_2 and 100% O_2 read 21% O_2 when exposed to pure N_2O (Orchard & Sykes, 1980). Pulse oximeters are also subject to calibration errors and have a variable speed of response (Severinghaus & Naifeh, 1987).

Problems at the patient interface are another frequent source of error. Thus, pulse oximeters may give a false reading if they are affected by movement, electrical interference, ambient light or infra-red radiation from a neonatal heating unit whilst non-invasive blood pressure monitors may give an aberrant reading if the cuff or tubing is moved during the measurement.

Yet another problem is that a device which monitors malfunction in one situation may not do so in another. For example, when the ventilation is controlled, rebreathing results in an increase in end-tidal CO_2 concentration. However, if the patient is breathing spontaneously and is lightly anaesthetized the retention of CO_2 may stimulate breathing so that there is little change in end-tidal CO_2.

These considerations indicate that there is not only a need for more reliable monitors with more sophisticated artefact rejection systems but that the inter-relationship between the individual monitors used in a system should also receive careful consideration. Ideally, monitors should complement each other: thus if the pulse plethysmograph shows that there is a forceful pulse and the automatic blood pressure reads zero it is likely that the latter is at fault.

The use of a number of separate monitoring devices results in scattered displays and difficulty in identifying alarms. Fortunately, manufacturers are now concentrating on integrated monitoring systems with a centralized display and alarm system. This has immense ergonomic advantages and enables alarms to be marshalled in a hierarchical manner so that attention is drawn to the most critical alarm should simultaneous alarm messages be generated.

A final criticism of present monitoring systems is that we are not yet able to monitor the variables which really matter. Thus we can monitor autonomic responses to surgery but not anaesthetic depth, and arterial oxygen saturation but not brain P_{O_2}. Although attempts are being made to monitor cellular function little success has so far been achieved (Jobsis-Vandervliet *et al.* 1987).

Alarms

One of the major problems in the design of a monitoring system is the provision of appropriate alarms. In the intensive care unit sophisticated monitoring techniques may be used for days or even weeks. During this period it is necessary to monitor not only the patient's condition, but also the performance of the various therapeutic devices employed. The information produced by the monitors is frequently displayed in different formats and in different sites around the patient, so that it is difficult for the physician or nurse to absorb the data whilst performing their other tasks. It has, therefore, been necessary to develop alarm systems which can alert the attendant to a significant apparatus malfunction or to a potentially dangerous change in the patient's condition.

ALARM LIMITS

It is convenient to categorize alarm messages according to their urgency (Schreiber, 1985). The first stage may be termed *advisory*. It signals a change in the measured variable which is not harmful to the patient but which could presage further changes of a more serious nature. The second stage is *caution* and signals a potentially serious change which requires a prompt action on the part of the attendant to avert serious injury to the patient. The third stage of *warning* indicates that damage to the patient is imminent and immediate action is required. Unfortunately, there is little agreement between physicians or manufacturers concerning the deviation from normality required to generate each of these categories of alarm and there is even greater confusion concerning the method of transmitting the alarm to the attendant, though most clinicians would feel that the caution and warning alarms should be accompanied by an audible signal. Some limits are generally agreed. For example, few physicians would wish to ventilate a patient with less than 21% oxygen and most would wish to be warned when the pulse rate fell below 45 beats per minute. However, an anaesthetist might well consider that a warning should be given when the inspired O_2 was less than 25% or more than 50%, whilst higher levels of inspired O_2 might be necessary to sustain life in a patient with severe abnormalities of lung function in an intensive care unit. There is, therefore, a strong case for providing alarm limits which can be adjusted to suit each patient. Unfortunately, this practice frequently leads to problems, for it is easy to forget to reset the alarm limits and those already set may not be appropriate for the next patient. Furthermore, the adjustment of limits on a number of monitors takes time and may distract the operator from the observation of the patient at a critical moment. Manufacturers have, therefore, tended to introduce default limits to which the alarms are automatically reset whenever the power is switched on.

Unfortunately, manufacturers must necessarily adopt limits which are close to normal values and this inevitably results in frequent alarms which, in turn, encourage the operator to inactivate them, so defeating the object of the alarm. Another approach employed in some instruments is for the alarms limits to be set on the basis of the initial values measured shortly after the power has been switched on. These 'intelligent alarm systems' examine the output over a variable period, compare the results with stored normal values and, provided the measured values are within a reasonable range, set the alarm limits to values which are statistically related to the initial measurements. This type of system obviates the need for the operator to set the alarms, enables the monitor to take account of pre-existing abnormalities such as hypertension and provides a warning of subsequent deviation from the initial values. However, if the initial values were substantially different from the normal (as they might be if the patient had displayed a hypertensive response to anxiety before induction) the alarm limits would subsequently have to be reset. To overcome this problem some instruments display the proposed limits but only put them into operation when the operator presses a button indicating that the limits are approved. Many other attempts are being made to improve the efficiency of alarms by using microprocessor technology. For example, some systems take into account the variability and the rate of change of a variable as well as its absolute level whilst other workers are examining the possibility of using artificial intelligence techniques which could use many different sources of information to help formulate the appropriate alarm limits.

ALARM SOUNDS

At the present time the large number of audible alarms within the operating theatre or intensive care environment causes unnecessary confusion (McIntyre, 1985). Furthermore there are a large number of false alarms which bear no relation to a deterioration in the patient's condition (Kestin *et al.* 1988). Bleeps, diathermy machines, patient monitors, infusion pumps, ventilators and many other therapeutic devices have high pitched alarms which are of similar sound and intensity. Because of their characteristics, these are very difficult to locate so that there are often unnecessary delays in identifying the source of the alarm. One proposal for overcoming this problem is to have a characteristic sound for each of the main categories of equipment found in a given environment (Kerr, 1985). Thus O_2 failure alarms would have one sound, infusion pumps another and so on. It is believed that six types of alarm would cover most of the types of equipment used in one environment. This is also the maximum number of sounds which can be remembered by the average person. The repetition frequency of the alarm could then indicate the degree of urgency, a single sound indicating caution and a more frequent repetition indicating warning.

INTEGRATED ALARM SYSTEMS

Further developments in monitoring will concentrate on the production of integrated monitoring systems with modular components. This type of system can provide a unified display with a single alarm sound. It has the additional advantage that the alarms can be prioritized so that attention is directed to the most acute problem if several

alarms are activated simultaneously. The origin of
the alarms can be identified by text messages on
the screen or by a synthesized voice, and alarm
limits may be set by any of the methods described
above. There is a wide choice of software which
permits sophisticated signal analysis or display, in
addition to the other functions, and many of the
units can be interconnected so that data from one
station can be displayed at another.

References

Jobsis-Vandervliet, F.F., Fox, E. & Sugioka, K. (1987)
Monitoring of cerebral oxygenation and cytochrome
aa$_3$ redox state. *International Anesthesiology Clinics* **25**,
209–230.

Kerr, J.H. (1985) Warning devices. *British Journal of
Anaesthesia* **57** 696–708.

Kestin, I.G., Miller, B.R. & Lockhart, C.H. (1988)
Auditory alarms during anesthesia monitoring. *Anesthesiology* **69**, 106–109.

McIntyre, J.W.R. (1985) Ergonomics: anaesthetists' use
of auditory alarms in the operating room. *Journal of
Clinical Monitoring* **2**, 47–55.

Orchard, C.H. & Sykes, M.K. (1980) Errors in oxygen
concentration analysis: sensitivity of the IMI analyzer
to nitrous oxide. *Anaesthesia* **35**, 1100–1103.

Schreiber, P., (1985) *Safety guidelines for anesthesia
systems.* North American Drager, Telford PA.

Severinghaus, J.W. & Naifeh, K.H. (1987) Accuracy of
response of six pulse oximeters to profound hypoxia.
Anesthesiology **67**, 551–558.

21: Monitoring during Anaesthesia

In the early days of anaesthesia the anaesthetist monitored the patient's condition and depth of anaesthesia by palpation of the pulse and by observation of the skin colour, ocular movements, pupil size and respiratory activity. The measurement of blood pressure during anaesthesia was introduced by Halstead in the early years of this century, but there was little further progress in this field until the 1940s and 1950s when the more widespread practice of thoracic and cardiac surgery stimulated the development of methods to assess cardiac and respiratory function. During the past 10 years there has been a marked increase in the use of monitoring devices. This has resulted, firstly, from the great improvements in reliability and artefact rejection associated with the widespread application of microprocessor technology and secondly, from the increasing frequency of malpractice litigation.

Unfortunately, there is little firm evidence that monitoring increases patient safety, and most studies of anaesthetic-related morbidity and mortality conclude that the major cause is lack of training or inexperience (Cooper *et al.* 1978; Lunn & Mushin, 1982). However, these studies and the recent confidential enquiry into perioperative deaths (Buck *et al.* 1987) have also revealed that little or no monitoring has been used in many of these patients, so that the true cause of the complication is often difficult to determine.

An analysis of critical incidents is probably a more realistic approach. A critical incident may be defined as any incident which, if uncorrected, will be potentially harmful to the patient. In a study of 8312 anaesthetics in a district general hospital, Craig and Wilson (1982) found an incidence of approximately 1% of which 65% were associated with human error and 12% with a combination of human error and equipment failure. Cooper *et al.* (1984) also concluded that human error was the major cause of anaesthetic mishaps, only 4% of the critical incidents in their series involving equipment failure. However, they also noted that additional monitoring might have helped to prevent 18 out of 70 incidents with substantive negative outcomes.

The practice of monitoring will be considered under three headings: monitoring the anaesthetist, monitoring the function of the anaesthetic or life support machine and monitoring of the patient.

Monitoring the anaesthetist

This is the most difficult to implement, but, if implemented successfully would have the greatest impact on patient safety. Every doctor should be prepared to submit to an audit of his or her practice by colleagues. Unfortunately, it takes courage to confess to mistakes and it is usually all too easy to hide all but the grossest errors of judgement or practice. Self-audit is a less satisfactory, but generally more acceptable, alternative. However, it can only be effective if all patients are visited in the post-operative period and if good clinical records are maintained.

Performance can be improved by a number of simple expedients. First, the anaesthetist should develop protocols and check lists for each of the procedures carried out during anaesthesia. For example, the anaesthetic machine should always be checked before each operating session; the names and doses of drugs used should always be carefully checked with the label on the bottle or ampoule and reliance should never be placed on the colour, size or shape of the drug container for identification. It is not sufficient to rely on movement of the chest or abdomen to verify correct placement of an endotracheal tube; one should always listen to ensure that there are breath sounds in each axilla (to exclude endobronchial intubation and possible obstruction of an upper lobe bronchus) and one should also check that there are no sounds of gas entering the stomach. Second, the anaesthetist should involve assistants as much as possible by encouraging them to check respiratory activity, pulse or blood pressure, whilst the anaesthetist is engaged in such tasks as endotracheal intubation or the insertion of an intravenous line. Thirdly, one should encourage a friendly dialogue with the surgeons so that the anaesthetist is given the earliest possible warning of cyanosis, bleeding or other possible complications.

Monitoring anaesthetic machine function

In recent years it has become customary to add sensing devices to anaesthetic machines to monitor various aspects of their function. There are two critical considerations in the design of such systems. The first is the delay between warning of malfunction and the occurrence of tissue damage, and the second is the integration of the monitoring devices to produce a comprehensive monitoring system.

The importance of the various delays between the onset and recognition of a fault is illustrated in Fig. 21.1 which depicts the processes involved in the delivery of O_2 to the patient. A sudden O_2 supply failure will be detected quite quickly by an O_2 monitor situated at the common gas outlet, but there will be a finite delay due to the time taken for the transit of the gas from the gas source to the common gas outlet (a function of the flow rate and the volume of the fresh gas circuit) and to the response time of the analyser. There will be a further delay before the fall in O_2 concentration can be detected by a sensor placed in the inspiratory tubing of the breathing system because of the time taken to wash out the breathing system and lung. For example, when a patient with an O_2 consumption of 300 ml·min^{-1} and functional residual capacity of 2 L breathes from a circle absorption system with a volume of 8 L, it may take 5 min for the inspired O_2 concentration to fall from 30 to 20% after a cessation of fresh gas inflow. The final stage in O_2 transport to the tissues may be monitored by the use of a pulse oximeter.

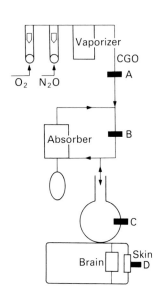

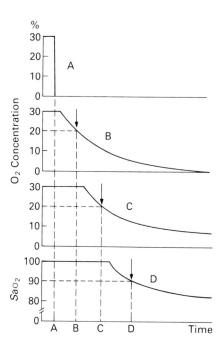

Fig. 21.1. Delays to be considered when designing a monitoring system. A sudden decrease in oxygen concentration (e.g. due to a pipeline disconnection) will be detected rapidly by a monitor at the common gas outlet (CGO) of an anaesthetic machine (A). However, the concentration in the breathing system (B) and alveolar gas (C) will decrease more slowly because of the time taken to wash out the breathing system and lungs. A pulse oximeter alarm (D) will be still further delayed because of the instrument response time and the lung-to-finger circulation time.

This introduces a further delay (which is greater with a finger probe than with an earpiece probe) so that it may be nearly 8 min before the pulse oximeter O_2 saturation reading falls to 90% in a patient who was initially breathing 30% O_2. However, since the arterial Po_2 is now on the steep part of the O_2 dissociation curve, the subsequent fall in saturation will be rapid, so that tissue damage from hypoxia may occur if remedial action is not taken immediately (Verhoeff & Sykes, 1990). However, even if the cause of the O_2 supply failure is discovered and rectified immediately, it may take another 5 min for the inspired oxygen concentration and arterial Po_2 is restored to normal. It is therefore essential to place the O_2 supply monitor as close to the gas source as possible and, if O_2 failure occurs, the patient must be disconnected from the breathing system immediately and ventilated with a separate source of fresh gas until the anaesthetic machine and breathing system have been flushed out with the restored gas mixture.

The second point to note is that the time course of blood gas changes in response to a change in inspired gas concentration is much quicker when the patient is being ventilated than when the patient is suddenly rendered apnoeic. As may be seen in Fig. 21.2, a sudden O_2 supply failure results in a dangerously low arterial oxygen saturation within one minute if ventilation is maintained, the

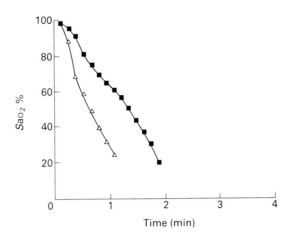

Fig. 21.2. Computer simulation of changes in arterial oxygen saturation (Sao_2%) after oxygen supply failure with continued ventilation with hypoxic gas mixtures in a non-rebreathing system ($\triangle$, FRC 1.5 L; $\blacksquare$, FRC 3.0 L). From Verhoeff & Sykes (1990).

rate of fall being accentuated by a high minute volume or reduced functional residual capacity (FRC). However, when the patient becomes apnoeic the rate of fall of alveolar Po_2 is governed mainly by the rate of oxygen consumption and the volume of oxygen in the FRC. Thus, if the patient has been breathing pure oxygen, full saturation may be maintained for many minutes and even with 30% inspired oxygen and an FRC of 1.5 L it

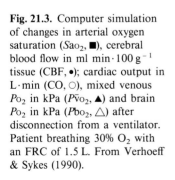

Fig. 21.3. Computer simulation of changes in arterial oxygen saturation (Sao_2, $\blacksquare$), cerebral blood flow in ml min·100 g⁻¹ tissue (CBF, $\bullet$); cardiac output in L·min (CO, $\circ$), mixed venous Po_2 in kPa ($P\bar{v}o_2$, $\blacktriangle$) and brain Po_2 in kPa (Pbo_2, $\triangle$) after disconnection from a ventilator. Patient breathing 30% O_2 with an FRC of 1.5 L. From Verhoeff & Sykes (1990).

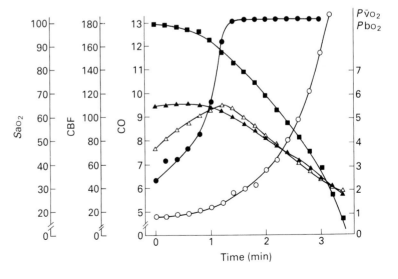

may take 1 min for the saturation to fall to 90%. It is, however, the brain P_{O_2} and not the arterial saturation which is the critical factor in the causation of hypoxic damage. During apnoea arterial P_{CO_2} rises and this results in a shift to the right of the O_2 dissociation curve (thus enhancing oxygen delivery), an increased cardiac output and a marked increase in cerebral blood flow. Thus during apnoea brain P_{O_2} actually increases whilst arterial P_{O_2} is decreasing and brain P_{O_2} may only fall to pre-existing levels when the arterial saturation has fallen to 60–70% (Fig. 21.3).

Monitoring the fresh gas supply

The first requirement is that there should be a device which provides an audible warning of a fall in pipeline pressure or reduced gas pressure between the O_2 regulators and the flowmeter. The requirements for such a device are that it should provide a distinctive audible warning which persists for a minimum of 10 s and which is loud enough to be heard against background noise levels commonly encountered in the theatre environment. The energy required to operate the device should be derived solely from the normal oxygen supply pressure and the device should be automatically tested whenever the oxygen supply is switched on or off. When used with a cylinder supply and set to alarm at half the normal reduced gas pressure, there will be enough oxygen remaining in the cylinder to power the device. However, if used with a pipeline it is necessary to provide a reservoir which is kept charged during normal operation of the machine but which contains sufficient gas to power the device if O_2 supply failure occurs (Memorandum, 1976). In many anaesthetic machines the oxygen pressure failure warning device is linked to a device which either reduces the flow of other gases in proportion to the reduction in O_2 flow or cuts off the supply of other gases completely.

The characteristics of the fresh gas supply which need to be monitored are fresh gas flow, O_2 concentration and vapour identity and concentration.

FRESH GAS FLOW

On most anaesthetic machines flow is displayed by rotameters and there is no audible warning of a reduction in flow. Furthermore there may be a leak between the flowmeters and the common gas outlet, particularly on machines with detachable vaporizers. Thus the only way of monitoring fresh gas flow into a breathing system is to monitor the performance of the breathing system itself.

O_2 CONCENTRATION

Current British and International Standards require an oxygen analyser to be fitted to every anaesthetic machine to monitor the oxygen concentration in the fresh gas supply. Polarographic analysers are subject to zero and calibration errors, battery failure, drying of the electrolyte and sensitivity to N_2O or halothane (pp. 258 and 289). Galvanic cells are not affected by N_2O but have a limited life, particularly if high O_2 concentrations are used regularly. Paramagnetic analysers are immune to these problems but are less robust. An oxygen analyser situated at the common gas outlet can provide warning of incorrect connection of the fresh gas supplies, a differential leak of oxygen at the flowmeters or flowmeter inaccuracy. However, an O_2 analyser may not gave a warning of O_2 supply failure if the machine is fitted with an N_2O cut-off device or proportional controller. With such devices, the fresh gas flow ceases when the O_2 supply fails but the O_2 concentration at the analyser may not change because the fresh gas flow stops before the hypoxic mixture reaches the sensor. Thus, if the machine is not fitted with an audible alarm for O_2 supply pressure failure, there will be no warning of fresh gas failure.

VAPOUR CONCENTRATION

At the present time the only vapour analysers which provide an indication of vapour identity are the mass spectrometer and the Raman scattering instrument ('Rascal'). However, if the identity of the vapour is known, the concentration can be determined by the use of ultraviolet or infra-red absorption analysers, or by the use of a piezo-electric device such as the Engstrom Emma, or by refractometry (see Chapter 17).

Monitoring the breathing system

Rebreathing may be caused by an inadequate fresh gas flow, valve malfunction, disconnection of the inner tube in a concentric Mapleson D (Bain) system or exhausted soda lime. This results in an increase in inspired and alveolar P_{CO_2} and a consequent reduction in inspired and alveolar P_{O_2}. Inspired P_{O_2} and vapour concentration may also differ from fresh gas concentration when the fresh gas flow is less than the minute volume owing to variations in oxygen, nitrous oxide and vapour uptake during an anaesthetic (Mushin & Galloon, 1960; Forbes, 1972).

OXYGEN CONCENTRATION

The inspired oxygen concentraton can be monitored by a slow response analyser in a non-rebreathing or circle CO_2 absorption system. However, a rapid analyser is required for measurements at the patient end of a Mapleson 'A' or 'D' system because of intermittent dilution by alveolar gas. In the latter systems it is possible to use a slow response oxygen analyser to warn of low inspired O_2 concentrations by placing the analyser downstream from the expiratory valve, but the analyser usually responds to the fluctuating concentration of oxygen in expired gas by producing a time-weighted average rather than a true mean. There are additional complications if the analyser is placed between the ventilator and bag mount on a Bain system, for the gas from the ventilator may mix with the expired gas coming from the patient. If the fresh gas flow into the breathing system ceases when a ventilator, such as the Nuffield 200, is being used with the Bain system, there will be an increase in the oxygen concentration recorded at the bag mount due to the mixing of the oxygen from the ventilator with the patient's expired gas. If, however, a ventilator which returns the patient's expired gas to the breathing system is used (e.g. the Penlon 400) then the oxygen concentration will fall in parallel with the O_2 concentration in the lungs.

CO_2 CONCENTRATION

During spontaneous ventilation rebreathing may result in an increase in end-tidal CO_2 or an increase in ventilation, so both a CO_2 analyser and expired volume meter are required to ensure that rebreathing is detected. If controlled ventilation is being used the onset of rebreathing causes an increase in both inspired and end-tidal CO_2, providing tidal volume and CO_2 production are unchanged. The increase in inspired CO_2 is clearly seen if the gas is thoroughly mixed within the breathing system. However, with some breathing systems (e.g. the Mapleson 'A'), the CO_2 trace may reach zero during inspiration, even though rebreathing is occuring (Fig. 21.4). With such systems it is therefore safer to rely on the end-tidal value since this represents the interaction between rebreathing and alveolar ventilation.

Unfortunately, there are a number of problems associated with the use of a rapid CO_2 analyser. First, it is important to ensure that the site of sampling is correct. A sample from the centre of the endotracheal tube provides an accurate measure of CO_2 but there is an increased risk of sample tube blockage due to the presence of secretions. Sampling between breathing system and endotracheal tube is satisfactory if the tidal volume is large, but an error may be introduced if the tidal volume is small or if there is a continuous flow of fresh gas diluting the end-tidal gas, as may occur with a Bain system. The optimal site for sampling is, therefore, at the top end of the endotracheal tube (p. 308). It is important to ensure that the frequency response of the CO_2 analyser is adequate and that the device is calibrated for use with the background gas used during anaesthesia.

EXPIRED VOLUME

It can be argued that expired volume monitoring is unnecessary during controlled ventilation if end-tidal CO_2 is being measured. However, the use of a volume monitor not only enables leaks and ventilator malfunction to be detected immediately but also provides additional information. For example, if the end-tidal CO_2 decreases whilst minute volume is unchanged, there must be either a decrease in CO_2 production (e.g. due to hypothermia) or an increase in alveolar dead space (e.g. due to hypovolaemia or pulmonary embolus). When a circle or non-rebreathing system is in use

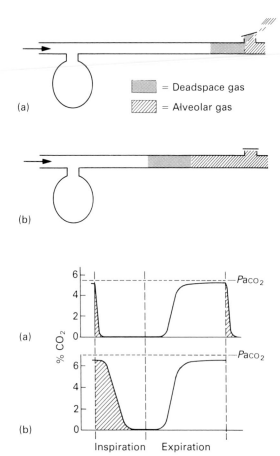

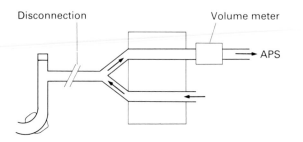

Fig. 21.5. A respirometer placed at the outlet from a ventilator and connected to an active antipollution system (APS) developing small sub-atmospheric pressure may record air passing through the expiratory pathway whenever the ventilator expiratory valve opens. Furthermore, if the respirometer has an inadequate frequency response, it may also not differentiate between a leakage of gas through the expiratory valve during inspiration and gas expired from the lung.

Fig. 21.4. Mapleson A breathing system (upper a & b) with CO_2 concentration recorded at the mouth (lower a & b). Normally the alveolar gas (shaded) is completely eliminated through the valve during the expiratory pause (a). However, when the fresh gas flow is inadequate there is incomplete washout of alveolar gas from the patient end of the reservoir tube during expiration. This gas is re-inhaled and followed by dead space gas and fresh gas containing no CO_2 (b). Since it is only possible to define the point at which inspiration starts by making a simultaneous measurement of flow and allowing for analyser sampling delays, it is not possible to detect the extent of rebreathing from a CO_2 trace alone. Note that the presence of zero CO_2 at some point in the cycle does *not* exclude the possibility of rebreathing. However, when rebreathing occurs the end-tidal and arterial P_{CO_2} (Pa_{CO_2}) will increase unless the patient compensates by hyperventilation.

the sensor can be placed in the expiratory pathway, but with the Mapleson 'A' and 'D' system it is necessary to place the sensor at the patient connection port because of the errors caused by the overflow of fresh gas. There are several other potential sources of error in expired volume measurement. For example, a slow response instrument placed close to the expiratory valve on a ventilator may fail to differentiate between expiratory flow and leakage through the expiratory valve during inspiration so that the expired volume measured may still correspond to the ventilator setting even though the volume delivered to the lungs is reduced. Another source of error is that a disconnection between the patient and breathing system may not be detected if the expiratory port of the ventilator is connected to an active anti-pollution system, for the sub-atmospheric pressure in the latter may cause air to flow through the sensor when the expiratory valve opens. Since this flow will only occur during expiration it may be mistaken for an expired tidal volume (Fig. 21.5). A somewhat similar problem may occur when the expired volume meter is placed in the expiratory limb of a circle CO_2 absorpton system which incorporates a ventilator with a falling bellows. If a disconnection occurs the weight in the bellows will draw in air via the expiratory tube and expel it via

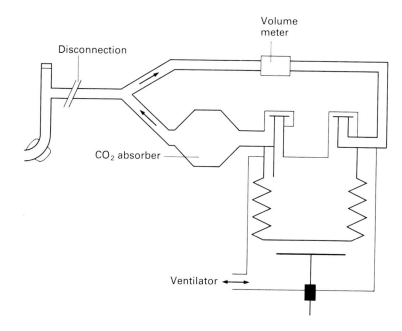

Fig. 21.6. A respirometer placed in the expiratory limb of a circle CO_2 absorption breathing system may fail to detect a disconnection at the patient Y-piece if used in conjunction with a ventilator with a hanging bellows since the latter will fill via the expiratory tube and empty via the inspiratory tube.

the inspiratory tube so that the expired volume displayed will equal that set on the bellows (Fig. 21.6).

AIRWAY PRESSURE

Another breathing system variable which requires monitoring is airway pressure. Ideally, the monitor should provide an analogue signal with two alarm limits, one for high peak pressure and one to warn of increased pressure during expiration. During mechanical ventilation airway pressure provides useful information concerning ventilator performance, lung compliance and airway resistance. High airway pressures are generated when airway resistance is increased or lung compliance is decreased and may also occur when there is obstruction to the outflow from the breathing system, e.g. during the application of positive end-expiratory pressure or when the expiratory valve has not been opened. Most ventilator disconnect alarms are activated by high peak pressures and by a failure to reach a pre-set pressure, such as 10–13 cmH$_2$O within a pre-determined time (20–30 s). However, the alarm may not be activated by a failure of fresh gas supply to a Bain breathing system since ap-

proximately half of the tidal volume is provided by the ventilator and this may provide a pressure which is adequate to satisfy the device.

Patient monitoring

The first essential is that ventilation and circulation should be monitored continuously, alarms being required if the anaesthetist is likely to be distracted from this task for more than 30 s. It is usually reasonable to rely on the observaton of chest wall movement and the excursion of the reservoir bag during spontaneous breathing or manually controlled ventilation. However, during mechanically controlled ventilation it is essential to monitor both airway pressure and expired volume, high/low alarms again being required if the anaesthetist cannot observe these monitors continuously. Since a rapid CO_2 analyser monitors both the breathing system and patient (Fig. 21.7) it is now considered to be an essential component of any monitoring system.

Until recently the only method of measuring inspired and expired gas and vapour concentrations was to use a mass spectrometer. Since these

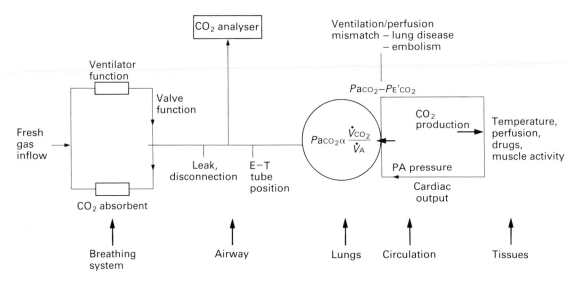

Fig. 21.7. Factors affecting end-tidal CO_2 concentration.

devices are bulky, expensive to run and complicated, a number of hospitals have utilised a multiplex system whereby one mass spectrometer serves up to 12 operating rooms (Ozanne *et al.* 1981). Each operating room is sampled in turn and the results displayed in either analogue or digital form on a panel in the appropriate anaesthetizing location. Such a system has a number of disadvantages (Gravenstein *et al.* 1984). First, there is a delay between sampling and analysis caused by the use of long, narrow sample tubes between the operating theatre and the analyser. Second, it is necessary to sample over at least two complete respiratory cycles in order to achieve signals which can be subjected to computer analysis for display of the digital values. With 12 operating rooms and a 15 s sampling period, the total delay may amount to 3 min, thus, reducing the utility of the instrument in diagnosing cardiac arrest or other acute emergencies.

With the advent of rapid paramagnetic O_2 and infrared CO_2, N_2O and vapour analysers, together with dedicated mass spectrometer or Raman scattering instruments, it is now possible to obtain breath-by-breath recordings of inspired and expired gas and vapour concentrations at the mouth. Such measurements represent the end product of

the anaesthetic machine-breathing system-patient interaction, and therefore, provide a useful monitor of the primary determinants of gas exchange. However, end-tidal samples are influenced by the magnitude of the arterial to end-tidal CO_2 tension difference which is increased by anaesthesia, hypotension and lung disease. Furthermore, there is an alveolar to arterial O_2 tension difference due to ventilation/perfusion inequalities and right-to-left shunt.

The circulation presents a greater problem because it is difficult to palpate the pulse continously for long periods, and it is difficult to estimate blood pressure by palpation of the pulse. Auscultation of the heart sounds by a precordial or oesophageal stethoscope is a valuable alternative particularly in neonatal anaesthesia when arterial pressure monitoring is more difficult. However, continuity of observation is rendered difficult by the discomfort of binaural ear pieces, whilst continous use of a monaural earpiece may lead to otitis externa in susceptible individuals. Pulse meters, which provide a visual indication of the heart rate, are of some help, but the best information is provided by an analogue display of pulse waveform measured with an optical finger plethysmograph or more sophisticated device (see below).

It is now generally accepted that the electrocardio-graph (ECG) should be displayed whenever possible. However, it is well known that normal ECG activity may be present, even though no pulse is palpable. The main use of the ECG should therefore be to monitor heart rate and to detect dysrhythmias, conduction defects or other alterations of electrical activity (e.g. myocardial ischaemia or changes in serum potassium).

Most indirect methods of measuring the blood pressure are subject to errors, and the correlation between diastolic pressure measured indirectly and directly is poor. Furthermore, the intermittent nature of such measurements may prove inadequate when the blood pressure is changing rapidly. Arterial pressure should therefore be measured directly in all patients undergoing major cardiac or vascular surgery and in patients in whom there are likely to be rapid fluctuations of blood pressure from any cause. Although methods for the continuous indirect measurement of arterial pressure are now becoming available commercially, they are still at an early stage of development and there is some doubt about their accuracy in the presence of peripheral vasoconstriction (see p. 183).

The recent development of pulse oximeters, which monitor both the heart rate and arterial saturation, represents an enormous advance in monitoring. The sensor may be placed on the finger, earlobe or nasal septum, though the earlobe is generally favoured because the delay in recording the change in saturation is shorter with the ear than with finger placement. Unfortunately, pulse oximeters are sensitive to motion artefacts and they may give inaccurate results in elderly patients with a poor peripheral circulation or when the pulse volume is reduced by blood loss or severe vasoconstriction. The sensors may also be affected by the presence of light or infrared radiation, bilirubin or extraneous dyes in the blood or marked venous pulsations. Furthermore, since the instruments measure the proportion of oxygenated and reduced haemoglobin there may be an error when methaemoglobin, carboxyhaemoglobin, or haemoglobin F is present (Chapter 18). However, these limitations should not be seen as contra-indications to their universal use during anaesthesia and recovery.

Monitoring of other therapeutic devices

HOT WATER HUMIDIFIERS

There are basically two designs in clinical use. In the older type the gas was passed over a water bath maintained at 55–60 °C. This heated and moistened the gas, though full saturation at this temperature was not achieved because of the relatively small water surface area. However, the gas cooled as it passed through the inspiratory tube so that relative humidity increased, even though absolute humidity was unchanged, and this resulted in the delivery of fully saturated gas to the patient at 32–37 °C. Full saturation at 32 °C represents an absolute humidity of $33\,mgH_2O\cdot L^{-1}$ which is equivalent to 75% relative humidity at 37 °C, and it is considered that this will provide adequate humidification for the majority of patients (Forbes, 1973). However, problems have been encountered because of a failure to provide adequate temperature control in the tank and because the rate of cooling along the inspiratory tube is dependent on the length and thermal conductivity of the tubing and on the rate of airflow through the tube. It is therefore vital to monitor the temperature of the water in the tank and the temperature of the inspired gas close to the patient.

In more recent designs of humidifiers, full saturation is achieved in the tank by the use of wicks and the temperature is maintained close to 37 °C throughout the delivery system. In these devices it is still necessary to monitor the gas temperature close to the patient whether the temperature is set manually or controlled by a sensor close to the patient.

INFUSION PUMPS AND INTRAVENOUS DRIP CONTROLLERS

These should be fitted with alarms which give warning of excessive or reduced fluid delivery. There should also be alarms which indicate an excessive line pressure due to obstruction of the venous access and devices which warn of the presence of air in the line.

BLOOD WARMERS

Accurate control of blood temperature is essential as there is an increased risk of haemolysis when the temperature exceeds 42 °C.

Conclusion

It is now generally accepted that appropriate standards of monitoring should be adopted during anaesthesia and intensive care (Eichorn *et al.* 1986; Sykes, 1987). There is general agreement on the minimum standards of monitoring required and many centres are now adopting standards based on those evolved in Boston, Massachusetts. Similar recommendations have recently been issued by the Association of Anaesthetists of Great Britain and Ireland (1988), However, when considering a monitoring system it is important to analyse the function of each monitor and how it relates to the other devices incorporated in the system. It is also important to decide on alarm limits and to ensure that these are set correctly at the beginning of each case. The use of a number of discrete monitors leads to poor display, and the most successful systems now incorporate the monitors in one single display panel, which also enables priorities to be set and confusion avoided.

References

Association of Anaesthetists of Great Britain and Ireland (1988) Recommendations for standards of monitoring during anaesthesia and recovery.

Buck, N., Devlin, H.B. & Lunn, J.N. (1987) *The report of a confidential enquiry into perioperative deaths.* The Nuffield Provincial Hospitals Trust, London.

Cooper, J.B., Newbower, R.S., Long, C.D. & McPeek, B. (1978) Preventable anesthesia mishaps: a study of human factors. *Anesthesiology* **49**, 399–406.

Cooper, J.B., Newbower, R.S. & Kitz, R.J. (1984) An analysis of major errors and equipment failures in anesthesia management: considerations for prevention and detection. *Anesthesiology* **60**, 34–42.

Craig, J. & Wilson, M.E. (1981) A survey of anaesthetic misadventures. *Anaesthesia* **36**, 933–936.

Forbes, A.R. (1972) Inspired oxygen concentrations in semi-closed absorber circuits with low flows of nitrous oxide and oxygen. *British Journal of Anaesthesia* **44**, 1081–1084.

Eichorn, J.H., Cooper, J.B., Cullen, D.J., Maier, W.R., Philip, J.H. & Seeman, R.G. (1986) Standards for patient monitoring during anesthesia at the Harvard Medical School. *Journal of the American Medical Associaton* **256**, 1017–1020.

Forbes, A.R. (1973) Humidification and mucus flow in the intubated trachea. *British Journal of Anaesthesia* **45**, 874–878.

Gravenstein, J.S., Gravenstein, N., van der Aa, J.J. & Paulus, D.A. (1984) Pitfalls with mass spectrometry in clinical anesthesia. *International Journal of Clinical Monitoring and Computing* **1**, 27–34.

Lunn, J.N. & Mushin, W.W. (1982) *Mortality associated with anaesthesia.* The Nuffield Provincial Hospitals Trust, London.

Memorandum (1976) Oxygen supply pressure failure warning and protection devices. *Anaesthesia* **31**, 316–318.

Mushin, W.W. & Galloon, S. (1960) The concentration of anaesthetics in closed circuits with special reference to halothane. III: clinical aspects. *British Journal of Anaesthesia* **32**, 324–333.

Ozanne, G.M., Young, W.G., Mazzei, W.J., & Severinghaus, J.W. (1981) Multipatient anesthetic mass spectrometry. *Anesthesiology* **55**, 62–70.

Sykes, M.K. (1987) Essential monitoring. *British Journal of Anaesthesia* **59**, 901–912.

Verhoeff, F. & Sykes, M.K. (1990) Delayed detection of hypoxic events by pulse oximeters: computer simulations. *Anaesthesia* **45**, 103–109.

22: Monitoring the Respiratory System

The monitoring of inspired and expired gas composition and the function of the anaesthetic machine, breathing system and ventilator has already been discussed (Chapter 21). This chapter is concerned with the measurement of CO_2 output and O_2 consumption as indices of tissue metabolism, the assessment of the efficiency of gas exchange in the lungs, and the measurement of lung volumes, lung mechanics and lung water.

Carbon dioxide output and oxygen consumption

There has recently been renewed interest in CO_2 output and O_2 consumption measurements since these can help to elucidate metabolic derangements in critically ill patients and can provide a guide to the need for nutritional support. There have also been a number of studies on the relationship between O_2 delivery and O_2 utilization in patients with septic shock or the respiratory distress syndrome and it has been suggested that O_2 consumption measurements may provide a useful guide to therapy in these conditions (Taylor *et al.* 1987; Shoemaker *et al.* 1987).

CO_2 output and O_2 consumption are indices of tissue metabolism and under resting, steady state conditions O_2 consumption is in the range $3–4 \, ml \cdot kg^{-1}$. It is increased by hyperthermia (about 7% per °C), increased muscle tone and shivering, and decreased by the administration of hypnotic drugs, hypothermia or inadequate tissue perfusion. Increases of up to 20% over resting levels may be induced by procedures such as turning or physiotherapy, and still greater increases are seen after trauma, surgery, burns, sepsis or the administration of inotropic drugs.

CO_2 output is greatly affected by changes in ventilation since these alter the CO_2 stores: mea-surements should therefore only be made when the patient has been in a steady state for 30–45 min. Under such conditions the ratio of CO_2 output to O_2 consumption at the mouth (R, the respiratory exchange ratio) equals the exchange at tissue level (RQ, the respiratory quotient). The RQ is determined by the principal energy source being utilized and is 0.7 for fat, 0.8 for protein and 1.0 for carbohydrate. An RQ of 0.6 may be encountered when there is ketosis whilst the RQ may increase to 1.2 or 1.3 during sodium bicarbonate infusion or hyperalimentation with carbohydrate solutions (Askenazi *et al.* 1980).

METHODS

CO_2 output ($\dot{V}\text{co}_2$) and O_2 consumption ($\dot{V}\text{o}_2$) can be measured by the application of the Fick equation:

$$\dot{V}\text{co}_2 = (C a \text{co}_2 - C \bar{v} \text{co}_2) \, \dot{Q}$$

$$\dot{V}\text{o}_2 = (C a \text{o}_2 - C \bar{v} \text{o}_2) \, \dot{Q}$$

where Ca and $C\bar{v}$ represent the CO_2 and O_2 contents of arterial and mixed venous blood whilst $\dot{Q}$ is the cardiac output. However, it is difficult to measure $\dot{Q}$ with an accuracy of better than $\pm 10\%$ and O_2 and CO_2 contents with an accuracy better than ± 0.3 vol.% so the accuracy of measurement of $\dot{V}\text{co}_2$ and $\dot{V}\text{o}_2$ is unacceptable. For this reason measurements are made by measuring the gas concentrations and volumes entering and leaving the lungs.

Carbon dioxide output

The patient breathes through a non-rebreathing valve which permits the expired gas to be collected in a large spirometer (e.g. Tissot) or Douglas bag for a period of 5–10 min. The expired gas is thoroughly mixed and a sample of known volume is then analysed with a Haldane apparatus or infra-red analyser to provide the mixed expired concentration ($F\bar{E}CO_2$). The Douglas bag is emptied through a gas meter and the expired minute volume ($\dot{V}E$) calculated after the addition of the sample volume. The CO_2 output is then calculated from the equation:

$$\dot{V}CO_2 = \dot{V}E \times F\bar{E}CO_2.$$

Since $\dot{V}E$ is fully saturated at ambient pressure and temperature it is necessary to measure ambient temperature and barometric pressure to correct the result to standard temperature and pressure dry (STPD).

The measurement of CO_2 output can only be equated with CO_2 production when $P_{a}CO_2$ does not change during the measurement. To ensure a steady-state the patient should breathe through the apparatus for 5–10 min before making the measurement. The gas expired during this period is used to wash out the Douglas bag or spirometer so that the gas in the connecting tubes and collecting device has the same composition as the true mixed expired gas.

When the patient is breathing spontaneously there are random variations in tidal volume and frequency which are averaged by the long period of gas collection. However, when the patient is ventilated mechanically, tidal volume and frequency are constant so that a satisfactory mixed expired sample can be obtained by passing the expired gas through a mixing box or through two anaesthetic reservoir bags connected in series. The bags are filled with nylon pot scourers and held partially inflated by a one-way valve on the exit (Fig. 22.1). When using this technique it is important to check

that mixing is complete by observing that the analyser gives a constant reading. The gas sample taken by the analyser should be returned to the circuit so that the gas meter measures the total expired volume.

Oxygen consumption ($\dot{V}O_2$)

In the *closed circuit technique* the patient re-breathes from a spirometer filled with 100% O_2. The expired CO_2 is absorbed by soda lime and the $\dot{V}O_2$ is then derived from the slope of the spirometer trace after correction from ambient temperature and pressure, saturated (ATPS) to STPD. The patient should breathe 100% O_2 for at least 10 min before being connected to the spirometer to minimize the error due to N_2 elimination from the blood. Continuous measurement can also be achieved by measuring the inflow of O_2 required to keep the volume of the system constant (Tsoi *et al.* 1982). This technique can be used with spontaneous or mechanical ventilation but can only be used with O_2 concentrations less than 100% when combined with continuous O_2 analysis.

The *open-circuit technique* described by Haldane is more accurate and more easily applied during anaesthesia and intensive care. The equation used is:

$$\dot{V}O_2 = (\dot{V}I \times FIO_2) - (\dot{V}E \times F\bar{E}O_2)$$

where $\dot{V}I$ and $\dot{V}E$ are the inspired and expired minute volumes, and FIO_2 and $F\bar{E}O_2$ are the inspired and mixed expired O_2 concentrations. $\dot{V}E$ and $F\bar{E}O_2$ are derived from expired gas collection as for $\dot{V}CO_2$ measurement. $\dot{V}I$ is greater than $\dot{V}E$ because of the unequal exchange of CO_2 and O_2 and is derived by measuring the difference in nitrogen concentration between inspired and

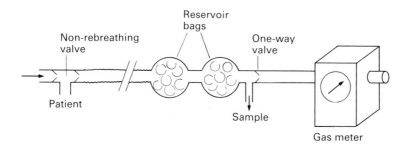

Fig. 22.1. Use of two reservoir bags filled with nylon pot scourers to mix expired gas.

mixed expired gas. Since N_2 is neither taken up nor excreted during the measurement:

$$\dot{V}_I \times F_{IN_2} = \dot{V}_E \times F_{\bar{E}N_2}$$

or

$$\dot{V}_I = \dot{V}_E \times \frac{F_{\bar{E}N_2}}{F_{IN_2}}$$

where

$$F_{IN_2} = 1 - F_{IO_2}$$

and

$$F_{\bar{E}N_2} = 1 - (F_{\bar{E}O_2} + F_{\bar{E}CO_2})$$

Again the use of a mixing unit greatly facilitates this measurement when the patient is on a ventilator.

There are many sources of error in the measurement of $\dot{V}_{CO_2}$ and $\dot{V}_{O_2}$ (Weissman, 1987). Extreme care must be taken to ensure that the patient is in a steady state, that there are no leaks in the breathing system, that the non-rebreathing valve is functioning perfectly and that the inspired gas is well mixed and of constant composition. The latter is often difficult to achieve if the patient is being mechanically ventilated. Whilst the Haldane transformation (the use of the N_2 concentrations to calculate the inspired volume) can be used with O_2 concentrations up to 50–60%, accuracy decreases as the concentration is increased (Ultman & Bursztein, 1981). It is particularly important to ensure that gas analysers are linear, provide accurate measurements of dry gas concentrations (better than $\pm 0.1\%$ v/v) and that volume measurements are accurate to within $\pm 1\%$.

There are now a number of commercially available 'metabolic carts'. These work on similar principles, are of variable accuracy and require careful use (Damask, 1986; Braun *et al.* 1989). In some devices direct connection to the patient is avoided by surrounding the patient's head with a plastic hood through which is drawn a high, constant flow of air. This captures the patient's exhaled gas but results in very small differences in gas concentration and increased difficulties in measurement. When using these devices it is important

to ensure that the O_2 concentration of the inspired air is not being augmented by spillage from nearby O_2 therapy devices.

The assessment of gas exchange in the lungs

While the arterial blood gas tensions may provide a useful guide to the patient's respiratory status, it must not be assumed that normal blood values preclude the presence of respiratory disease. For example, chronic obstructive airway disease results in ventilation/perfusion inequalities with ratios ranging from infinity (ventilation but no blood flow) to zero (perfusion but no ventilation). Alveoli which are ventilated but not perfused excrete no CO_2 and therefore their ventilation is completely wasted. In alveoli with some perfusion but with a high ventilation/perfusion ratio, the alveolar P_{CO_2} is below normal, so that each unit of ventilation results in the elimination of fewer CO_2 molecules than in normally perfused and ventilated units. This again, necessitates an increase in total ventilation in order to maintain the same total CO_2 elimination. Both these sources of inefficiency in CO_2 elimination may, therefore, be equated with the effects of an added dead space, the so-called alveolar (or parallel) dead space which must be added to the anatomical (or series) dead space of the conducting airways. The sum of the two, *the physiological dead space* is normally one-third of the tidal volume in patients with normal lungs but when alveolar dead space is increased, the dead space/tidal volume ratio may increase to 0.6–0.7. In the normal patient a minute volume of approximately 6 L will provide 4.3 L of alveolar ventilation when the dead space/tidal volume ratio is 0.3: this is sufficient to keep the P_{CO_2} at normal levels with a basal CO_2 production of $200\ ml \cdot min^{-1}$. However, if the dead space tidal/volume ratio increases to 0.6 a total ventilation of 11 L is required to maintain the same alveolar ventilation. It is difficult for most patients to sustain higher levels of ventilation than this for prolonged periods and, therefore, it is rare to be able to wean a patient from mechanical ventilation when the dead space/tidal volume ratio exceeds 0.6 (Fig. 22.2).

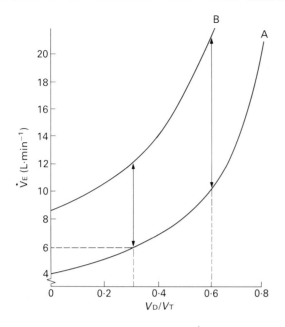

Fig. 22.2. Increase in minute volume ($\dot{V}_E$) required to compensate for increased deadspace/tidal volume ratio (V_D/V_T). Curve A: $\dot{V}_{CO_2}$ 200 ml·min^{-1}, P_{CO_2} = 5.3 kPa (40 mmHg). Curve B: $\dot{V}_{CO_2}$ 400 ml·min^{-1}, P_{CO_2} 5.3 kPa (40 mmHg).

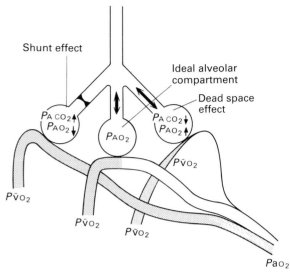

Fig. 22.3. The three compartment model used to quantify abnormalities of lung function. The composition of the gas in the ideal alveolar compartment (P_{AO_2}) is determined by the inspired P_{O_2}, the alveolar P_{CO_2} (equated with arterial P_{CO_2}) and the respiratory exchange ratio. Inefficiencies in CO_2 elimination due to alveoli with high ventilation/perfusion ratios are equated with an imaginary alveolar dead-space and inefficiencies in O_2 transfer due to alveoli with low ventilation/perfusion ratios are equated with an imaginary right-to-left shunt.

Blood flowing through completely non-ventilated alveoli takes up no oxygen and so constitutes a right-to-left shunt. Blood flowing through alveoli with a low ventilation/perfusion ratio has a low P_{O_2} and a high P_{CO_2} and, therefore, contributes to arterial hypoxaemia. Whilst the increased P_{CO_2} of blood leaving low ventilation/perfusion ratio alveoli may be compensated by the increased CO_2 elimination from high ventilation/perfusion ratio alveoli, there can be no compensation for the desaturated blood entering the left heart, because it is not possible for the high alveolar P_{O_2} in the high ventilation/perfusion alveoli to add significant extra quantities of oxygen to the blood once the red cell is fully saturated. Thus, ventilation/perfusion ratios are always associated with an increase in dead space ventilation and arterial hypoxaemia, though arterial P_{CO_2} usually remains within normal limits until the disease is severe and the patient can no longer compensate for the wasted ventilation by an increase in minute volume.

Although there are techniques which enable the full spectrum of ventilation/perfusion ratios to be quantified, these are technically difficult to perform and the results are open to criticism (Lee *et al.* 1987; Kaufman *et al.* 1987). For clinical purposes it is therefore usual to quantify gas exchange by modelling the lung as though it consisted of three compartments (Fig. 22.3):

1 An ideal alveolar compartment in which ventilation and blood flow are considered to be ideally matched and in which the alveolar P_{O_2} is determined by the inspired P_{O_2}, the alveolar P_{CO_2} and the respiratory exchange ratio.

2 A dead space compartment which is ventilated but has no blood flow.

3 A shunt compartment which is perfused but not ventilated.

Thus the dead space compartment includes alveoli which are overventilated in relation to the perfusion and ventilated alveoli with no perfusion, whilst the shunt compartment includes alveoli with a low ventilation/perfusion ratio, non-ventilated alveoli and any right-to-left shunts which bypass the lungs. Since a moderate increase in inspired oxygen concentration (30–35%) can increase the Po_2 in alveoli with low ventilation/perfusion ratios to normal levels, and so eliminates hypoxaemia due to this cause, it is possible to separate the effects of low ventilation/perfusion ratio alveoli from right- to-left shunts by making measurements on air and oxygen breathing. However, the results may be affected by changes in the distribution of blood flow resulting from the increase in alveolar oxygen concentration.

Since end-tidal gas is derived from alveoli with a wide spectrum of ventilation/perfusion ratios, it is not representative of gas in the ideal alveolar gas compartment. It is, therefore, customary to calculate the ideal alveolar gas composition from the inspired oxygen concentration and the respiratory exchange ratio assuming that the ideal alveolar Pco_2 is equal to arterial Pco_2. The difference between the calculated ideal alveolar Po_2 and arterial Po_2 may then be used to quantify the defect in oxygen transfer between gas and blood whilst the difference between arterial Pco_2 and end-tidal Pco_2 provides information about inefficiencies in CO_2 elimination.

Alveolar ventilation and dead space

The arterial Pco_2 is determined by the relationship between CO_2 production ($\dot{V}co_2$) and alveolar ventilation ($\dot{V}_A$) and so defines the adequacy of ventilation:

$$Paco_2 \text{ (kPa)} = \frac{\dot{V}co_2 \text{ (ml·min}^{-1}\text{ STPD)}}{\dot{V}_A \text{ (L·min}^{-1}\text{ BTPS)}} \times 0.115^{\dagger}$$

However, arterial puncture carries a risk and should only be carried out when there is an appro-

---

† The factor 0.115 converts fractional concentration to partial pressure and corrects for the different conditions under which gas volumes are expressed. If $Paco_2$ is in mmHg the factor is 0.863.

priate indication. Arterialized venous or capillary samples (obtained from veins on the back of the hand or a finger prick after heating a limb) can be used when the circulation is adequate but these yield inaccurate results when vasoconstriction is present. Various alternative estimates of the adequacy of ventilation are available.

MINUTE VOLUME

Nomograms are available which relate CO_2 production (predicted from age, weight, body temperature and sex) to the alveolar ventilation required to produce a normal $Paco_2$ (Radford 1955; Engstrom & Herzog, 1959). These nomograms use assumed values for the patient's dead space, and the latter also makes an allowance for the gas compressed in the ventilator tubes and humidifier, since this reduces the tidal volume delivered to the alveoli. Whilst such nomograms enable ventilation to be set with reasonable accuracy in patients with normal lungs they are liable to be inaccurate in the presence of lung disease because of an increase in alveolar dead space.

END-TIDAL CARBON DIOXIDE

In the conscious patient with healthy lungs the alveolar plateau of CO_2 is almost horizontal and the end-tidal Pco_2 approximates closely to arterial Pco_2 (Fig. 22.4). However, when there are ventilation/perfusion inequalities there is an increase in alveolar dead space and an increase in the arterial to end-tidal Pco_2 difference (a–APco_2). The increase in alveolar dead space is due to regional increases in ventilation relative to perfusion. This may be caused by areas of reduced perfusion (e.g. due to pulmonary embolus or a reduction in pulmonary artery pressures resulting from drugs or hypovolaemia) or to the maldistribution of ventilation (e.g. due to the presence of lung disease or the use of high airway pressure during controlled mechanical ventilation). When perfusion is reduced the alveolar plateau tends to be horizontal since the non-perfused alveoli empty synchronously with the perfused alveoli. However, when lung disease is present well ventilated areas of lung

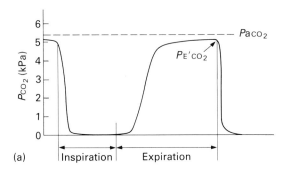

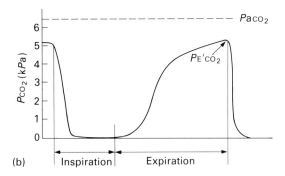

Fig. 22.4. Capnograms. (a) The small difference between arterial P_{CO_2} (Pa_{CO_2}) and end-tidal P_{CO_2} ($P_{E'CO_2}$) in the normal lung. (b) The increased slope of the CO_2 plateau and increased arterial-to-end-tidal P_{CO_2} difference in patients with chronic obstructive lung disease.

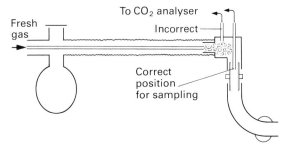

Fig. 22.5. Dilution of end-tidal gas by fresh gas in a Mapleson D (Bain) breathing system.

tend to empty early in expiration whilst poorly ventilated areas empty late, so causing an upwardly sloping alveolar plateau.

During anaesthesia in patients with normal lungs the a–AP_{CO_2} difference averages 0.8 kPa (5 mmHg). The difference increases during severe hypovolaemia or in patients with severe obstructive airways disease and may be as much as 3–4 kPa (20–30 mmHg). The difference is decreased by prolonging inspiration but may increase if alveolar pressure is increased by the use of high positive end-expiratory pressure levels.

The most representative end-tidal sample is obtained by sampling from the lumen of the endotracheal tube, but this increases the chances of aspirating secretions into the analyser. It is therefore customary to site the tip of the sampling catheter close to the endotracheal tube connection. When using the concentric Mapleson D breathing system (the Bain) it is important to insert a right-angled connector between the breathing system and sample point to prevent dilution of the end-tidal sample by the jet of fresh gas (Fig. 22.5). This precaution is also necessary with in-line CO_2 analysers (Gravenstein *et al.* 1985). The sampling flow rate in some analysers may exceed 500 ml·min^{-1}. If these are used with paediatric or other low flow systems they may distort the breathing system characteristics and produce significant operating theatre pollution. Under these circumstances the effluent from the analysers should be returned to the breathing system. Some infra-red analysers reset the electronic zero with every breath when the minimum concentration is recorded during inspiration. These devices should obviously not be used with breathing systems such as the Mapleson D in which the rebreathing of CO_2 is a normal feature, or when the inspired CO_2 concentration is deliberately increased in order to prevent hypocapnia during controlled ventilation. Errors in end-tidal CO_2 measurement also arise from interference by N_2O (p. 236) and by an inadequate frequency response (Brunner & Westenskow, 1988). Partial blockage of the sampling line is not uncommon in clinical practice and errors due to this cause can only be avoided if the response time is checked at regular intervals (p. 224).

TRANSCUTANEOUS P_{CO_2}

This technique can provide useful trend information in the neonate where there is a reasonable correlation with arterial P_{CO_2}. However the technique does not work well in adults because the thicker skin limits the diffusion of CO_2.

REBREATHING CARBON DIOXIDE

If a gas mixture containing 5–7% CO_2 in O_2 is rebreathed from a bag it will equilibrate with the mixed venous blood entering the lungs. Since the mixed venous to arterial P_{CO_2} difference is relatively constant (0.9 kPa or 6 mmHg), the arterial P_{CO_2} can be derived by subtracting this difference from the measurement of the CO_2 concentration of the gas in the bag after equilibration. The problem is to achieve equilibration of the gas in the bag, lungs and venous blood within one circulation time (20 s), for recirculation of blood which has not given up its CO_2 in the lungs will result in an increase in mixed venous P_{O_2}. Several techniques have been used. In one the patient rebreathes from a 2 L bag containing 1 L of 5% CO_2–O_2 mixture for several periods of 15 s, the bag being disconnected for 1–2 min between each period of rebreathing to allow the arterial P_{CO_2} to return to the pre-existing level. In another technique 1 L of O_2 is rebreathed for 90 s and the bag then re-applied for two periods of 15–20 s (Campbell & Howell, 1962). If the gas in the bag is analysed by a simple analyser such as the modified Haldane (Chapter 17) attainment of equilibrium is demonstrated by similar CO_2 concentrations in successive rebreathing periods. However, if a rapid analyser is available equilibration is verified by the development of a plateau when inspired and rapid concentrations are equal (Fig. 22.6).

The technique provides P_{CO_2} measurements with an accuracy of ± 0.4 kPa (± 3 mmHg) as long as the cardiac output is within 50% of normal limits, the accuracy of measurement being improved by multiplying the mixed venous P_{CO_2} by 0.8 rather than assuming a fixed venous–arterial difference (McEvoy *et al.* 1974). The technique has been widely used in exercise testing and has proved useful for determining P_{CO_2} in neonates and adults on mechanical ventilation when other forms of blood gas analysis were not available (Sykes, 1960; Heese & Freeseman, 1964). In the latter circum-

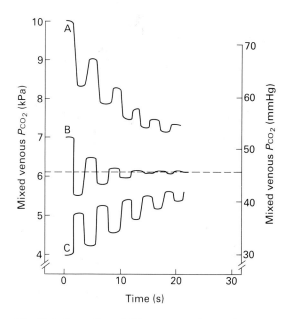

Fig. 22.6. Recording of CO_2 concentration at the mouth during rebreathing. The bag concentration (7%) is initially higher than alveolar concentration and equilibrium is shown by the presence of a plateau (B). Gas mixtures A and C do not reach equilibrium within 20 s.

stances the bag size is matched to the size of patient and mixing is achieved by manual compression of the bag.

MEASUREMENT OF DEAD SPACE

Physiological dead space is measured by using the Enghoff modification of the Bohr equation:

$$V_D = \frac{V_T (Pa_{CO_2} - P\bar{E}_{CO_2})}{Pa_{CO_2}} .$$

Thus, dead space/tidal volume ratio

$$(V_D/V_T) = \frac{Pa_{CO_2} - P\bar{E}_{CO_2}}{Pa_{CO_2}} .$$

$P\bar{E}_{CO_2}$ (the mixed expired CO_2) can be obtained by collecting mixed expired gas in a Douglas bag and subjecting this to analysis after further mixing. When the patient is on controlled ventilation, the expired gas may be passed through a mixing unit and the CO_2 concentration measured with an infra-red analyser. The arterial sample for P_{CO_2}

should be drawn slowly whilst the mixed expired gas is being collected and tidal volume may be derived from a gas meter or other accurate volume measuring device. If the patient is being ventilated mechanically, it is important to either use a special valve to separate the gas compressed in the ventilator tubes from the true expired gas or to make the appropriate correction for dilution of the mixed expired gas.

Arterial oxygenation

When monitoring the transport of oxygen from the inspired gas to the tissues one must consider the factors governing the alveolar O_2 tension (P_{AO_2}), the alveolar to arterial P_{O_2} difference (A–aP_{O_2}), the arterial O_2 content (C_{aO_2}), the cardiac output ($\dot{Q}_T$) and the mixed venous oxygen content ($C_{\bar{v}O_2}$). These factors are summarized in Fig. 22.7.

ALVEOLAR P_{O_2}

Since the ideal alveolar compartment is an imaginary entity it is necessary to calculate the ideal alveolar P_{O_2} from the inspired P_{O_2}, the alveolar P_{CO_2} (which dilutes the inspired gas) and the overall respiratory exchange ratio (which deter-

mines the change in gas volume in the alveolus during the respiratory cycle). Whilst the inspired P_{O_2}, CO_2 output and O_2 consumption can be measured one cannot measure ideal alveolar P_{CO_2}. It is therefore customary to assume that the arterial P_{CO_2} will provide the best estimate of the average P_{CO_2} at which the lung is working. By substituting this value in the simplified form of the alveolar air equation one can then calculate ideal alveolar P_{O_2}:

$$\text{ideal alveolar } P_{O_2} = \text{inspired } P_{O_2} - \frac{\text{arterial } P_{CO_2}}{R}$$

where

$$R = \frac{CO_2 \text{ output}}{O_2 \text{ consumption}} = 0.8 \text{ normally.}$$

This relationship is plotted in Fig. 22.8.

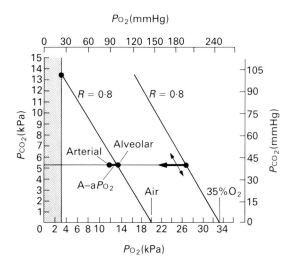

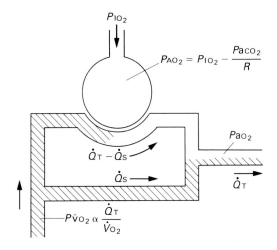

Fig. 22.7. Factors affecting the delivery of oxygen to the tissues. $\dot{Q}s$ is the shunt component which bypasses the lungs and $\dot{Q}_T$ is the cardiac output.

Fig. 22.8. O_2–CO_2 diagram illustrating the relationship between alveolar P_{O_2} and P_{CO_2} when breathing air ($F_{IO_2} = 20$ kPa or 150 mmHg) and approximately 35 per cent oxygen ($F_{IO_2} = 33.3$ kPa or 250 mmHg). The slope of the line depends on the respiratory exchange ratio, here assumed to be 0.8. The arterial P_{O_2} is less than the alveolar P_{O_2}, the magnitude of the A–aP_{O_2} being dependent on the percentage venous admixture, the mixed venous oxygen content and the slope of the oxygen dissociation curve between the alveolar and arterial P_{O_2}. The shaded area to the left of the diagram represents the range of arterial oxygen tensions normally incompatible with prolonged survival.

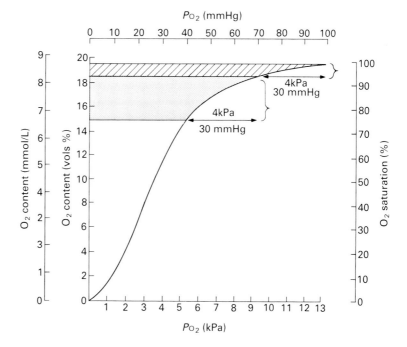

Fig. 22.9. Oxygen dissociation curve to show relationship between P_{O_2} and percentage saturation and oxygen content. The differences in oxygen content resulting from an A–aP_{O_2} of 4.0 kPa (30 mmHg) at different levels of alveolar P_{O_2} are illustrated by the shaded areas.

ALVEOLAR–ARTERIAL P_{O_2} DIFFERENCE

If all the alveoli were perfectly ventilated and perfused, there would be little difference between ideal alveolar and arterial P_{O_2}. In practice there is always a difference between these two values, there being three potential mechanisms. First, there may be a block to the diffusion of O_2 through the alveolar–capillary membrane. This factor is now believed to be of negligible importance when the alveolar P_{O_2} exceeds about 8 kPa. Second, in alveoli with a decreased ventilation/perfusion ratio, there is an increase in alveolar P_{CO_2} and reduction in alveolar P_{O_2} so that blood leaving these alveoli has a P_{O_2} lower than ideal alveolar P_{O_2}. Hypoxaemia due to ventilation/perfusion inequalities can be minimized by increasing the inspired O_2 concentration to 30–35% since this increases the alveolar P_{O_2} to normal values in the majority of alveoli with low ventilation/perfusion ratios. The third mechanism is an intrapulmonary shunt resulting from continued perfusion of collapsed or consolidated alveoli. A shunt is quantified by calculating the proportion of mixed venous blood which would have to be added to the oxygenated blood leaving

the well ventilated alveoli in order to produce the observed A–aP_{O_2}. It is, therefore, calculated from the oxygen contents of the arterial and mixed venous blood and the oxygen content of blood having the same blood gas tensions as those existing in the ideal alveolar compartment. Unfortunately, P_{O_2} is not linearly related to content and so the oxygen content difference associated with a given A–aP_{O_2} depends on its position on the oxygen dissociation curve (Fig. 22.9). Similarly, the arterial P_{O_2} resulting from a given shunt will be affected by the mixed venous P_{O_2}, a reduction in mixed venous P_{O_2} and consequently in mixed venous saturation, resulting in a reduction in arterial P_{O_2} and saturation. Thus the magnitude of the alveolar–arterial P_{O_2} difference cannot be used as a quantitative index of O_2 transfer in the lungs.

VENOUS ADMIXTURE AND SHUNT

When breathing air the calculated value includes the effects of ventilation/perfusion inequality and true right-to-left shunt. This is usually, termed the total venous admixture ($\dot{Q}_{va}/\dot{Q}_T$) in the British

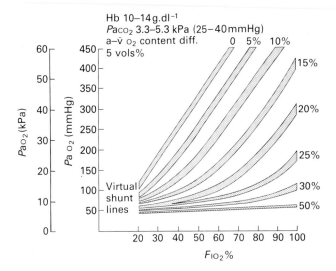

Fig. 22.10. Iso-shunt diagram (Benatar *et al.* 1973) relating inspired oxygen concentration (F_{IO_2}), arterial Po_2 and percentage shunt. The shaded areas include variations in Hb from 10 to $14\,g\cdot dl^{-1}$ and $Paco_2$ from 3.5–5.3 kPa (25–40 mmHg).

literature and physiologic shunt in North American publications. When the measurement is made on inspired O_2 concentrations above about 30% only the true shunt component is quantified ($\dot{Q}_s/\dot{Q}_T$).

To perform the calculation it is necessary to determine the O_2 content of the end-pulmonary capillary blood from the ideal alveolar compartment ($Cc'o_2$) and to measure the arterial and mixed venous O_2 contents (Cao_2, $C\bar{v}o_2$). Then

$$\frac{\dot{Q}_s}{\dot{Q}_T} = \frac{Cc'o_2 - Cao_2}{Cc'o_2 - C\bar{v}o_2} \, .$$

$Cc'o_2$ cannot be measured and is therefore calculated from the ideal alveolar Po_2, the haemoglobin concentration and the oxyhaemoglobin dissociation curve assuming that the pH of the end-capillary blood is the same as arterial pH:

$$Cc'o_2 \,(vol.\%) = (Hb \times 1.34 \times Sc'o_2) + (Pao_2 \times f)$$

where Hb is the haemoglobin concentration ($g\cdot dl^{-1}$), 1.34[†] is the factor for the O_2 combining power of Hb in $ml\cdot g^{-1}$, $Sc'o_2$ is the percentage saturation of the end-capillary blood and ($Pao_2 \times f$) is the quantity of dissolved O_2 in

---

[†] The theoretical factor based on the molecular weight of Hb is $1.39\,ml\cdot g^{-1}$. However, most studies suggest that values between 1.32 and 1.36 are usually found in patients.

$ml\cdot dl^{-1}$. If Pao_2 is in kPa $f = 0.0004\,ml\cdot dl^{-1}$ but if Pao_2 is in mmHg $f = 0.003\,ml\cdot dl^{-1}$.

Cao_2 and $C\bar{v}o_2$ may be derived similarly from the measured Pao_2 and $P\bar{v}o_2$ but are best measured directly (e.g. by the Lex-O_2-Con) or calculated from the measured O_2 saturations to eliminate errors due to shifts of the O_2 dissociation curve. When the arterial Po_2 is on the upper part of the dissociation curve, errors are minimized by using values of $Cc'o_2$ and Cao_2 calculated from the O_2 dissociation curve for the ($Cc'o_2 - Cao_2$) difference and directly measured values for the ($Cao_2 - C\bar{v}o_2$) difference in the following form of the shunt equation:

$$\frac{\dot{Q}_s}{\dot{Q}_T} = \frac{(Cc'o_2 - Cao_2)}{(Cc'o_2 - Cao_2) + (Cao_2 - C\bar{v}o_2)} \, .$$

It may be seen that if the Pao_2 is high enough to produce full saturation of the red cell (>25 kPa) ($Cc'o_2 - Cao_2$) = $f(Pao_2 - Pao_2)$.

If mixed venous Po_2 cannot be measured an arterio-venous O_2 content difference of $5\,ml\cdot100\,ml^{-1}$ may be assumed. The equation then simplifies to

$$\frac{\dot{Q}_s}{\dot{Q}_T} = \frac{f(Pao_2 - Pao_2)}{f(Pao_2 - Pao_2) + 5} \, .$$

These calculations are greatly facilitated by using the nomograms generated by Bird (1971) or a computer program. The iso-shunt diagram of Benatar *et al.* (1973) provides a useful alternative which is sufficiently accurate for clinical purposes (Fig. 22.10).

The cardiac output may be derived from the Fick equation:

$$\dot{Q}_T \, (\text{L} \cdot \text{min}^{-1}) = \frac{\dot{V}_{O_2} \, (\text{ml} \cdot \text{min}^{-1} \, \text{STPD})}{(Ca_{O_2} - C\bar{v}_{O_2})}$$

where $(Ca_{O_2} - C\bar{v}_{O_2})$ is expressed in $\text{ml} \cdot \text{L}^{-1}$ blood at STPD.

However, in clinical practice cardiac output is usually measured directly by the thermodilution technique (p. 217).

A rearrangement of the Fick equation indicates that the mixed venous O_2 content or saturation can provide a useful guide to the adequacy of O_2 delivery to the tissues (Schweiss, 1987):

$$C\bar{v}_{O_2} = Ca_{O_2} - \frac{\dot{V}_{O_2}}{\dot{Q}_T} \, .$$

Mixed venous O_2 saturation can be continuously measured *in vivo* by fibre-optic catheters thus enabling Q_T to be optimized by the suitable use of blood volume expansion and inotropic or vasodilator drugs. However, mixed venous P_{O_2} may not be reduced when cardiac output is markedly decreased since there may be a regional redistribution of blood flow towards the vital organs. Under these circumstances O_2 consumption will also be reduced.

Continuous monitoring may be achieved by using fibre-optic catheters but drift is a problem unless a three-wavelength catheter is used (p. 264). Fibrin deposition on the catheter tip also degrades the signal. For this reason discrete samples are usually analysed *in vitro*.

Alveolar P_{O_2}

The end-tidal P_{O_2} differs from the ideal alveolar P_{O_2} because it is affected by the presence of ventilation/perfusion inequalities. The end-tidal P_{O_2} is reduced by a decrease in inspired P_{O_2} or an increase in P_{CO_2}. Until recently end-tidal P_{O_2} could only be measured by mass spectrometer. However, there are now rapid response analysers using the Raman scattering or paramagnetic principles.

Transcutaneous P_{O_2}

This technique is widely used in neonatology where accurate and rapid control of P_{CO_2} is essential to minimize the risk of developing retrolental fibroplasia (Lubbers, 1987). However, it is important to calibrate the electrode against arterial samples at regular intervals. Transcutaneous P_{O_2} has been used in adults to provide a warning of transient dips in Pa_{O_2} during surgical procedures within the chest or airways, during suction in the intensive therapy unit etc., but is being replaced by pulse oximetry (Tremper & Barker, 1987). Conjunctival P_{O_2} monitoring has also been used for following rapid changes in arterial P_{O_2} but has not achieved widespread clinical application (Abraham, 1987).

Oxygen saturation

Reflection and transmission oximeters have been used to measure oxygen saturation for over 40 years. However, with the exception of one device which had a bulky earpiece and measured light absorption at eight different wavelengths, no absolute calibration could be obtained.

In 1973 a new device was described — the pulse oximeter. This has a small probe which can be attached to the ear, finger or nasal septum and provides an absolute measure of saturation. However, the accuracy of the device depends on the algorithms used by the manufacturer and there are marked variations in the accuracy and speed of response of the individual instruments. A satisfactory signal can only be obtained if there is an adequate degree of pulsation at the probe site. The transducer is affected by motion artefact, infra-red or visible light sources, large venous pressure swings, some diagnostic dyes and nail polishes, bilirubin, carboxy- and methaemoglobin. Most oximeters display some indication of pulse amplitude but this information may be rendered useless by the incorporation of automatic gain controls which adjust the output signal strength to match the full scale reading of the display.

The use of pulse oximeters is likely to expand considerably as they become cheaper. However, it must be remembered that the reduction in the Sa_{O_2} at the periphery represents the final change in a series of linked systems and may not be noted for several minutes after a failure of the O_2 supply. For this reason it is essential to use monitors at all stages of the O_2 delivery system and if a fall in Sa_{O_2} is noted it is important to disconnect the patient and to ventilate with a separate O_2 delivery system to minimize the delay in restoring a normal Pa_{O_2} (Verhoeff & Sykes, 1990).

Other aspects of lung function

LUNG VOLUME

Acute increases in lung volume may be produced by bronchospasm, by the application of PEEP or by the use of high frequency ventilation. With ventilation at normal frequencies, intra-alveolar pressure at the end of expiration is closely related to the pressure measured in the airways. However, during high frequency ventilation, or when expiration is shortened in relation to inspiration, alveolar pressure may be higher than airway pressure because of incomplete emptying of the alveoli during the short expiratory period. Under these circumstances, a measure of lung volume may be necessary to detect over-inflation.

The simplest technique is to measure chest circumference with a tape measure or a bellows pneumograph (p. 193). An inductance plethysmograph provides a better estimate of an acute increase in volume and can be calibrated to provide an accurate measure of tidal volume (p. 194). Lung volume may also be measured directly by open or closed circuit techniques (p. 195). The recent development of an automated technique utilizing sulphur hexafluoride washout enables functional residual capacity (FRC)

measurements to be made without altering ventilator therapy (East *et al.* 1987).

LUNG MECHANICS

Changes in lung mechanics during spontaneous ventilation are rarely measured since it is necessary to measure transpulmonary pressure with an oesophageal balloon. During paralysis and controlled ventilation, however, the airway pressure may be related to flow rate and volume change to yield values of airway resistance and total thoracic compliance.

The simplest method of assessing both variables is to use a constant flow generator type of ventilator (Fig. 22.11). With this pattern of air flow the initial rise in airway pressure or the subsequent fall (during a zero flow interval at the end of inspiration) represents the pressure drop down the airways. By relating this to the flow rate (either set on the ventilator or measured with a pneumotachograph) airway resistance (R_A) can be measured:

$$R_A \text{ (cmH}_2\text{O}\cdot\text{L}^{-1}\cdot\text{s)} = \frac{\text{pressure drop (cmH}_2\text{O)}}{\text{flow rate (L}\cdot\text{s}^{-1})}.$$

Total thoracic compliance may be derived from the airway pressure during the zero flow interval (= alveolar pressure) divided by the expired volume:

$$C_T \text{ (ml}\cdot\text{cmH}_2\text{O}^{-1}) = \frac{P \text{ (cmH}_2\text{O)}}{V_E \text{ (L)}}.$$

'Static' pressure volume curves may also be recorded by injecting 100–200 ml increments of volume into the lungs with a 2 L syringe. After each aliquot is injected the volume is held constant for 2–3 s and the pressure recorded. Such *P/V* curves are a useful guide to the progression of lung changes in the acute respiratory distress syndrome (ARDS) (Fig. 22.12). In the early stages of this disease an inflection point is often seen on the inspiratory curve. This is believed to represent the point at which collapsed alveoli are recruited and may help in setting an appropriate PEEP level (Matamis *et al.* 1984).

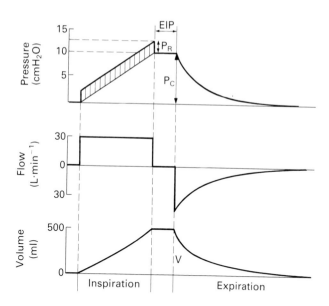

Fig. 22.11. Measurement of total thoracic compliance and airway resistance using a constant flow pattern of ventilation. Compliance can be calculated from the airway pressure (P_c) measured during the period of zero flow associated with an end-inspiratory pause (EIP) and the expired volume (V). The sudden increase or decrease in pressure at the onset or cessation of inspiratory gas flow (P_R) can be related to the inspiratory flow rate to provide a measure of airway resistance. In the above example compliance = 500 ml ÷ 10 cmH$_2$O = 50 ml·cmH$_2$O^{-1} and airway resistance = 2.5 cmH$_2$O per 30 L·min flow = 5 cmH$_2$O·L^{-1} s.

LUNG WATER AND PULMONARY OEDEMA

In patients with a normal alveolar capillary membrane the capillary transmural pressure gradient is opposed by the osmotic pressure gradient developed by the plasma proteins so that there is relatively little filtration of fluid from the capillaries into the interstitial space and lymphatics.

However, filtration will increase if there is an increase in pulmonary microvascular pressure or if the plasma protein concentration is reduced. This leads to an increase in extravascular lung water (EVLW) which may be increased to three times the normal value without clinical signs of pulmonary oedema. These two causes of increased filtration

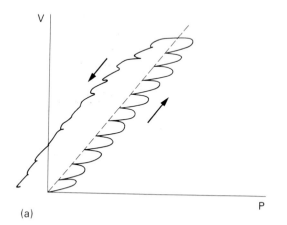

(a)

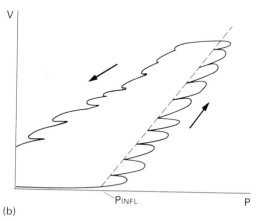

(b)

Fig. 22.12. A pressure–volume curve produced by injecting sequential aliquots of O$_2$ into the lungs from a syringe. (a) Normal. (b) In this patient with the adult respiratory distress syndrome, there is an inflection on the inspiratory curve (P_{INFL}). This is believed to represent the point at which the majority of the collapsed alveolar units re-open and may be used as a guide to the level of PEEP required to maintain optimal lung expansion. The hysteresis between the inspiratory and expiratory curves is largely due to oxygen consumption during the measurement. (Gattinoni *et al.* 1987.)

result in a filtrate which is low in protein. This lowers the osmotic pressure of the interstitial fluid, thus tending to further reduce filtration. The third cause of increased filtration is an increase in permeability due to sepsis, acid aspiration or other causes of damage to the alveolar–capillary membrane. This results in a filtrate rich in protein at normal microvascular pressures.

The lymphatic drainage system of the lung is remarkably effective and in the early stages of pulmonary oedema the only signs of fluid accumulation are cuffs of oedema around the small bronchi and pulmonary arteries. In the second stage crescentic areas of fluid appear in the alveoli. This is followed by the stage of alveolar flooding and finally by the spread of fluid to the airways with the production of frothy, blood-stained sputum. There is usually little interference with gas exchange when oedema is limited to the interstitial space but an increase in respiratory rate and a reduction in Pa_{CO_2} and Pa_{O_2} often accompany the alveolar accumulation of fluid. It is probable that the increased respiratory drive results from stimulation of the J-receptors due to changes in interstitial pressure whilst the reduction in Pa_{O_2} is due initially to inequalities of ventilation and perfusion and later to increases in shunt from the flooded alveoli. The increase in interstitial pressure results in narrowing of the smaller airways and increases the work of breathing, but in the later stages, mucosal oedema may occur in larger bronchi and may be accompanied by a wheezing type of respiration. Fine crepitations at the lung bases are often present in the early stages of oedema but these give way to course rhales as fluid accumulation increases.

Assessment of lung water accumulation

The earliest signs of lung water accumulation are the signs of pulmonary congestion on the X-ray. Later there is a diffuse shadowing in the lung parenchyma followed by the appearance of patchy opacities. The X-ray changes are accompanied by dyspnoea, wheezing, a fall in arterial Po_2 and Pco_2, crepitations or rales and, later, cyanosis and the production of frothy, pink sputum.

Measurement of EVLW

There are two approaches to the clinical measurement of EVLW. The first is based on the inhalation of three gases, one of which is insoluble, the second of which is soluble in blood, and the third which is soluble in both blood and water. The gases may be rebreathed or delivered as a single breath and the changes in concentrations measured. Unfortunately, these techniques are subject to a number of errors, the most important being that much of the water is present in areas of lung which are not ventilated (Dennison *et al.* 1980).

The second approach is based on the use of two indicators, one of which is confined to the circulation and the second of which diffuses throughout the water in the lung. The intravascular indicators have included dyes such as Evans Blue or Indocyanine Green, whilst the diffusible indicators have included tritiated water or heat. The use of liquid indicators has given disappointing results, not only because they only a measure a fraction of the EVLW present but also because the fraction measured depends on the volume of lung perfused and so varies with factors such as exercise, perfusion pressures, cardiac output and the distribution of the oedema. However, heat is many times more diffusible than molecular tracers and is thus more likely to provide a reliable measurement. Noble and Severinghaus (1972) described a technique with injection of a bolus of cold solution into the pulmonary artery with detection in the femoral artery and similar techniques have subsequently been shown to be relatively independent of changes in cardiac output or quantity of oedema (Holcroft *et al.* 1978). However, heat is distributed to parts of the lung other than the EVLW compartment and there is still some doubt concerning the validity of the technique. Since the technique requires femoral and pulmonary artery cannulation and the interpretation of the results is open to question, it is not much used clinically.

Respiratory studies during sleep or sedation

It is now recognized that many patients show periodic dips in arterial saturation during sleep or sedation, saturation levels often falling to 70–80% when the patient is breathing air. When the patient has a reduced saturation in the conscious state (e.g. due to the presence of lung disease or post-operative pulmonary complications) the saturation may fall to much lower levels. The decreases in saturation are associated with periodic hypo-ventilation or apnoea of central origin or with partial or complete airway obstruction. The respiratory disturbances seem to be most frequently associated with the deeper or rapid eye movement (REM) stages of sleep so it is often necessary to correlate the respiratory disturbances with sleep staging.

Partial airway obstruction is usually manifested by snoring but it is more difficult to differentiate between central or obstructive apnoea. It is, therefore, usual to employ a combination of monitors which are adapted to the clinical circumstances in which the study is carried out. Arterial saturation is now almost invariably monitored with a pulse oximeter attached to a finger or earlobe whilst heart rate is derived from the oximeter or from a standard electrocardiograph (ECG). Thoracic and abdominal movements provide useful information because these tend to become asynchronous or in opposite phase when obstruction develops. Movements may be recorded by bellows pneumographs, mercury in rubber strain gauges, linear displacement transducers or a respiratory inductance plethysmograph (Catling *et al.* 1980). These signals may be correlated with airflow at the mouth sensed by an oro/nasal thermistor or with a CO_2 trace obtained from a facemask or catheter inserted into the nasopharynx through a nostril. Oesophageal pressure measurements are extremely helpful to differentiate between central and obstructive apnoea, as large negative intra-thoracic pressures may be generated during obstruction. When these are observed there are usually large changes in heart rate and arterial pressure which may be observed by continuous recording from a finger cuff with a Finapres device (p. 183). In order to derive sleep stages it is necessary to record the electroencephalo-gram (EEG), electromyogram (EMG) and electro-oculogram (EOG).

There are a number of major problems in carrying out such studies. First, it is necessary to ensure that the electrodes and other sensors are firmly attached to the patient. It is also helpful to have a low-light video of the patient synchronized with the recordings so that movements and other sources of artefact can be detected. The second problem is that an immense amount of data is generated. This must be stored on an FM or videorecorder or computer so that it can be subjected to later analysis. Automated analysis of the heart rate, blood pressure, oxygen saturation and other changes is obviously desirable so that the frequency, duration and severity of changes can be documented in a standardized manner, and doubtful data later re-examined by the investigator. Preliminary studies using these techniques in patients recovering from surgery are yielding much useful information (Catley *et al.* 1985) and it seems likely that such monitoring will be used more widely in the future.

References

Abraham, A. (1987) Conjunctival oxygen tension monitoring. *International Anesthesiology Clinics* **25**, 97–112.

Askenazi, J., Carpentier, Y.A. and Elwyn, D.H. (1980) Influence of total parenteral nutrition on fuel utilization in injury or sepsis. *Annals of Surgery* **191**, 40–46.

Benatar, S.R., Hewlett, A.M. & Nunn, J.F. (1973) The use of iso-shunt lines for control of O_2 therapy. *British Journal of Anaesthesia* **45**, 711–718.

Bird, C.C. (1971) Oxygen tension and blood oxygen tension, oxyhaemoglobin saturation, haemoglobin concentration and oxygen tension of blood. *Anaesthesia* **36**, 192–198.

Braun, U., Zundel, J., Freiboth, K., Weyland, W., Turner, E., Hedelmeyer, C.F. & Hellige, G. (1989) Evaluation of methods for indirect calorimetry with a ventilated lung model. *Intensive Care Medicine* **15**, 196–202.

Brunner, J.X. & Westenskow, D.R. (1988) How the rise time of carbon dioxide analysers influences the accuracy of carbon dioxide measurements. *British Journal of Anaesthesia* **61**, 628–638.

Campbell, E.J.M. & Howell, J.B. (1962) Rebreathing method for measurement of mixed venous P_{O_2}. *British Medical Journal* ii, 630–633.

Catley, D.M., Thornton, C., Jordan, C., Lehane, J.R., Royston, D. & Jones, J.G. (1985) Pronounced episodic desaturation in the postoperative period: its association with ventilatory pattern and analgesic regime. *Anesthesiology* **63**, 20–28.

Catling, J.A., Pinto, D.M., Jordan, C. & Jones, J.G. (1980) Respiratory effects of analgesia after cholecystectomy: comparison of continuous and intermittent papaveretum. *British Medical Journal* **281**, 478–480.

Damask, M.C. (1986) Metabolic measurements during mechanical ventilation. *IEEE Engineering in Medicine and Biology* **5**, 30–35.

Dennison, D.M., Davies, N.J.H. & Brown, D.J. (1979) A theoretical comparison of single breath and rebreathing methods of studying soluble gas exchange in the lung. In Cumming, G. & Bonsignore, G. (eds) *The pulmonary circulation in Health and Disease*, pp. 139–160. Plenum Press, Oxford.

East, T.D., Andriano, H.P. & Pace, N.L. (1987) Automated measurement of functional residual capacity by sulfur hexafluoride washout. *Journal of Clinical Monitoring* **3**, 14–21.

Engström, C.G. & Herzog, P. (1959) Ventilation nomogram for practical use with the Engström respirator. *Acta Chirurgica Scandinavica* (Suppl.) **245**, 37–42.

Gattinoni, L., Mascheroni, D., Basilico, R.E., Foti, G., Pesenti, A. & Avalli, L. (1987) Volume/pressure curve of total respiratory system in paralysed patients: artefacts and correction factors. *Intensive Care Medicine* **13**, 19–25.

Gravenstein, N., Lampotang, S. & Benekin, J.E.W. (1985) Factors influencing capnography in the Bain Circuit. *Journal of Clinical Monitoring* **1**, 6–10.

Heese, H. de V. & Freeseman, C. (1964) Determination of mixed venous P_{CO_2} in infants and children. *British Medical Journal* i, 1290–1292.

Holcroft, J.W., Trunkey, D.D. & Carpenter, M.A. (1978) Excessive fluid administration in resuscitating baboons from hemorrhage shock, and an assessment of the thermodye technique for measuring extravascular lung water. *American Journal of Surgery* **135**, 412–416.

Kaufman, R.D., Patterson, R.W. & Lee, A.St.J. (1987) Derivation of $\dot{V}_A/\dot{Q}$ distribution from blood–gas tensions. *British Journal of Anaesthesia* **59**, 1599–1609.

Lee, A.St.J., Patterson, R.W. & Kaufman, R.D. (1987) Relationships among ventilation–perfusion distribution, multiple inert gas methodology and metabolic blood–gas tensions. *British Journal of Anaesthesia* **59**, 1579–1598.

Lubbers, D.W. (1987) Theory and development of transcutaneous oxygen pressure measurement. *International Anesthesiology Clinics* **25**, 31–65.

McEvoy, J.D.S., Jones, N.L. & Campbell, E.J.M. (1974) Mixed venous and arterial P_{CO_2}. *British Medical Journal* **4**, 687–690.

Matamis, D., Lemaire, F., Harf, A., Brun-Buisson, C., Ansquer, J.C. & Atlan, G. (1984) Total respiratory pressure-volume curves in the adult respiratory distress syndrome. *Chest* **86**, 58–66.

Noble, W.H. & Severinghaus, J.W. (1972) Thermal and conductivity dilution curves for rapid quantitation of pulmonary edema. *Journal of Applied Physiology* **32**, 770–775.

Radford, E.P. (1955) Ventilation standards for use in artificial respiration. *Journal of Applied Physiology* **7**, 451–460.

Schweiss, J.F. (1987) Mixed venous hemoglobin saturation: theory and application. *International Anesthesiology Clinics* **25**, 113–136.

Shoemaker, W.C., Appel, P.L. & Kram, H.B. (1987) The role of oxygen transport patterns in the pathophysiology, prediction of outcome and therapy of shock. In Bryan-Brown, C. & Ayres, S.M. (eds), *Oxygen transport and utilisation*, pp. 65–92. Society of Critical Care Medicine, Fullerton, California.

Sykes, M.K. (1960) Observations on a rebreathing technique for the determination of arterial P_{CO_2} in the apnoeic patient. *British Journal of Anaesthesia* **32**, 256–261.

Taylor, A.E., Hernandez, L., Perry, M., Smith, M. & Womack, W. (1987) Overview of tissue oxygenation. In Bryan-Brown, C. & Ayres, S.M. (eds) *Oxygen transport and utilisation*, pp. 13–24. Society of Critical Care Medicine, Fullerton, California.

Tremper, K.K. & Barker, S.J. (1987) Transcutaneous oxygen measurement: experimental studies and adult applications. *International Anesthesiology Clinics* **25**, 67–96.

Tsoi, C.M., Raemer, B. & Westenskow, D.R. (1982) Instrumentation for simultaneously measuring $\dot{V}_{CO_2}$ and $\dot{V}_{O_2}$ in humans using titration methods. *Journal of Applied Physiology* **52**, 786–791.

Ultman, J.S. & Bursztein, S. (1981) Analysis of error in the determination of respiratory gas exchange at varying $F_{I_{O_2}}$. *Journal of Applied Physiology* **50**, 210–216.

Verhoeff, F. & Sykes, M.K. (1990) Delayed detection of hypoxic events by pulse oximeters: computer simulations. *Anaesthesia* **45**, 103–109.

Weissman, C. (1987) Measuring oxygen uptake in the clinical setting. In Bryan-Brown, C. & Ayres, S.M. (eds), *Oxygen transport and utilisation*, pp. 25–64. Society of Critical Care Medicine, Fullerton, California.

23: Monitoring the Cardiovascular System

This will be considered under six headings: electrical activity of the heart; pulse and arterial pressure; heart filling pressures; ventricular volumes and wall motion; cardiac output; and regional blood flow.

The electrocardiograph (ECG)

The ECG displays the surface potential changes from the electrical activity in the heart. Whilst it may provide useful information concerning the rate, rhythm, propagation of the excitation wave, heart position, muscle hypertrophy and regional ischaemia, it gives no information concerning pump function. Cardiac anaesthetists are only too familiar with the sight of a virtually motionless heart despite a relatively normal ECG trace!

For maximum diagnostic information it is necessary to use a 12-lead ECG. However, this would prove too cumbersome for the average operating theatre environment so a two- or three-lead display is usually chosen. Whilst leads I, II or III provide the most useful information on rhythm abnormalities, it is now generally agreed that information on the development of regional myocardial ischaemia is equally important. This is best detected by the V_5 configuration where the left leg lead is placed in the fifth left interspace at the anterior axillary line. A useful alternative is the CM_5 configuration, the right arm lead being placed over the right sternomanubrial junction and the left leg lead in the fifth left interspace at the anterior axillary line. The indifferent lead can be placed at any convenient site, such as below the left clavicle. Another useful configuration is the CB_5. This is a bipolar lead with the positive electrode in the fifth left interspace at the anterior axillary line and the negative electrode over the centre of the right scapula. It provides good information on rhythm changes and also

enables regional myocardial ischaemia to be detected (Bazaral & Norfleet, 1981; Griffin & Kaplan, 1987).

Care is required to obtain an optimal ECG signal (Gardner & Hollingsworth, 1986). Modern disposable electrodes perform surprisingly well and produce minimal skin irritation, even when left in place for long periods. However, it is important to ensure that the electrode is placed in close contact with the skin and to remember that the signal improves with time as the skin becomes wetted by the electrode jelly. It is generally unwise to use needle electrodes since the small surface area of the electrode results in a high current density and increased likelihood of burns if there is a fault in the diathermy or ECG amplifier, and they also distort the waveform. Full precautions should also be taken to minimize the risk of electroshock (Chapter 11).

Pulse and arterial pressure

Current recommendations for monitoring place great emphasis on the use of some form of continuous monitor which indicates that the heart is beating and that a pulse is being produced. The instruments used include the precordial or oesophageal stethoscope, the pulse plethysmograph, the pulse oximeter or a direct display of the arterial pressure waveform. Most indirect methods of measuring the blood pressure provide intermittent readings. However, the recently introduced Penaz technique (Chapter 14) produces a continuous arterial pressure waveform from a finger cuff.

HEART SOUNDS AND PULSE

The *precordial stethoscope*, strapped tightly to the chest over the apex beat, provides a simple means of monitoring the rate and rhythm of the heart. In the neonate a decrease in intensity and muffling of the heart sounds occurs when cardiac output is reduced by hypovolaemia or deep anaesthesia. The *oesophageal stethoscope* is less affected by movement artefacts and may be positioned so that breath sounds are heard simultaneously. It is particularly valuable for detecting the presence of secretions, bronchospasm or the coarse rhonci often associated with misplacement of an endotracheal or endobronchial tube. Both types of stethoscope may be fitted with binaural or monaural earpieces. The former exclude other sounds and are uncomfortable to wear for long periods. In the US most physicians have their own monaural stethoscope which is moulded to fit their ear and is thus more comfortable; however, prolonged use may lead to otitis externa in susceptible individuals. An alternative is to amplify the sound for transmission by loudspeaker. This has the advantage that all those close to the loudspeaker can hear the output but the wide range of frequencies encompassed by breath and heart sounds necessitates the use of a high quality amplifier and speaker.

The *pulse plethysmograph* is a most useful monitor because it provides a continuous visual display of pulse amplitude. It consists of a finger or ear probe containing a light emitting diode (LED) and a photodiode to sense the pulsatile variations in the intensity of the transmitted or reflected light. In a normal or dilated vascular bed the signal is similar to the arterial pressure waveform but when there is vasoconstriction or a reduction in cardiac output the amplitude decreases and the waveform appears to become damped (Fig. 23.1). If placed on the same limb as the blood pressure cuff the return of

pulsations during cuff deflation may be taken to indicate the systolic point. However, the method may be inaccurate in the overweight or elderly when the elbow is bent to allow the hand to rest on the chest.

Some form of plethysmographic display is now incorporated in most pulse oximeters but in some the amplitude information is of little value since an automatic gain is incorporated to ensure that the pulse waveform fills the whole of the display.

ARTERIAL PRESSURE MEASUREMENT

It is now accepted that arterial pressure should be measured at appropriate intervals in all but the most minor interventions. The arterial pressure depends on both cardiac output and peripheral resistance and there are many physiological mechanisms which tend to maintain arterial pressure in the presence of changes of blood volume or cardiac output. It is therefore only a crude index of the state of the circulation and should be interpreted in the light of observed changes in blood volume, filling pressures and vascular tone. It should also be remembered that the recorded pressure varies with the site of measurement, the systolic and pulse pressure being greater in the peripheral vessels due to reflected waves and other factors: thus a pressure of 110/80 in the aorta may be recorded as 130/70 in the dorsalis pedis artery. It is also important to take account of the difference in height between the cuff or pressure transducer and the heart, the blood pressure reading decreasing by approximately 10 mmHg for every 13 cm that the transducer is above the heart and vice versa. It is, of course essential to ensure that the recording system is adjusted to produce an optimal response (Gardner & Hollingsworth, 1986).

The measurement of blood pressure by normal non-invasive means, whether by the Riva-Rocci method or any of the automated devices, is subject to large errors particularly in diastolic pressure. Care in placement of a cuff of appropriate width and length and slow deflation (not more than 3–4 mmHg·s^{-1}) are essential to optimize accuracy.

Instruments based on the Penaz technique (p. 83) now provide a continuous display of the

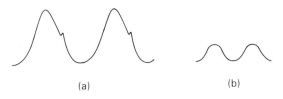

(a)   (b)

Fig. 23.1. Pulse plethysmograms. (a) Normal trace. (b) Low cardiac output and/or vasoconstriction.

pulse waveform from a cuff placed round a finger. Whilst this technique is capable of displaying changes in arterial pressure accurately, the absolute values are more variable. Much of this variability is associated with the position and tensioning of the cuff. Improved accuracy can be obtained by comparing the instrument with some other non-invasive method after initiating recording.

As with all finger cuff methods it is important to ensure that the cuff is at heart level or a correction for the difference in height applied. Since the pressure in the cuff is continuously adjusted to match the intravascular pressure the finger tends to become blue, congested and painful after 30–40 minutes use, and ischaemic damage has been reported. This problem can be obviated by deflating the cuff for several minutes every 30 min.

Direct arterial pressure measurement is indicated in cardiac and major thoracic surgery, neuro-surgery, the extremely obese and in situations where rapid fluctuations in blood pressure may occur (major arterial surgery, major trauma, surgery for a phaeochromocytoma or the use of controlled hypotension).

Arterial puncture

The complications resulting from the placement of an arterial cannula are haematoma formation, infection, thrombosis, embolism and skin necrosis over the site of the cannula (Bedford & Wollman, 1973). There is also the risk of kinking of the cannula, which leads to degradation of the pressure signal, and of exsanguination if a disconnection occurs. The incidence of these complications is least with a single puncture with a small needle and greatest with prolonged cannulation. Gillies *et al.* (1979) assessed the complications of a single puncture by a 23 or 21 standard wire gauge (SWG) needle at 580 sites in 282 patients, and found bruising present in 176, tenderness in 87 and haematoma formation in 31 of the sites even though the operators were experienced and used a standard technique with 5 min compression of the puncture site after removal of the needle. Bedford (1977) found a 34% incidence of radial artery thrombosis after 24 h of cannulation with an

18-gauge cannula, but showed that this could be reduced to about 5% if a 20-gauge Teflon cannula was used for the same length of time (Bedford, 1975, 1985). Similar findings were recorded by Davis and Stewart (1980). Although thrombosed arteries appear to recanalize in time, many patients have decreased pulsation in an artery which has been cannulated and subsequent cannulation of the same artery or a distal branch may lead to inaccurate recordings of pressure.

Choice of puncture site

Any palpable artery may be cannulated, the choice being governed mainly by the ease of maintaining the cannula in position.

The radial artery of the non-dominant arm is the obvious first choice because the artery is relatively superficial, the cannula can be fixed securely to the wrist and the patient can move the arm joints without dislodging the cannula. It is generally unwise to cannulate a radial artery if the patient has had a previous brachial artery catheterization on that side (since the arterial pressure may be incorrect) and it is logical to use the right radial artery for thoracic aneurysm surgery where the left subclavian artery is often occluded. The right radial artery should also be used in premature infants with a patent ductus arteriosus, since the left side may receive desaturated blood from the ductus arteriosus. Finally, it is important to ensure that there is an adequate ulnar artery collateral circulation. This is customarily assessed by performing Allen's test in which both radial and ulnar arteries are occluded while the patient squeezes the hand to blanch the skin. The patient then opens the hand and the pressure on the ulnar artery is released. A satisfactory collateral circulation results in a flushing of the skin over the fingers within 5 s (Bedford, 1977). However, there is some evidence that a slower return of colour (7–10 s) is associated with an inadequate blood flow to the thenar area. The test is difficult to interpret in patients who are cold, burned, pale or jaundiced and hyperextension of the digits may also delay the restoration of the colour. Simple alternative tests are to feel for the presence of a pulse in the radial artery distal to an occluding finger or the use of a pulse plethysmo-graph to detect pulsation of the thumb, while the radial artery is occluded with digital pressure.

The radial artery is usually cannulated at the wrist joint where it is easily palpable. However, its course is somewhat tortuous and difficulty is some-times encountered in threading the cannula up the artery. This difficulty is usually due to failure to place the needle centrally in the vessel lumen but may also be caused by arterial wall disease in patients with a tortuous artery. In such circum-stances a technique utilizing a flexible guide-wire is often more successful because this can negotiate the bends more easily than the standard cannula or needle device.

It is technically more difficult to cannulate the ulnar artery because it is not as superficial as the radial artery and it tends to be tortuous as it passes the wrist joint. The brachial artery has the advan-tages of being larger and closer to the heart so that there is less systolic pressure augmentation due to reflection of the pulse pressure wave from distal branching. There are usually abundant collateral vessels about the elbow so that occlusion of the artery rarely results in distal vascular ischaemia (Barnes et al. 1976). However, the artery has gained a bad reputation for complications because of its frequent use for cardiac catheterization. Median nerve damage may occur secondary to direct trauma or haematoma formation but the main difficulty with brachial artery cannulation is the difficulty in splinting the arm to prevent dislodgment of the cannula.

Theoretically, cannulation of the axillary artery should have even greater advantages since the artery is large and closer to the aorta. Furthermore, the axillary pulse is often palpable in severe shock and the patient is able to use the arm normally when the cannula is in place. However, the axillary artery is situated within a neurovascular sheath and haematoma formation may result in neuro-logical sequelae. The approach to the axillary artery is similar to that for an axillary nerve block but it is preferable to use a flexible guide-wire to intro-duce the cannula (Adler & Bryan-Brown, 1973). Since the cannula is close to the arch of the aorta

it is important to take extreme care to avoid air embolism from small bubbles in the flush solution.

The femoral artery was widely used for monitor-ing in the early days of open heart surgery but it has been reported that approximately 1% of can-nulations required an embolectomy for ischaemia. This is probably associated with the high incidence of arteriosclerotic lesions in this artery. Haem-atoma formation and infection are also problems (Gurman & Kriemerman, 1985). Cannulation of the dorsalis pedis artery is difficult because of the relatively small size of the artery and the fact that it is often occluded in patients with arterial disease. Because of its distal situation, systolic pressures typically read 10–15 mmHg higher than brachial pressures, whilst diastolic readings are 15–20 mmHg lower (Spoerel et al. 1975; Youngberg & Miller, 1976). Mean pressure in this artery should be more closely related to mean aortic pressure but there may be a discrepancy between the two if there is significant arterial disease in the lower extremities. Because of the narrow lumen there is a high incidence of post-cannulation occlusion so the collateral circulation should be tested before can-nulation. A suggested technique is to occlude both the dorsalis pedis and posterior tibial arteries with digital pressure and then blanch the patient's great toe with direct compression. The toe colour should return within 5 s of release of tibial artery pressure. Cannulation of the superficial temporal artery is frequently used in infants.

Cannula care

The cannula should be inserted with full aseptic precautions and fixed firmly in place so that it cannot slide in and out of the skin. There is evidence that an iodine-containing preparation applied to the puncture site can reduce the inci-dence of skin infection, and a similar solution should be applied to blood sampling ports or injection sites. The cannula should be connected to a continuous flushing device (e.g. the Sorensen Intraflo, which delivers approximately $3 \text{ ml} \cdot \text{hr}^{-1}$ of heparinized saline and which permits a rapid flush after blood sampling). Blanching of the skin during rapid flushing with 1–2 ml of flush solution suggests that the artery distal to the cannula is blocked and removal of the cannula should be considered. The cannula should also be removed if skin infection develops or if a large haematoma forms. Proximal occlusion of the artery and aspiration of the cannula by a syringe during removal may help to remove any thrombus formed during the period of cannulation.

Heart filling pressures

CENTRAL VENOUS PRESSURE (CVP)

The systemic venous system contains about 70% of the total blood volume and is under strong neurogenic control. When venous tone is normal a 10% change in blood volume results in little change in CVP, but more extensive losses or gains result in a fall or an increase in CVP (p. 163).

The absolute level of CVP is somewhat variable. Part of the reason for this is that the surface marking of the right atrium (the intersection of the mid-axillary line with a perpendicular drawn through the fourth interspace at the sternum) may not be accurately related to its true position. Furthermore, vascular tone may vary with temperature, sympathetic activity and body position. Whilst very high or very low CVP values are diagnostic of heart failure or hypovolaemia, the main value of CVP measurement is in following the response to therapy (Poole-Wilson, 1978).

The most common routes for insertion of the central venous catheter are the median basilic vein at the elbow or the internal jugular vein in the neck (Rosen *et al.* 1981). The femoral and external jugular veins can also be used but it is often difficult to thread a cannula from the latter into a central vein. Cannulation via the cephalic vein in the arm is also unlikely to lead to central cannulation because of its tortuous course in the upper arm. Cannulation of the median basilic vein is technically simple, but the tip of the cannula frequently passes into the neck veins or the innominate vein rather than the superior vena cava. Satisfactory placement is most easily achieved if the arm is abducted to a right angle, to straighten the axillary vein, and the head turned towards the

same side. Puncture of the internal jugular vein is technically more difficult and it is not uncommon to puncture the carotid artery with the possible formation of a large haematoma. Cannulation must be performed with the patient in a head-down position, since this distends the vein and minimizes the chances of air embolus. Cannulation of the right side is preferred owing to the danger of thoracic duct damage on the left side. The length of cannula in the vein should be checked by laying the guide-wire along the course of the vein and a chest X-ray taken whenever possible to confirm the position of the tip of the catheter. Cannulation of a central vein should result in a respiratory swing on a saline manometer and characteristic venous pulsations if the pressure is recorded by a transducer. An initial reading of more than 20 cmH$_2$O should raise the possibility that the catheter has entered the right ventricle or pulmonary artery.

Indications for CVP measurement

The three main indications are as follows:
1 To monitor the right heart filling pressure during transfusion in patients with cardiovascular disease or severe anaemia.
2 To monitor right heart filling pressure in patients with potential massive blood loss.
3 To elucidate the cause of sudden, unexplained hypotension.

The normal CVP is 0–6 cmH$_2$O when referred to the right atrium. A CVP of more than 10–12 cmH$_2$O suggests that there is an imbalance between venous return and cardiac output, i.e. that is there is either right sided heart failure or a transfusion overload. A very low CVP suggests hypovolaemia or a decrease in peripheral vascular tone. The most valuable information from the CVP trace can be obtained by observing the response to a brisk transfusion of 100–200 ml of fluid (Fig. 23.2). If the patient is hypovolaemic the CVP will change little. If normovolaemic, the CVP will increase by 1–2 cmH$_2$O and return to the pre-existing level immediately the transfusion ceases. If the patient is overloaded or in heart failure the CVP will increase by 3–4 cmH$_2$O and will then remain high or only fall slowly towards its

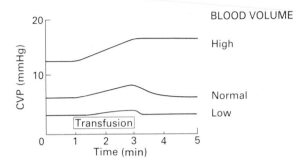

Fig.23.2. Response of CVP to transfusion of 200 ml fluid over 2 min. Bottom trace: reduced blood volume. Middle trace: normal blood volume. Top trace: increased blood volume or right-sided cardiac failure.

previous level. The measurement of the response of the CVP to transfusion is particularly valuable when transfusing patients with diminished cardiac reserve due to anaemia or heart failure.

PULMONARY CAPILLARY WEDGE PRESSURE

When the heart is normal there is little difference between right and left heart filling pressures. However, when cardiac disease is present there may be a marked disparity between right and left atrial pressures. Under these circumstances the passage of a balloon-tipped flotation catheter (Swan–Ganz) may provide valuable extra information which will enable left ventricular function to be optimized (O'Quin & Marini, 1983). When the catheter is wedged in a branch of the pulmonary artery and the balloon inflated, a measurement of pulmonary capillary wedge pressure (PCWP) is obtained which, under most circumstances, closely approximates to mean left atrial pressure. When the balloon is deflated pulmonary artery pressure can be recorded. However, the technique is invasive and there are many possible complications, particularly if the catheter is left *in situ* for several days.

Various types of Swan–Ganz catheter are available depending on the measurements which need to be made. The simplest is a double lumen catheter, one lumen being used for inflation of the balloon and the other to measure pressures and withdraw blood samples. Triple lumen catheters, with a side-hole at the level of the right ventricle,

are usually associated with a thermistor at the tip of the catheter and are used to make thermodilution measurements of cardiac output.

The catheter is passed through a sheath inserted into the internal jugular or median basilic vein and threaded into a position near the right atrium. This position is reached when the catheter has passed about 15 cm from the jugular or subclavian veins, 40 cm from the right antecubital fossa and 30 cm from the femoral vein. The balloon is then inflated with the recommended volume of saline (usually 0.8–1.5 ml) and the catheter advanced slowly. The balloon is carried in the direction of the blood flow and so passes through the right atrium and right ventricle into the pulmonary artery, the position being detected by observation of the pressure trace (Fig. 23.3). When the balloon has reached the wedge position (in an artery about 1 cm in diameter) it is deflated to check that pulmonary artery pressure can be recorded. This indicates that blood can flow past the catheter, thus minimizing the chance of pulmonary infarction. As the catheter softens after insertion there is a tendency for the tip to migrate more peripherally. Inflation of the balloon should therefore be performed slowly. If occlusion occurs at a volume of less than 75% of the recommended volume the catheter should be withdrawn 2–3 cm and the inflation repeated.

The most frequent complications associated with the use of the Swan–Ganz catheter are dysrhythmias, air embolism, coiling in the right ventricle with the possibility of knotting, thrombosis round the catheter, infection, rupture of the balloon and rupture of the pulmonary artery due to excessive inflation of the balloon. The catheter must be attached to a continuous flush system to ensure patency, and the balloon should only be inflated

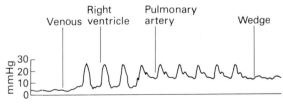

Fig. 23.3. Pressure trace recorded during insertion of Swan–Ganz catheter into the pulmonary artery.

intermittently for brief periods to enable wedge measurements to be made. Care is necessary to ensure that the catheter is not wedged when blood samples are withdrawn, for it is easy to withdraw left atrial blood (which is fully oxygenated) rather than pulmonary artery blood when the catheter is close to a wedge position.

The major source of error with the wedge measurement is the position of the catheter. If the tip is wedged in the upper zones of the lung there may be no fluid connection between the catheter and left atrium, since alveolar pressure may exceed capillary pressure. The area of lung subjected to these conditions may be increased if positive end-expiratory pressure is applied so that the pressure recorded may be alveolar rather than left atrial. It is therefore important to check that the catheter tip lies in the lower lung zones, by observing its position on an X-ray, and to take all readings at the end of expiration whether ventilation is spontaneous or controlled.

If the balloon ruptures or a satisfactory wedge position cannot be obtained, a good estimate of left atrial pressure can be obtained from the pulmonary artery end-diastolic pressure. This is similar to left atrial pressure in the absence of increased pulmonary vascular resistance or a heart rate above 120 beats per minute (Lappas et al. 1973; Buchbinder & Ganz, 1976). However, it is important to ensure that the recording system has a good dynamic response to ensure that the measurement is accurate.

The interpretation of the pulmonary capillary wedge pressure is the subject of much controversy (see Nadeau and Noble, 1986 for a comprehensive review). The normal pressure is 8–12 mmHg. The mean PCWP correlates well with left ventricular end-diastolic pressure (LVEDP) over a wide range of filling pressures in patients who have normal left ventricular and mitral valve function but may be greater than LVEDP when there is mitral stenosis, a left atrial myxoma or during the application of PEEP. In left ventricular failure the elevated LVEDP may exceed the mean left atrial and mean PCWP. A similar error may arise when there is aortic regurgitation. The main indications for Swan–Ganz catheterization are as follows:

1 To assess left ventricular function in patients with left-sided heart disease.
2 To eliminate a raised left atrial pressure as a cause of pulmonary oedema.
3 To optimize left ventricular filling pressure in patients with coronary artery disease or with shock due to sepsis or haemorrhage (Kaplan & Wells, 1981).
4 To enable thermal dilution cardiac output measurements to be made when these are considered essential for patient management.

The initial enthusiasm for the use of flow directed pulmonary artery catheters is now being tempered by the frequent incidence of complications and the resultant morbidity and mortality (Sise et al. 1981; Robin, 1985). There are also technical problems which reduce the accuracy of wedge pressure measurements (Morris et al. 1985) and under some circumstances there is a poor correlation between wedge pressure and left ventricular end-diastolic volume (Calvin et al. 1981; Hansen et al. 1986). Although a number of early studies suggested that the use of flow directed catheters decreased the incidence of perioperative myocardial infarction (Weintraub & Barash, 1987) a recent prospective study showed that their use had no major impact on outcome (Tuman et al. 1989).

Ventricular volumes and ejection fraction

Atrial pressures correlate poorly with end-diastolic volumes when ventricular compliance is altered by changes in pleural pressure, afterload, ventricular hypertrophy, myocardial disease, or constrictive pericarditis, and also when there is tricuspid or mitral valve disease. Ventricular compliance may also be affected by drugs. For example, catecholamines, calcium ions and sodium nitroprusside appear to increase compliance whilst cyclopropane has been shown to decrease compliance. It has, therefore, been suggested that measurements of right ventricular volume and ejection fraction can provide a better guide to fluid replacement than measurement of atrial pressures (Martyn et al. 1981). However, the main use of measurements of ejection fraction is in pre-operative evaluation. Left ventricular ejection fraction is normally 55–65%. A value of less than 35% in the conscious patient suggests severe impairment of cardiac function and is associated with a poor response to anaesthesia and surgery (Kazmers *et al.* 1988). Right and left ventricular volumes and ejection fractions are usually measured by radionuclear techniques. However, right ventricular volumes can also be measured by thermodilution. Two-dimensional echocardiography has been used but is subject to errors in the critically ill (Kaul *et al.* 1984).

RADIONUCLEAR TECHNIQUES

Techniques utilizing radioisotopes are the 'gold standard' against which other techniques are judged. However, there are many assumptions involved in the calculation of volumes from one or two dimensional views, even if the outline of the chambers can be clearly demonstrated, and in single pass techniques, where count rates are low, it is often difficult to identify the position of the ventricular walls (see Chapter 10).

First pass studies

A bolus of radioactive tracer such as technetium-99m is injected into the right side of the circulation and its transit through the heart is recorded by sequential images obtained by a gamma camera. The technique thus resembles angiocardiography (see p. 123). The advantage of the technique is that it is rapid and it is also possible to identify intracardiac shunts. However, accuracy is limited by the short time available for accumulation of counts, and repeated measurements are restricted by the radiation dose.

Gated cardiac blood pool imaging

The injected radionuclide is allowed to equilibrate throughout the blood pool and images are then accumulated at a given point in the cardiac cycle by 'gating' the gamma camera to the ECG. The technique thus provides a static image of the heart chambers at a given point in the cardiac cycle. Ejection fraction (EF) can then be calculated:

$$EF = \frac{\text{end-diastolic volume} - \text{end-systolic volume}}{\text{end-diastolic volume}}$$

Alternatively, images may be accumulated at more frequent intervals throughout the cycle so that the pattern of contraction of each part of the ventricular wall can be visualized and quantified. This enables wall motion abnormalities to be identified.

Although the best images are obtained by using a gamma camera, a single nuclear probe has been used with success in the anaesthetized patient (Giles *et al.* 1982).

THERMODILUTION MEASUREMENT

A modified Swan–Ganz catheter is required. This has an injection port with three holes situated 21 cm from the tip to allow injection just above the tricuspid valve and the thermistor has a very rapid response (90% in 50 ms) so that beat-by-beat differences in temperature can be recorded from the pulmonary artery (Vincent *et al.* 1986). The position of the injection ports is checked by pressure measurement during withdrawal from the ventricle and the cold saline is injected in the normal manner at the end of expiration. The descending limb of the curve shows beat-by-beat variations in temperature. Since the descending limb of the curve is exponential in character ejection fraction can be calculated from the ratio of the heights of successive plateaux of temperature from the baseline (Fig. 23.4). The technique has been validated by Kay *et al.* (1983), the normal value of the right ventricular ejection fraction being 40–45%. Errors may arise when there is tricuspid incompetence or cardiac dysrhythmias are present. However, the latter error may be reduced by averaging measurements over several beats.

The technique has the advantage that repeated measurements can be made. It has been used as a guide to fluid therapy in burned patients (Martyn *et al.* 1981) and it has also been suggested that an increase in right ventricular end-diastolic pressure in the presence of a decreased right ventricular ejection fraction is a useful index of myocardial ischaemia in patients with right coronary artery disease (Hines & Barash, 1986).

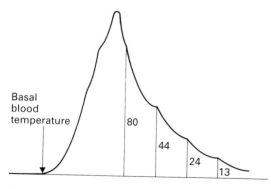

Fig. 23.4. Record of PA temperature after RV injection of cold saline to show how RV ejection fraction is calculated from beat-by-beat changes in temperature.

Mean residual fraction RF_1 = 44/80 = 0.55; RF_2 = 24/44 = 0.55; RF_3 = 13/24 = 0.54.

Ejection fraction = 1 – RF = 0.45.

RV stroke volume = cardiac output ÷ heart rate.

RV end-diastolic volume = RV stroke volume ÷ RV ejection fraction.

RV end-systolic volume = RV end-diastolic volume – RV stroke volume.

ECHOCARDIOGRAPHY

Two-dimensional echocardiography can be carried out by placing transducers on the chest wall or within the oesophagus. The latter route is frequently used for monitoring during anaesthesia, although the size of the probe precludes placement in the conscious patient. The transducer is mounted at the tip of a gastroscope and manipulated into the appropriate position by the operator. The most frequently used view provides a short-axis cross-sectional view of the left ventricle which allows visualization of the myocardium within the distribution of the major epicardial arteries: cross-sections at papillary level have proved best for diagnosis of regional wall motion abnormalities secondary to myocardial ischaemia.

Although ECG changes in the V_5 and II leads enable over 90% of ischaemic events to be detected, they are a relatively late sign of ischaemia. Since changes in ventricular compliance and wall motion usually precede S–T changes attempts are now being made to use trans-oesophageal echocardiography to detect regional wall motion abnormalities. Present studies suggest that this technique is superior to

the ECG in detecting myocardial ischaemia and infarction (Smith *et al.* 1985; Clements & de Bruijn, 1987).

Further developments such as colour flow mapping, which enables blood flow patterns in the cardiac chambers to be determined, will greatly increase the potential of this technique in the future. However, the technology is very expensive and the results are greatly dependent on the skill and experience of the operator. For a further review of the use of echocardiography in monitoring see Seward *et al.* (1988) and Lamantia *et al.* (1989).

Cardiac output

Of the three techniques for measuring cardiac output directly (Fick, dye-dilution and thermal-dilution) only thermal-dilution is widely used in clinical practice. The Fick method requires measurements of oxygen consumption and arterial and mixed venous O_2 contents and thus imposes a major technical load. Dye-dilution outputs require withdrawal of 30–50 ml of arterial blood through a cuvette and hence cannot be repeated often unless the blood is returned to the patient. Furthermore, the quality of the dye curve deteriorates when cardiac output is low, particularly if the dye injection is made peripherally.

Thermal-dilution cardiac output measurements can be made repeatedly and automated analysis of the curve recorded from a thermistor in the pulmonary artery can yield a value for cardiac output within seconds of the injection. However, the accuracy of the thermal technique is critically dependent on the time of injection during the respiratory cycle, variations of up to 50% of the value being obtained between injections made during the inspiratory or expiratory phases of mechanical ventilation. To minimize this error injections are made at end-expiration.

There are two non-invasive techniques for measuring cardiac output which produce satisfactory indications of trends, but they are difficult to calibrate accurately. The Doppler technique, which measures the velocity of flow in the arch of the aorta or descending aorta, can only produce a measurement of volume flow if the cross sectional diameter of the aorta is known (see p. 218), whilst the impedance technique can only be calibrated accurately by comparing it with another standard method (see p. 219).

The main indications for cardiac output measurement are (1) to assess left ventricular function during treatment with inotropic or vasodilator drugs and (2) to optimize oxygen transport during septic shock or during mechanical ventilation with positive end-expiratory pressure.

MEASUREMENTS OF MIXED VENOUS P_{O_2},
CONTENT OR SATURATION

As shown by the Fick equation mixed venous oxygen content ($C\bar{v}_{O_2}$) depends on the arterial oxygen content (Ca_{O_2}), the cardiac output ($\dot{Q}_T$) and the tissue oxygen consumption ($\dot{V}_{O_2}$):

$$\dot{Q}_T = \frac{\dot{V}_{O_2}}{Ca_{O_2} - C\bar{v}_{O_2}}$$

or

$$C\bar{v}_{O_2} = Ca_{O_2} - \frac{\dot{V}_{O_2}}{\dot{Q}_T}.$$

Since oxygen content = (saturation × 1.34 × Hb) + (dissolved O_2) it is apparent that a reduction in mixed venous P_{O_2}, saturation or content will occur if there is a reduction in arterial P_{O_2}, saturation or content or cardiac output, or if there is an increase in tissue oxygen consumption. Since mixed venous P_{O_2} is believed to provide the best estimate of the actual P_{O_2} driving oxygen into the cells this would appear to be the most appropriate measurement for assessing tissue oxygenation (Schweiss, 1987). However, there are advantages in measuring saturation rather than P_{O_2} in venous blood. First, a change in P_{O_2} from 5.3 (40) to 2.6 kPa (20 mmHg) corresponds to a change in saturation from 75 to 33% at a pH of 7.40. In this range measurements of saturation are, therefore, a more accurate measure of oxygenation than are measurements of P_{O_2}. Secondly, although intravascular measurements of P_{O_2} can be made by intravascular electrodes these are less accurate and drift more than devices which

measure saturation *in vivo*. With modern fibre optic systems satisfactory measurements of saturation can be made over periods of hours or even days.

Mixed venous saturation measurements are most useful when there are acute changes in the circulation. Thus, they have been used as a guide to therapy with inotropes or vasodilators, as a guide to blood volume replacement in haemorrhage and in the setting of optimal PEEP levels. Continuous monitoring also detects acute falls in saturation due to transient increases in oxygen consumption, e.g. due to shivering or physiotherapy. However, it must be remembered that the measurement is affected not only by the relationship of oxygen consumption to cardiac output but also by all the factors which affect the supply of oxygen to the tissues (inspired oxygen fraction, ventilation, haemoglobin, oxygen dissociation curve shift, abnormal haemoglobin, etc.). Furthermore, in situations where marked vasoconstriction exists (e.g. after cardiopulmonary bypass or in severe hypothermia) the mixed venous saturation may be normal despite a severe fall in cardiac output because much of the tissue mass is not being perfused. The controversies currently surrounding mixed venous saturation monitoring are thoroughly discussed by Norfleet and Watson (1985).

Regional blood flow

The methods of assessing regional blood flow are essentially clinical, for most of the measurement techniques are too complicated to use in clinical practice. The presence of consciousness and responsive pupil reflexes usually indicates that cerebral blood flow is adequate. During anaesthesia devices such as the cerebral function monitor have been utilized to monitor blood flow over the critical points at the junctions of various arterial territories (p. 65). In the case of the coronary circulation ECG changes in the precordial leads are the main indication of regional ischaemia. In the kidney the most useful clinical monitor of blood flow is the urine output, which should be at least 30 ml·hr^{-1}.

References

Adler, D.C. & Bryan-Brown, C.W. (1973) Use of the axillary artery for intravascular monitoring. *Critical Care Medicine* **1**, 148–150.

Barnes, R.W., Foster, E.J., Janssen, G.A. & Boutros, A.R. (1976) Safety of brachial artery catheters as monitors in the intensive care unit — prospective evaluation with the Doppler ultrasonic velocity detector. *Anesthesiology* **44**, 260–264.

Bazaral, M.G. & Norfleet, E.A. (1981) Comparison of CB_5 and V_5 leads for intraoperative electrocardiograhic monitoring. *Anesthesia and Analgesia* **60**, 849–853.

Bedford, R.F. (1975) Percutaneous radial artery cannulation — increased safety using Teflon catheters. *Anesthesiology* **42**, 219–222.

Bedford, R.F. (1977) Radial artery function following percutaneous cannulation with 18 and 20 gauge catheters. *Anesthesiology* **47**, 37–39.

Bedford, R.F. (1990) Invasive blood pressure monitoring. In Blitt, C.D. (ed.) *Monitoring in anesthesia and critical care medicine* 2nd edn. pp. 93–134. Churchill Livingstone, London.

Bedford, R.F. & Wollman, H. (1973) Complications of percutaneous radial artery cannulation: an objective prospective study in man. *Anesthesiology* **38**, 228–236.

Buchbinder, N. & Ganz, W. (1976) Hemodynamic monitoring: invasive techniques. *Anesthesiology* **45**, 146–155.

Calvin, J.E., Driedger, A.A. & Sibbald, W.J. (1981) Does the pulmonary capillary wedge pressure predict left ventricular preload in critically ill patients? *Critical Care Medicine* **9**, 437–443.

Clements, F.M. & de Bruijn, N.P. (1987) Review article. Perioperative evaluation of regional wall motion by transesophageal two — dimensional echocardiography. *Anesthesia and Analgesia* **66**, 249–261.

Davis, F.M. & Stewart, J.M. (1980) Radial artery cannulation: a prospective study in patients undergoing cardiothoracic surgery. *British Journal of Anaesthesia* **52**, 41–47.

Gardner, R.M. & Hollingsworth, K.W. (1986) Optimizing the electrocardiogram and pressure monitoring. *Critical Care Medicine* **14**, 651–658.

Giles, R.W., Berger, J.H., Barash, P., Tarabadkar, S., Marx, P.G., Hammond, G.L., Geha, A.S., Laks, H. & Zaret, B.L. (1982) Continuous monitoring of left ventricular performance with the computerised nuclear probe during laryngoscopy and intubation prior to coronary bypass surgery. *American Journal of Cardiology* **50**, 735–741.

Gillies, I.D.S., Morgan, M., Sykes, M.K., Brown, A.E. & Jones, N.O. (1979) The nature and incidence of complications of peripheral arterial puncture. *Anaesthesia* **34**, 506–509.

Griffin, R.M. & Kaplan, J.A. (1987) Myocardial ischaemia during non-cardiac surgery. A comparison of different lead systems using computerised ST segment analysis. *Anaesthesia* **42**, 115–159.

Gurman, G.M. & Kriemerman, S. (1985) Cannulation of big arteries in critically ill patients. *Critical Care Medicine* **13**, 217–220.

Hansen, P.M., Viquerat, C.E., Matthay, M.A., Wiener-Kronish, J.P., DeMarco, T., Bahtia, S., Marks, J.D., Botvihik, E.M. & Chatterjee, K. (1986) Poor correlation between pulmonary arterial wedge pressure and left ventricular end-diastolic volume after coronary bypass graft surgery. *Anesthesiology* **64**, 764–770.

Hines, R. & Barash, P.G. (1986) Intraoperative right ventricular dysfunction detected with a right ventricular ejection fraction catheter. *Journal of Clinical Monitoring* **2**, 206–208.

Kaplan, J.A. & Wells, P.M. (1981) Early diagnosis of myocardial ischemia using the pulmonary arterial catheter. *Anesthesia & Analgesia* **60**, 789–793.

Kay, M., Afshari, M., Barash, P., Weber, W., Iskandrian, A., Bemis, C., Hakki, A.H. & Mundth, E.D. (1983) Measurement of ejection fraction by thermal dilution techniques. *Journal of Surgical Research* **34**, 337–346.

Kaul, S., Hopkins, J.M., Shah, P.M. (1984) Assessment of right ventricular function using two-dimensional echocardiography. *American Heart Journal* **107**, 526–531.

Kazmers, A., Cerqueira, M.D. & Zierlev, R.E. (1988) The role of preoperative radionuclide left ventricular ejection fraction for risk assessment in carotid surgery. *Archives of Surgery* **123**, 416–419.

Lamantia, K.P., Hines, R. & Barash, P.G. (1989) Monitoring the cardiovascular system: current status and future directions. In Foëx P. (ed) *Ballière's clinical anaesthesiology*, vol. **3.1**, Anaesthesia for the compromised heart, pp. 103–129. Baillière Tindall, London.

Lappas, D., Lell, W.A., Gabel, J.C., Civetta, J.M. & Lowenstein, E. (1973) Indirect measurement of left-atrial pressure in surgical patients — pulmonary-capillary wedge and pulmonary-artery diastolic compared with left-atrial pressure. *Anesthesiology* **38**, 394–397.

Martyn, J.A.J., Snider, M.T., Farrago, L.F. & Burke, J.F. (1981) Thermodilution right ventricular volume: a novel and better predictor of volume replacement in acute thermal injury. *Journal of Trauma* **21**, 619–626.

Morris, A.H., Chapman, R.H. & Gardner, R.M. (1985) Frequency of wedge pressure errors in the ICU. *Critical Care Medicine* **13**, 705–708.

Nadeau, S. & Noble, W.H. (1986) Misinterpretation of pressure measurements from the pulmonary artery catheter. *Canadian Anaesthetist's Society Journal* **33**, 352–63.

Norfleet, E.A. & Watson, C.B. (1985) Continuous mixed venous oxygen saturation measurement: a significant advance in hemodynamic monitoring? *Journal of Clinical Monitoring* **1**, 245–258.

O'Quin, R. & Marini, J.J. (1983) Pulmonary artery occlusion pressure: clinical physiology, measurement and interpretation. *American Review of Respiratory Disease* **128**, 319–326.

Poole-Wilson, P.A. (1978) Clinical physiology. Interpretation of haemodynamic measurements. *British Journal of Hospital Medicine* **20**, 371–382.

Robin, E.D. (1985) The cult of the Swan–Ganz catheter — overuse and abuse of pulmonary flow catheters. *Annals of Internal Medicine* **103**, 445–449.

Rosen, M., Latto, I.P., Ng, W.S. (1981) *Handbook of percutaneous central venous catheterization.* WB Saunders & Co., London.

Schweiss, J.F. (1987) Mixed venous hemoglobin saturation: theory and application. *International Anesthesiology Clinics* **25**, 113–136.

Seward, J.B., Khandheria, B.K., Oh, J.K., Abel, M.D., Hughes, R.J., Edwards, W.D., Nicholas, B.A., Freeman, W.K. & Tajik, A.J. (1988) Transesophageal echocardiography: technique, anatomic correlations, implementation and clinical applications. *Mayo Clinic Proceedings* **63**, 649–680.

Sise, M.J., Hollingsworth, P., Brimm, J.E., Peters, R.M., Virgilio, R.W. & Shackford, S.R. (1981) Complications of the flow-directed pulmonary artery catheter: a prospective analysis in 219 patients. *Critical Care Medicine* **9**, 315–318.

Smith, J.S., Cahalan, M.K., Benefiel, D.J., Byrd, B.F., Lurz, F.W., Shapiro, W.A., Roizen, M.F., Bouchard, A., & Schiller, N.B. (1985) Intraoperative detection of myocardial ischaemia in high-risk patients: electrocardiography versus two-dimensional echocardiography. *Circulation* **72**, 1015–1021.

Spoerel, W.E., Deimling, P. & Aitken, R. (1975) Direct arterial pressure monitoring from the dorsalis pedis artery. *Canadian Anaesthetists' Society Journal* **22**, 91–99.

Tuman, K.J., McCarthy, R.J., Spiess, B.D., DaValle, M., Hompland, S.J., Dabir, R., & Ivankovich, A.D. (1989) Effect of pulmonary artery catheterization on outcome in patients undergoing coronary artery surgery. *Anesthesiology* **70**, 199–206.

Vincent, J.-L., Thirion, M., Brimioulle, S., Lejeune, P. & Kahn, R.J. (1986) Thermodilution measurement of right ventricular ejection fraction with a modified pulmonary artery catheter. *Intensive Care Medicine* **12**, 33–38.

Weintraub, A.C. & Barash, P.G. (1987) A pulmonary artery catheter is indicated in all patients for coronary artery surgery. *Journal of Cardiothoracic Anesthesia* **1**, 358–361.

Youngberg, J.A. & Miller, E.D. (1976) Evaluation of percutaneous cannulations of the dorsalis pedis artery. *Anesthesiology* **44**, 80–83.

24: Monitoring the Nervous System

As general anaesthetics produce their principal effects through the central nervous system (CNS), it would be surprising if monitoring its function were not of prime interest. In practice, however, fairly crude and indirect indices have been utilized and indeed found satisfactory for most clinical purposes. The responses to verbal or painful stimuli have been used to assess the presence or absence of consciousness; the muscular response to a painful stimulus, and the presence or absence of autonomic responses such as sweating, tachycardia and pupil size as a guide to the depth of anaesthesia. Guedel (1937) classified such indicators into stages and planes of anaesthesia, which were reasonably coherent as long as single inhalational agents were used.

With the evolution of modern techniques of anaesthesia involving the administration of muscle relaxants and intravenous analgesics, the need for better indicators of CNS function has gradually become apparent. Anaesthetists have become concerned to be sure that, as well as being paralysed and immobile, the patient is unconscious, but at the same time not excessively anaesthetized for the surgical procedure. Thus, better quantification of the depth of anaesthesia and reliable warning signs of impending consciousness have been sought by research workers.

Apart from this general interest, there has developed a need to assess brain function during neurovascular surgery and other situations in which brain perfusion may be compromised, e.g. during profound hypotension and during cardiopulmonary bypass. Finally, monitoring has proved to be of value in the intensive management of brain trauma and some kinds of therapy such as barbiturate brain protection. For these purposes, various indicators have been investigated. Most have been derived from the electroencephalogram (EEG), but also under study and development for clinical purposes are evoked potentials (EPs) and lower oesophageal contraction (LOC), both of which are thought to indicate levels of central nervous system activity as well as a more quantitative approach to signs of autonomic activity.

Depth of anaesthesia

CLINICAL SCORING

This is based on a signal summation approach for use in paralysed, ventilated patients and was described by Evans *et al.* (1983). Four indices of autonomic over-activity were selected for integration: systolic blood pressure (P), heart rate (R), sweating (S), and tear formation (T), and scores for each of these are added to give the PRST score. The weightings are described in Table 24.1 and lead to a range of scores from 0 to 8. This score has been used to trigger the administration of bolus doses of an agent when a particular score is exceeded, or can be used to control the rate of a suitable continuous infusion. The weakness of relying on the PRST score lies in the many drugs which may be given concomitantly and the diseases which may also co-exist. Amongst the former, anticholinergics, antihypertensives, adrenergic blockers and agonists, psycho-active drugs, some analgesics and ophthalmic drugs come to mind. Amongst the latter, some kinds of heart disease, diabetic neuropathy, eye disease and endocrine diseases may affect the responses. Such a score, therefore, requires intelligent interpretation and its principal use may be to supplement conventional manual records.

Table 23.1. The PRST score

Index	Condition	Score
Systolic pressure (mmHg)	<control + 15	0
	<control + 30	1
	>control + 30	2
Heart rate	<control + 15	0
	<control + 30	1
	>control + 30	2
Sweating	nil	0
	skin moist to touch	1
	visible beads of sweat	2
Tears	no excess of tears in open eye	0
	excess of tears in open eye	1
	tear overflow from closed eye	2

The electroencephalogram (EEG)

The most easily accessible non-invasive sign of brain activity is the EEG. This is the summated effect, recorded from the scalp, of post-synaptic action potentials in nearby underlying neurones. These potentials bear a general relationship to the level of cerebral blood flow and to oxygen consumption. They are small voltages, of the order of $10-100\,\mu V$, and so require high amplification. However, the signal is complex and non-specific, and by long tradition, certain characteristics of the amplifying system have become accepted. These were originally developed to aid the visual differentiation of awake, sleeping and comatose patterns, and the diagnosis of abnormal electrical activity. This led to certain frequency bands being characterized: α activity is in the range 8–13 Hz, β is activity above 13 Hz, θ is 4–7 Hz and δ is below 4 Hz. In the resting awake state, the predominant frequency is around 10 Hz, and alpha components are blocked by eye opening.

The EEG undergoes characteristic changes with various drugs. For example, barbiturates initially increase fast activity but bigger doses produce slow activity. As coma deepens periods of high voltage, low frequency activity alternate with electrical silence (burst suppression), and eventually there is loss of all electrical activity (see Fig. 24.1). Inhalation agents also produce sequential changes which are broadly similar, although each agent has certain unique features.

Unfortunately, identifying and recording these in a meaningful way during anaesthesia is impracticable. Large quantities of paper containing many traces need to be scanned to pick out relevant features and little progress in the use of the EEG for monitoring was achieved until data compression techniques were applied. These inevitably lose some potential information, but in practice also cut out great masses of irrelevant information, allowing the user to concentrate on a few relevant features. Several clinical instruments have been introduced including the cerebral function monitor (CFM), the cerebral function analysing monitor (CFAM) and the activity of brain monitor (ABM—Datex Ltd). In addition there is interest in other derivatives of the EEG such as the median frequency and the spectral edge frequency. The latter is displayed in some clinical instruments. A fuller account of the techniques used to generate these special displays is given on p. 164 *et seq.* In this chapter their value in monitoring is considered.

Recording techniques

The most difficult part of any EEG monitoring technique is the recording of the potentials. Scalp electrodes with low contact impedance ($<5000\,\Omega$)

Althesin : induction

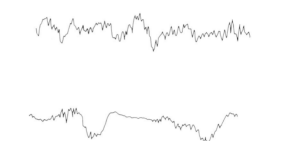

[50 μV

1 s

Fig. 24.1. Changes in the EEG with depth of anaesthesia. Note transition from fast to slower waves during induction, with a mixture of slow and fast waves during moderate anaesthesia and burst suppression during deep anaesthesia.

Moderate

Deep

are essential and are usually chlorided silver discs fixed to the scalp with collodion. Good technique is especially important when using data compression monitoring systems that do not allow visualization of the raw EEG, for in this situation artefacts may not be recognized.

The cerebral function analysing monitor (CFAM)

This is a development of the cerebral function monitor, which was one of the first instruments to

present EEG data in the form of a simple display (p. 64). The EEG is recorded from three, or preferably four, electrodes using bilateral centro-parietal placements (positions C3-P3 and C4-P4 in the 10:20 system — See Fig. 24.2). These positions avoid the frontal and temporal regions where there is more likelihood of picking up slow waves due to eye movement or fast components from scalp or facial musculature.

The display is divided into two sections. The upper trace is similar to that utilized in the CFM.

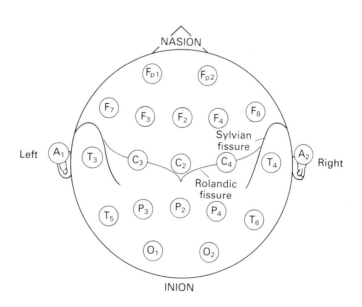

Fig. 24.2. EEG electrode positions used in the 10–20 system.

The signal is first filtered to exclude frequencies outside the 2–15 Hz range, thus eliminating low frequency artefacts due to sweating and high frequency artefacts due to radio-frequency or mains interference. It is then subjected to logarithmic amplitude compression and envelope detection so that the resulting trace shows the mean amplitude and variation in amplitude (10th to 90th centile values) on the y-axis and time on the x-axis. Maximum and minimum values outside this range are superimposed every 2 s to highlight brief peaks or periods of burst suppression. The lower section of the trace displays the percentage of activity in each of the conventional frequency bands, and periods of suppression and very low frequency (<1 Hz) are also shown (Fig. 24.3). The electrode contact resistance is displayed continuously and the presence of scalp muscle potentials or other artefacts is also detected and displayed.

It has been claimed that the CFAM is a comprehensive monitoring system which allows visual and quantitative definition of depth of anaesthesia, controlled sedation and coma, and that it can give warning of imminent arousal. It can also be used to monitor the increased cerebral activity of status epilepticus and the effectiveness of anti-convulsant activity.

The CFAM trace bears a fairly consistent relationship with blood levels or doses of intravenous agents, whether given by boluses or infusions. Onset of anaesthesia is accompanied by a sharp rise in the amplitude signal and this is then followed by a steady decline. As the concentration of drug rises, there is a progressive shift of the power spectrum towards the lower frequencies. At even greater concentrations, burst suppression is associated with a widening of the amplitude trace and the appearance of very low frequency activity. The CFAM is also claimed to be able to detect inadequate anaesthesia in response to a stimulus and impending awakening, both situations being associated with a rise in the power spectrum trace.

The principal disadvantage of the CFAM is that it is only a general indicator of metabolic activity and this may be depressed by a variety of causes including brain oedema, resulting from hypoxia, or trauma, hypotension or metabolic encephalopathies, any of which may be being treated by barbiturate-induced metabolic cerebral depression. It can clearly indicate a deep level of anaesthesia if other causes of depression can be excluded and likewise that too light a level is present. Apart from this, the machine can only indicate that something has changed or that something is not normal, but

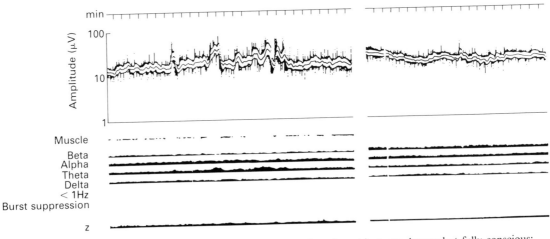

Fig. 24.3. Two CFAM traces. The one on the left was obtained when the subject was drowsy but fully conscious: the one on the right was taken during light enflurane anaesthesia. This trace shows loss of scalp muscle action potentials and less variability in amplitude and per cent frequency content. (z is the electrode impedance.) (From Prior, 1987.)

Fig. 24.4. ABM tracing obtained during arthroscopy performed under continuous propofol infusion anaesthesia, following an induction bolus dose of 2 mg·kg^{-1} and supplemented by boluses of alfentanil. From top to bottom: (a) administration of propofol and alfentanil; (b) systolic and diastolic blood pressures (lines) and heart rate (dots); (c) spontaneous EMG; (d) EEG: above zero line — zero crossing frequency; under zero line — mean integrated voltage; (e) inspired and expired P_{CO_2} (mmHg). The frontalis EMG trace increases in amplitude after painful stimuli and decreases again after the administration of the analgesic. It also increases after the infusion is stopped and consciousness is regained. (From Herregods & Rolly, 1987.)

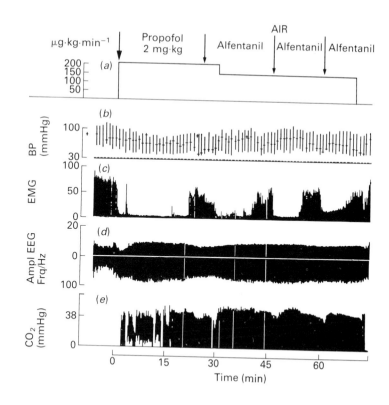

not which of several possible causes is responsible. Its principal usage is in the detection of the onset of brain ischaemia during operations which affect cerebral blood supply and during cardiopulmonary perfusion.

The brain activity monitor (ABM)

This instrument analyses the potentials obtained from three electrodes placed on the mid-forehead and behind each ear. The signal is subjected to high pass filtering (70–300 Hz) to obtain the frontalis muscle electromyogram (EMG), whilst low pass filtering (1.5–25 Hz) is used to produce the EEG signal (Fig. 24.4). The number of times the EEG signal crosses the baseline is then analysed to give the zero crossing frequency. Utilizing the same signal, negative voltages are rectified to make all the voltages positive and the area under the curve is integrated. This gives the mean integrated voltage (i.e. the mean amplitude of the EEG signal) which is expressed on a non-linear scale as a

voltage between 0 and 50 μV. The device also measures end-tidal carbon dioxide, blood pressure and pulse rate, and the neuromuscular response to train-of-four (TOF) stimulation (see below). The principal value of the device has been in the detection and display of frontalis muscle activity. The EEG related displays have not been found very useful.

The Surface EMG trace. Surface electromyography can be obtained from any group of muscles. However, the frontalis muscle has come to be regarded as of special relevance. This is because the muscle not only has voluntary innervation but also has autonomic (involuntary) innervation, each nerve supply travelling by separate neural pathways. It thus provides a simple non-invasive indicator of autonomic activity. There does not seem to be any point in trying to distinguish between 'spontaneous' and 'evoked' surface EMGs in this situation because 'spontaneous' may indicate only that the nature of the evoking stimulus is internal and has not been correctly detected, since the frontalis EMG has been found to be affected by levels of vigilance, altered emotional state, noise, and cerebral ischaemia. In the unconscious patient, of course, volitional activity is absent. The EMG scale on the ABM is also expressed in arbitrary units of 0–100 and corresponds to a non-linear scale of 0–15 μV. The frontalis muscle, like any other, can be influenced by neuromuscular drugs, but is relatively less sensitive than the hypothenar muscles. Thus the activity can still be interpreted, with some caution, even in the presence of muscle relaxants. However, the simultaneous display of the TOF responses of the hypothenar muscles is advisable.

The mean amplitude of the frontalis EMG decreases during physiological sleep to about one-third of its awake value and falls further to about 10–15% of the awake value under anaesthesia. Surgical stimuli in the absence of adequate anaesthesia are associated with a sharp increase in activity (see Fig. 24.4). Responses can also be observed to loud noises, even in adequately anaesthetized patients. Rapid rises to almost near normal levels occur as patients regain consciousness and precede the onset of awareness by a short interval.

Interpreting the ABM. Having further dimensions of monitoring obviously enhances the ability to interpret the derived EEG parameters. The TOF from the hypothenar muscles indicates whether or not the frontalis muscle EMG activity is likely to have been suppressed by muscle relaxants: the frontalis trace helps to differentiate between mean power values which are compatible with impending awareness or with adequate but light anaesthesia. As with the CFAM, however, some skill in interpretation is needed, based on experience. There are no characteristic values which can be utilized as alarms.

Power spectrum displays

The changes in the EEG which such machines try to encapsulate can be visualized more comprehensively by expressing the EEG power at each frequency as a percentage of the total EEG power, and expressing the result as a percent power–frequency spectrum (Rampil, 1987). Many such spectra, each representing EEG activity over some short epoch (usually 5–10 s), can be displayed as a single plot by writing out successive horizontal traces with upward and outward displacement. By blanking out overlapping traces, a three-dimensional effect can be produced which looks like a range of hills and mountains in a landscape (see Figs 24.5 & 5.6.). A number of instruments are now commercially available. Such a trace will display the changes that occur as the patient progresses from awake to natural sleep, to anaesthesia, and back to recovery of consciousness. Broadly speaking, spectral displays merely demon-

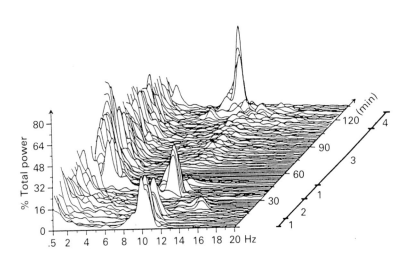

Fig. 24.5. EEG power spectrum during clinical anaesthesia with enflurane in 60% N_2O and O_2. Natural sleep and anaesthesia show similar power spectra. (1) awake; (2) asleep; (3) anaesthetized; (4) return to consciousness. (From Stoeckel & Schwilden, 1987.)

strate the same phenomenon of a shift of power to low frequencies with increasing depth of anaesthesia. However, the additional information they contain makes it more likely that, for example, ischaemic changes can be detected during carotid endarterectomy, than can be detected by the CFM (Rampil *et al.* 1983).

Median EEG frequency. The consistent tendency for the power spectrum to shift towards lower frequencies with deepening anaesthesia has fed the hope that one or more numerical indices might be derived from the EEG which would relate to the 'depth' of anaesthesia. Such an idea is obviously problematic with such a complex waveform, since different frequency distributions, having quite different clinical implications, may have the same mean frequency.

Fast Fourier analysis of the raw EEG signal can be followed by partitioning the total amount of electrical power to each of the commonly defined frequency bands, and thus the power spectrum can be transformed into a set of numbers corresponding to the four conventional frequency bands (β, α, θ, δ). However, one has to remember that these conventional bands may not necessarily represent a natural decomposition of the frequency spectrum for the purpose of assessing anaesthetic effects, since they were originally derived as useful descriptors for analysing the EEG of the resting awake subject. Because the partitioning into different frequencies changes with anaesthesia, the selection of any one frequency band for monitoring would be likely to be quite inappropriate.

Thus, any suitable quantification of the EEG power spectrum must be independent of frequency and in a multi-modal distribution such as the EEG, the median of the distribution (the 50% quantile) is the most insensitive with respect to outliers and represents the best single measure of central tendency (Fig. 24.6).

Clinical assessments of the depth of anaesthesia derived from the normal EEG have shown excellent correlation with the median of the power spectrum of the EEG (Doenicke *et al.* 1982). Good correlation of the median frequency with the blood level of etomidate has also been demon-

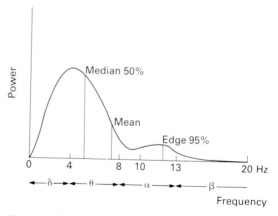

Fig. 24.6. EEG power spectrum showing three variables that have been used to describe EEG frequency shifts during anaesthesia. The four standard frequency bands are also shown (α, β, θ, δ).

strated in volunteers (Schwilden *et al.* 1985). Other agents, such as methohexitone (Schwilden *et al.* 1987), ketamine (Schüttler *et al.* 1987), propofol (Schüttler *et al.* 1985) and thiopentone (Hudson *et al.* 1983), have also been studied and the median frequency has shown a progressive fall with rising drug concentrations to levels where burst suppression appeared on the EEG.

Unfortunately, the correlation between median frequency and the conventional signs of depth of anaesthesia is not consistent even within a single subject. Characteristically, any particular clinical sign is associated with a higher median frequency during emergence from anaesthesia than during induction. Fortunately, these differences are not great. Induction of sleep occurs at a median frequency of approximately 5 Hz and responsiveness is regained at about the same level. Median values above 5–6 Hz are likely to be associated with awareness. Burst suppression (i.e. deep anaesthesia) is associated with a median frequency in the range of about 1.6–2 Hz. Loss and recovery of the eyelash reflex and other clinical signs are associated with intermediate values. Table 24.2 shows some typical values from Stoeckel and Schwilden (1987).

Spectral edge frequency. This is the frequency below which 95% of the power in the processed

Table 24.2. Relationship between clinical signs and median EEG frequency in six volunteers during infusions of etomidate which produced three different blood concentrations.*

	Increasing concentration		Decreasing concentration	
signs	median (SD) (Hz)		median (SD) (Hz)	signs
Baseline (awake)	9.5 (0.4)		6.6 (0.6)	Full orientation
Falling asleep	4.8 (0.8)		4.7 (0.7)	Responsive
Corneal reflex	2.0 (0.4)		2.0 (0.3)	Corneal reflex
Burst suppression	1.6 (0.3)		1.8 (0.3)	Burst suppression

* Data from Stoeckel and Schwilden (1987).

EEG lies (Fig. 24.6). Its value is about 25 Hz in the awake state, and progressively falls with increasing concentrations of anaesthetics. However, the correlation between the blood level of drugs and spectral edge frequency is not as good as with the median EEG frequency (Arden *et al.* 1986). The changes are more marked and clinically useful when the adequacy of the blood supply to the brain

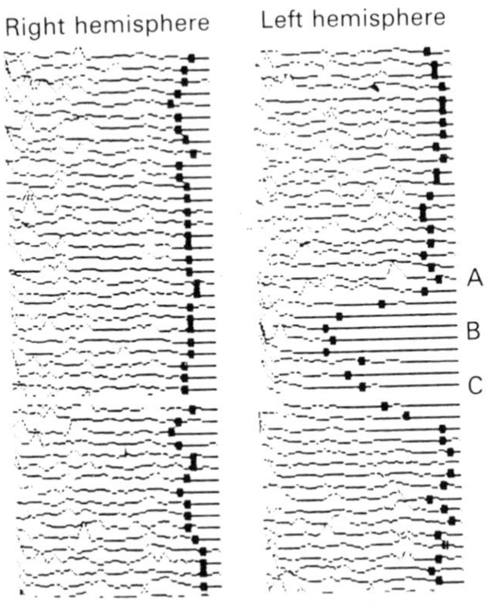

Fig. 24.7. Compressed spectral arrays from both cerebral hemispheres, with the spectral edge frequency. At (A), a shunt in the left carotid artery was removed after endarterectomy had been completed but while the common carotid artery was still clamped. At (B), the external carotid artery clamp was removed, with little improvement. At (C), the reconstructed internal carotid artery was unclamped, leading to rapid return of the spectral edge frequency to its previous value. (From Hug, 1986.)

is being assessed. Figure 24.7 shows such a tracing associated with carotid endarterectomy.

Evoked responses (evoked potentials–EPs)

These are electrical responses in the nervous system which are linked in time with a stimulus. For example, a cortical evoked potential is an EEG manifestation of the response of the cortex of the brain to some external stimulus. A visually evoked potential (VEP) may actually be large enough to be seen as a wave in the EEG if it is measured directly over the visual cortex in the occipital region. However, evoked potentials produced from discrete stimuli are usually very much smaller than the 'noise' of the spontaneous EEG and to identify such an evoked potential, averaging is necessary. After a brief stimulus, a short epoch (<100 ms) of EEG signal is stored in an electronic memory. This process is repeated many times, with each successive record being superimposed upon the preceding ones. The evoked potential always comes at the same time after the stimulus and is thus recorded in the same part of the memory. These potentials are therefore summated, whereas all the random activity which is unrelated to the stimulus is averaged, and approaches zero. The number of responses which have to be averaged depends on the strength of the signal and varies from several hundred for early cortical waves to several thousand for brain stem responses (p. 46).

Evoked potentials can be induced by visual, somatosensory or auditory stimuli. Somatosensory EPs can also be recorded from the brain stem or from a peripheral nerve. The potentials induced are usually complex waves whose configuration is much affected by electrode position.

Somatosensory brain stem evoked potentials have been used to check for potential cord damage during operations such as insertion of Harrington rods (Bradshaw *et al.* 1984). The more general interest of EPs to an anaesthetist lies in the fact that either the latency or the amplitude of the waves show characteristic changes related to drug effects. In general, volatile agents produce increases in the latency of brain-stem waves and changes in both the latency and the amplitude of cortical waves. For recent reviews see Jones (1987), Thornton and Newton (1989), and Sebel (1989).

Of the various sensory modalities which have been explored, auditory evoked responses seem to be the most promising in that they are not only related to drug dosage but also to the degree of surgical stimulus (Fig. 24.8). Up till now, no instru-

ment based on this technology has been marketed for routine monitoring, although instruments are available for research purposes. They are sometimes referred to as CATs, an acronym for computer of average transients. The progressive changes with deepening anaesthesia are seen in the medium latency waves (Fig. 24.9). There is a progressive reduction in the amplitude of the first positive wave (Pa) and the first negative wave (Nb), and an increasing latency of the peaks of both waves. Thornton *et al.* (1983) noted that loss of consciousness in volunteers seemed to be associated with a change from a three-wave to a two-wave pattern in the middle latency waves, and that the best correlate of this change was the latency of the peak of the Pa wave. When this exceeded 42 ms the volunteer did not respond to requests to squeeze the experimenter's hand. This is the nearest that anyone has yet come to developing a

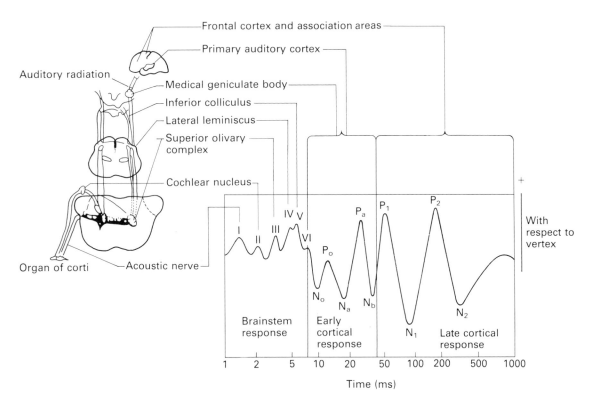

Fig. 24.8. The pathway of the evoked auditory response from the cochlea to the cortex with the recorded response. (From Thornton & Newton, 1989.)

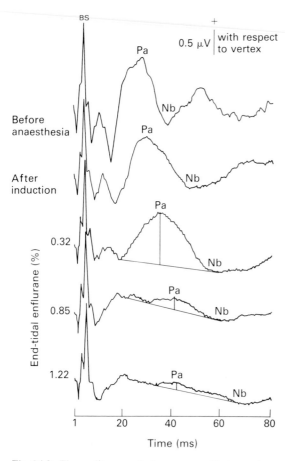

Fig. 24.9. The auditory evoked response with increasing end-tidal concentrations of enflurane. The compressed brain-stem response (BS) remains unchanged whilst the latencies of the early cortical responses (Pa & Nb) increase and the amplitudes decrease with increasing enflurane concentrations. (After Thornton *et al.*, 1983.)

'number' which can be interpreted as indicating lack of awareness in any particular individual.

Lower oesophageal contractility

The oesophagus demonstrates three kinds of muscular activity. Primary peristalsis is initiated in the striated muscle of the upper oesophagus and produces the propulsive activity of swallowing. Secondary peristaltic activity arises spontaneously and is probably triggered to remove food particles. Tertiary activity is non-propulsive. This tertiary

activity appears to be under the control of an oesophageal motility centre facilitated from higher centres and can be provoked in the conscious individual by emotion and stress.

Under anaesthesia, voluntary activity is suppressed. In the relaxed ventilated patient, respiratory pressure waves and cardiac impulses can be identified as artefacts in oesophageal pressure traces. Superimposed on this external activity are the spontaneous tertiary contractions within the lower oesophagus itself. It has been observed that the frequency with which spontaneous lower oesophageal contractions (SLOCs) occur is related to depth of anaesthesia, whether produced by inhalational agents or intravenous agents. There is a tendency for them to occur with greater frequency as patients approach consciousness, and to diminish in frequency and eventually disappear altogether as anaesthesia deepens.

If a balloon is placed in the oesophagus and suddenly inflated, a secondary contraction is induced and can be detected lower down the oesophagus by a second balloon (Fig. 24.10). This phenomenon is also progressively depressed by increasing the depth of anaesthesia but, in contrast to spontaneous contractions, it is the amplitude of the provoked response which is related to the degree of anaesthesia. It seems likely that there is a common co-ordinating centre in the brain-stem for both responses.

Both spontaneous contractions (SLOCs) and provoked contractions (PLOCs) can be used as a guide to the depth of anaesthesia and have been employed in a closed feedback mechanism for controlling the depth of anaesthesia (Evans *et al.* 1983). They have also been evaluated as a test for the onset of awareness. Whilst there is certainly a good correlation between anaesthetic depth and the frequency of SLOCs and the amplitude of PLOCs, neither are reliable for detecting awareness. In some individuals, oesophageal activity is atypical. On rare occasions, the direction of change has been in the reverse direction. There is certainly no numeric or absolute value of either SLOCs or PLOCs which can be correlated with normal indicators of consciousness (Isaac & Rosen, 1988).

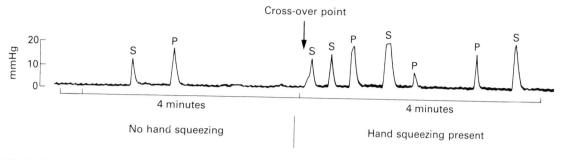

Fig. 24.10. Spontaneous (S) and provoked (P) contractions in the lower oesophagus. The arrow marks the point at which the subject stopped responding to verbal instructions. (Read from right to left.)

It has been claimed that spontaneous activity is lost whilst provoked contractions are still elicited in head injury patients who are subsequently diagnosed as clinically brain dead (Sinclair & Suter 1987), although Aitkenhead and Thomas (1987) claimed that spontaneous contractions were still observed in some clinically brain dead patients. This observation throws doubt on the absolute adequacy of the current criteria for diagnosing brain stem death, although perhaps not for predicting that there is no hope of recovery.

Measurement of neuromuscular function

Neuromuscular blockade has become a cornerstone of modern anaesthetic practice and blocking drugs have been used successfully by countless anaesthetists without regular monitoring of their action for many years. However, a new generation of drugs has been introduced with not only a shorter duration of action, but a greater rate of recovery once recovery begins. This means that there are now more opportunities for the clinician to make errors of judgement and a greater need for monitoring the action of these drugs more closely.

Both the extent and nature of neuromuscular blockade can be assessed by stimulating a motor nerve and observing the response of one or more of the affected muscles. Although, it is the muscles of respiration and the abdominal wall which require relaxation, it has become conventional to stimulate the ulnar nerve at the wrist, and then measure the response of either *adductor pollicis* or the combined hypothenar muscles. There are several methods of

assessment, which include measurement of responses to single stimuli, trains of stimuli and tetanic bursts.

NERVE STIMULATION

An essential pre-requisite for accurate assessment of neuromuscular function is that the nerve concerned must be stimulated in a standard manner. An ideal nerve stimulator would have the following characteristics:

1 The stimulator should be battery powered and entirely insulated from all earthed objects. This ensures that the contact electrodes cannot present a hazard, either through electrocution or radio-frequency burns from surgical diathermy. If battery operation is not feasible, the output circuits must be isolated from all grounded parts within the instrument (see Chapter 11).

2 Since the neural response is a direct function of current *density*, it is the delivered current that matters, not the voltage. Therefore, it is essential that the stimulator can deliver a pulse which is more powerful than that required to produce a maximal response.

3 For a given output setting the stimulator must always produce the same current density in the nerve. If this were not the case, changes in skin impedance would cause variation in current output and changes in muscular response. Therefore, the stimulator must deliver pulses of *constant current* at any given output setting.

4 So as to ensure a standardized pattern of stimulation, the output waveform should maintain a rectangular form, regardless of load impedance.

5 It should be possible to deliver pulses as single events, at a regular rate (1 Hz) or in train of four (TOF) pulses, delivered at 2 Hz with 10 s pauses between trains. The latter arrangement has been found to be particularly useful, since the fade observed with successive pulses has been found to correlate well with the degree of block. This means that the 'pre-relaxation' control measurements are less important or may be dispensed with altogether.

6 Pulse width is also important. Very short pulses may require very high currents to achieve maximal responses, while excessively long pulses may cause repetitive neuronal firing and misleadingly large compound responses. The optimal pulse length is approximately 200 μs.

7 It is also important that the stimulator can deliver tetanic bursts; usually 50 Hz for 5 s.

These requirements are of practical importance, since not all the currently available devices can meet them, and therefore cannot be expected to produce reliable results (Mylrea *et al.* 1984).

STIMULATING NEEDLE ELECTRODES

It might be expected that needle electrodes which place the stimulating current very close to the nerve would be desirable, but in fact there are several disadvantages:

1 The electrode may be placed *through* rather than alongside the nerve, and either direct trauma or the high current density may damage the nerve.

2 Needle electrodes have been implicated in causing burns in association with surgical diathermy (Finlay *et al.* 1974; Lippmann & Fields, 1974) in instruments that did not meet all the criteria recommended above.

3 Because of unnecessarily high current density, needle electrodes may cause more discomfort to a volunteer or patient than surface electrodes.

Surface stimulating electrodes

Conventionally, two surface electrodes are placed immediately over the ulnar nerve immediately proximal to the wrist joint. It is important to realize that the motor supply to the muscles of the hand is supplied almost entirely by the deep terminal branch, which leaves the nerve distal to the pisiform. (Palmaris brevis is sometimes supplied by the palmar cutaneous branch, which leaves the nerve at mid-forearm level.) If, therefore, the electrodes are placed over the ulnar nerve at the wrist the motor branches to flexor carpi ulnaris and flexor digitorum profundus, together with many of the sensory branches can be avoided. It is, of course, difficult to avoid stimulation of the dorsal branch, which leaves the nerve only 5 cm proximal to the wrist joint. It is important that reversible Ag:AgCl electrodes are used and many disposable electrocardiograph (ECG) electrodes are suitable. The best stimulating arrangement is provided by a pair of electrodes mounted on a single 'patch'; this allows both electrodes to be placed as distal as possible.

Under anaesthesia, the wrist is rarely as accessible as the face, and for clinical monitoring without quantitation many anaesthetists utilize a facial response, placing the two stimulating electrodes over the ramus of the mandible and the temporomandibular joint and observing the movement of the corner of the mouth.

Establishing control conditions

Ideally, the electrodes are positioned and the stimulator connected before the induction of anaesthesia. It is not generally possible to establish 'control' responses at this stage, because the stimuli cause discomfort to many patients. These control responses are best elicited immediately following induction but prior to the administration of a muscle relaxant. The stimulator is set to deliver pulses at 1 Hz and the output intensity increased gradually until a maximal response is observed. Then a further increase is applied to ensure that the stimulus is supramaximal. This is essential, since sub-maximal stimuli will leave some motor units unaffected. Since very small changes (such as in electrode impedance and geometry) will alter the current field in individual neurones, the number of neurones carrying action potentials will also vary.

This variation makes accurate assessment of neuro-muscular transmission impossible.

Finally, a series of 'control' stimuli are applied in the same manner as those to be used during anaesthesia. During the monitoring period it is essential that conditions remain as constant as possible. Thus the patient should, where possible, be in the operating position with the monitored arm in the position in which it is to remain. It should be wrapped in 'Gamgee' or similar insulating material so that the muscles are not affected by changing skin temperature.

Measurement of muscle response

The muscular response to nerve stimulation can be assessed by a variety of means. The simplest method is that most frequently used by clinical anaesthetists while monitoring uncomplicated cases. The observer simply holds the patient's thumb and assesses the strength of the 'twitch' response (caused largely by the contraction of adductor pollicis). When monitoring single pulses this is of limited value, since all such responses must be compared with those observed prior to the administration of the relaxant. This crude method can, however, be used fairly effectively with a TOF by counting how many responses there are. This is virtually the only means of quantitation when using facial electrodes. If there is only one twitch this almost invariably correlates with satisfactory abdominal relaxation. For deeper levels of block it may be necessary to abolish all the responses, but if a 5 s tetanic burst is given, one or more responses may be detectable for a few seconds, due to post-tetanic potentiation.

The mechanogram

The force of thumb movement can be assessed more efficiently by attaching some kind of force transducer to the thumb, and connecting this to a rapid response pen recorder. This allows quantitative comparisons to be made. Such transducers can be as simple as a handgrip fitted with a force sensitive button, to which the hand is securely

taped. The transducer measures compressive force as the thumb flexes. In more sophisticated systems the hand is taped securely to a baseplate and the adducted thumb attached to a force transducer which measures the tension produced by the isometric contraction of adductor pollicis (Fig. 24.11).

Tension transducers of this type can also be arranged to apply a degree of pre-tension (up to 300 g) before stimuli are applied. This results in more consistent muscular responses.

Although the mechanical response can be said to indicate the aspect of muscular contraction which is most physiologically significant, the accurate measurement of that response presents many practical difficulties, not least the time consuming process of hand immobilization, preloading and protection from physical interference. Furthermore, the strength of muscle contraction may be greatly affected by physical influences such as temperature.

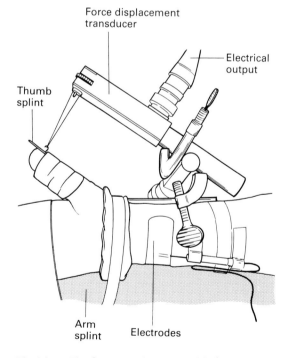

Fig. 24.11. The force transducer assembly for measuring thumb adduction in response to stimuli of the ulnar nerve.

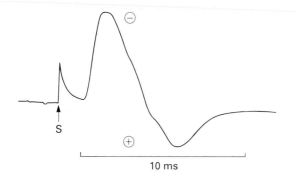

Fig. 24.12. Evoked compound action potential. S = stimulus artefact. The signal is integrated over a 10 ms period starting 3 ms after the stimulus.

The integrated electromyogam

Many of these problems may be overcome by measuring the compound action potential from the muscles concerned, and this can be achieved using simple surface electrodes. There are two favoured arrangements (Kalli, 1989). Two electrodes can be placed so as to detect the electrical activity of adductor pollicis, usually on the palmar and dorsal surfaces of the hand overlying the muscle. However, a larger and more reliable signal can be obtained by two electrodes on the hypothenar eminence. Unlike the first arrangement, this configuration detects the aggregate activity of at least two muscles, and there is no evidence that the results are in any way less significant. The detected signal is biphasic, preceded by a stimulus artefact and immediately followed, unless the muscle is paralysed, by a large movement artefact (Fig. 24.12).

Because of the very high frequency components in the signal, it is more convenient to integrate it within a brief time 'gate' (10 ms) which excludes the stimulus artefact. The output then is an indication of the total electrical activity of the muscle over a short time period (Carter *et al.* 1986).

Despite initial optimism that the technique could not only eliminate transducers, but also the need for careful immobilization of the hand, it has become clear that changes in hand position affect the electrode geometry sufficiently to alter the measured response, and it remains necessary to immobilize and insulate the monitored limb if accurate quantitative data are required.

MONITORING NEUROMUSCULAR BLOCK

While it is perfectly satisfactory to monitor the response to single twitches at, say, 10 s intervals, it is more informative to observe the effects of TOF stimuli (Ali *et al.* 1971). This is expressed as the ratio of the fourth response as a fraction of the first, the so-called T4 ratio, which is independent of control values (Fig. 24.13). This ratio is particularly useful while monitoring recovery from neuromuscular blockade. Such is the sensitivity of the T4 index that clinical recovery can usually be demonstrated when T4 is still in the range 0.6–0.8 (Ali *et al.* 1971; Ali *et al.* 1975).

As discussed earlier, the fourth response is rarely detectable at clinically satisfactory levels of blockade, so that T4 remains zero throughout, and the TOF count must then be used instead. When there is a more intense block there may be no response, in which case a 'post-tetanic count' may be useful. It may be asked why, if the single pulse block is greater than 100%, is there any need to bother to measure it? The answer is simple: we need to know not only how deep the block is, but also whether it is recovering or getting deeper. When using an

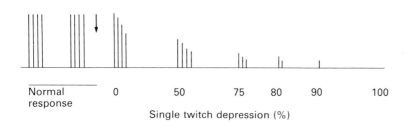

Normal
response

Single twitch depression (%)

Fig. 24.13. Pattern of train-of-four responses during onset of neuromuscular block.

automatic, EMG-based monitor, the clinician can observe (Fig. 24.14) the progress of neuromuscular block in terms of both TOF and single twitch data, the latter provided by the first response in each group.

Diagnosis of unknown neuromuscular problems

Not infrequently, a patient is suspected of having residual neuromuscular blockade when the clinician would have expected otherwise. If only non-depolarizing drugs have been used, then straightforward monitoring to recovery may be all that is required. However, if the patient has been given suxamethonium at some point, it is pertinent to consider whether the problem is due to persistent depolarization or whether the block has altered and become a phase II block. Here, it is conventional to observe the response to a tetanic burst, followed by a series of single stimuli, so that an assessment of tetanic fade and post-tetanic facilitation may be made (Ali & Savarese, 1976). In most cases, a

simple stimulator with palpated responses is adequate to establish the type of block involved.

If the T4 ratio is monitored throughout the conduct of suxamethonium blockade, the transition to phase II block is easily detected by a marked transition from well-sustained responses in phase I to steeply fading responses at the onset of phase II (Lee, 1975).

ASSESSMENT OF DIAPHRAGMATIC PARALYSIS

The responses of the adductor pollicis do not accurately reflect the degree of neuromuscular block in the principal muscle of respiration, the diaphragm. However, not only is there no motor nerve in a conveniently superficial and accessible place, but there is no easy method by which the diaphragmatic responses can be recorded. There have been several descriptions of experimental methods. Briefly, the technique depends upon a hand-held electrode being manoeuvred into the optimum position before the administration of

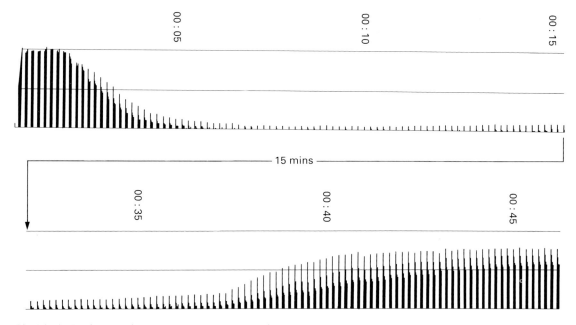

Fig. 24.14. Tracing showing the onset and recovery of neuromuscular block using train-of-four (TOF) stimuli. The dark area shows the fourth response. (Reproduced by courtesy of Dr C.E. Blogg.)

muscle relaxants, and the position maintained. The diaphragmatic twitch causes pressure gradients between the middle third of the oesophagus and the stomach, which are detected by two balloon catheters connected to a differential pressure transducer.

These contractions are best recorded when the abdomen is closed, which is, unfortunately, not the period of greatest interest. Furthermore, they disturb a surgeon working in the upper abdomen. The technique is of greater interest in research applications, since it allows the effects of drugs on the hand muscles and the diaphragm to be compared directly.

It is also possible to monitor the diaphragmatic EMG using carefully placed needle electrodes (Fink, 1960). The integrated diaphragmatic EMG is a good indicator of returning respiratory activity, and may become of greater interest now that an increasing number of anaesthetists aim to maintain the arterial P_{CO_2} at a physiological level during intermittent positive pressure ventilation rather than using hyperventilation which inhibits spontaneous diaphragmatic muscle activity (Fig. 24.15).

Monitoring in neurosurgery

There are two major problems in anaesthesia for craniotomy. The first is the need to prevent any increase in intracranial pressure and the second is the maintenance of an adequate cerebral perfusion pressure.

In most patients, the presence of a raised intracranial pressure is deduced from the history (confusion, headache and vomiting), clinical examination (especially papilloedema), and other investigations designed to reveal the nature, site and size of the lesion (Teasdale *et al.* 1984). In patients with a raised intracranial pressure it is vital to maintain a constant arterial and venous pressure and a lower than normal arterial P_{CO_2} until the dura is opened. When the dura is opened the intracranial pressure approaches atmospheric and further steps may then be taken to reduce brain tension by removing fluid from the ventricular system. In patients with a vascular tumour or in those undergoing clipping of a cerebral aneurysm, induced hypotension may then be required.

Arterial pressure may be monitored intermittently non-invasively but in the majority of patients continuous direct arterial pressure monitoring is advisable since this enables the anaesthetist to detect changes in pressure immediately and so speeds up the therapeutic response. It also enables samples to be taken for blood gas analysis. The use of small transducers attached to the patient at right atrial level facilitates pressure monitoring since zero adjustments are not required if the table is raised, lowered or tilted. A continuous flushing device is highly desirable.

Central venous pressure (CVP) is measured through a line inserted from the antecubital fossa, since neck lines often intrude on the surgical field. It is useful if the tip of this line can be situated in

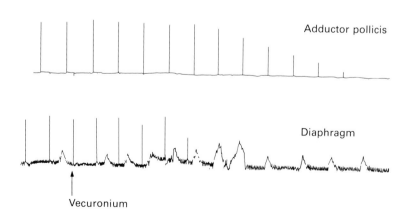

Adductor pollicis

Diaphragm

Vecuronium

Fig. 24.15. Tracings of the diaphragm integrated EMG (below) to show the development of diaphragmatic paralysis compared with the response of the adductor pollicis as measured by a force transducer. (From Chauvin *et al.* 1987.)

the right atrium since it may then be advanced into the right ventricle to aspirate air should air embolism occur. The position can be checked either by the pressure waveform and advancing the catheter into the right ventricle and then withdrawing it, or by connecting the saline-filled catheter to an EEG lead and observing the characteristic biphasic P-wave on entry into the right atrium (Michenfelder *et al.* 1969; Martin, 1970). Display of the venous pressure waveform is useful to differentiate a raised venous pressure due to air embolus from inadvertent migration of the catheter tip into the right ventricle or pulmonary artery.

The ECG should be displayed continuously since dysrhythmias may result from raised intracranial pressure or surgical retraction, in addition to the usual causes encountered during anaesthesia. A precordial or oesophageal stethoscope provides useful information on air entry and added sounds and may reveal the typical mill-wheel murmur if there is a large air embolus.

In some units anaesthesia with spontaneous ventilation is preferred for posterior fossa surgery since changes in respiratory pattern are believed to be a reliable and sensitive indication of brain stem disturbance due to surgical manipulation. These changes can be displayed by a spirometer connected to the breathing system or by a pneumotachograph. However, many anaesthetists now believe that continuous monitoring of the cardiovascular system yields as much information as respiratory monitoring and that there are major advantages in using controlled ventilation.

Another major problem in neurosurgery is the detection and prevention of air embolus. Air tends to enter through veins in the neck or skull when the patient is in the sitting position, particularly if the venous pressure is low due to preoperative dehydration. The air passes to the right atrium, ventricle and pulmonary arteries and obstructs pulmonary blood flow. This results in hypotension, dysrhythmias and a sudden reduction in end-tidal CO_2, usually with a horizontal alveolar plateau. The theoretical treatment is to place the patient in the head-down, left lateral position to try and move the air to the apex of the right ventricle so that cardiac output may be maintained while the air is

aspirated through the central venous catheter. However, this is often impossible when the surgical field is exposed.

A reduction in end-tidal CO_2 or an increase in the arterial to end-tidal CO_2 difference may result from pulmonary fat or thromboembolism but also from a reduction in pulmonary artery pressure or blood flow, due to blood loss or peripheral pooling of blood. Thus it is not diagnostic of pulmonary air embolus.

An alternative method of detection is the use of Doppler ultrasound. A transducer is fixed to the chest wall over the right atrium or right ventricle, just to the right of the sternum, between the fourth and sixth intercostal spaces. Correct positioning is checked by the intravenous injection of 0.5–1 ml of CO_2 which produces a characteristic change of sound in the headphones. The Doppler system is extremely sensitive and detects very small air bubbles. It is also affected by diathermy (Maroon & Albin, 1974).

The key to successful neurosurgical anaesthesia is careful monitoring and control of the respiratory and cardiovascular systems. It is therefore essential to monitor arterial saturation with a pulse-oximeter and ventilation with a capnograph and to ensure that there is no obstruction to expiration by displaying airway pressure.

Intracranial pressure monitoring

The indications for intracranial pressure (ICP) monitoring are not generally agreed. There are technical difficulties in making the measurement, its use is not without risk and there are no studies which demonstrate a significant increase in survival in patients in whom the technique has been used. The most common indication at the present time is for the management of head injury where the technique is used to measure not only the level of pressure but also the response to treatment. It is particularly useful if clinical signs of CNS activity are masked by the use of sedation or muscle relaxants. It may also be used to measure the changes in pressure in normal or high pressure hydrocephalus and in monitoring the performance of ventriculo-atrial shunts. It has also been

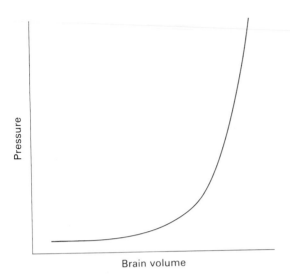

Fig. 24.16. Pressure – brain volume relationship.

suggested that monitoring may improve survival when arterial spasm gives rise to cerebral oedema after aneurysm surgery.

Since the volume of the cranium is fixed, any increase in the volume of cerebrospinal fluid, blood or brain substance must result in a decrease in volume of the other two. In the early phase of brain swelling there is a compensatory decrease in blood volume, cerebrospinal fluid volume or both, so that the increase in pressure is small. However, there is a limit to the extent of this compensation and when this is exceeded there is a much greater increase in pressure for a given increase in volume (Fig. 24.16). The increase in pressure is often accompanied by circulatory and respiratory effects. When cerebral blood flow is decreased, ischaemia may occur. This may stimulate the cardiovascular centres with the production of hypertension and bradycardia. Medullary herniation may also occur. This usually produces hypertension and bradycardia but may be accompanied by respiratory irregularities and apnoea.

The major determinant of cerebral blood flow is cerebral perfusion pressure which is the difference between mean arterial pressure and intracranial pressure. Normally, this is greater than 60 mmHg. A cerebral perfusion pressure of less than 40 mmHg is often associated with cerebral ischaemia.

METHODS

Since there may be obstruction to the flow of CSF from the brain to the spinal cord it is necessary to measure intracranial pressure rather than spinal CSF pressure. There are four methods of measurement: (i) via an intraventricular catheter, (ii) with a subarachnoid screw, (iii) with an extradural transducer, and (iv) with a catheter tip transducer.

Intraventricular catheter

This is the standard by which other methods are judged. A catheter is inserted into a lateral ventricle through a burr hole. The catheter is filled with saline and connected to a standard pressure transducer which is zeroed with reference to a fixed point on the patient's head, e.g. the external auditory meatus. Catheter-tip transducers have also been used. When the brain is swollen it is often difficult to locate the ventricle though the availability of computerized axial tomography (CAT) scans now minimizes this problem. The catheter may become obstructed by pieces of brain tissue or by pressure from the surrounding brain; infection is a major problem even when prophylactic antibiotics are used. However, the presence of the catheter facilitates therapeutic withdrawal of CSF and it is easy to recalibrate the pressure transducer. Intracranial compliance may also be measured by injecting 1 ml of saline or withdrawing 1 ml of CSF and observing the change in pressure. If compliance is normal this should produce a pressure rise of less than 2 mmHg.

Subarachnoid screw

This consists of a hollow bolt which is screwed through a burr hole made through the fronto-parietal suture line. The tip of the bolt passes through the dura and the interior is filled with saline so that there is a liquid bridge between the CSF and the pressure transducer. The latter may be fixed directly to the bolt or connected to it by a length of plastic tubing. The transducer must be zeroed with some fixed point on the head and it is important to exclude all air bubbles and to ensure

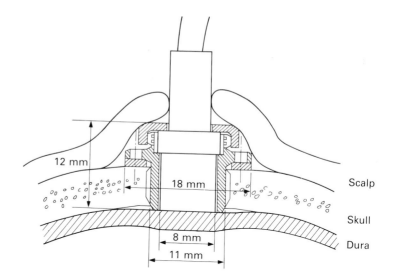

Fig. 24.17. Extradural pressure transducer. (After Koster & Kuypers, 1980.)

that the whole system is completely leakproof. Again, the major problem is infection, though blockage of the orifice by brain tissue may produce false readings. Since the tip of the bolt rests on or close to the brain, aspiration of CSF is not possible.

Extradural transducers

Three different types of transducer are in use. All measure ICP through the intact dura and avoid the use of a fluid connecting path between the CSF and the transducer.

In one system an external collar is inserted through the bone and pushed inwards until the dura bulges into it. A transducer is then inserted through the collar until the dura is just flattened (Fig. 24.17). At this point the forces on each side of

the dura are equal so that the subdural pressure may be measured (Koster & Kuypers, 1980).

In the second type of transducer there is a small disc covered by a membrane which is placed in contact with the dura. The membrane is connected to the control box by a tube which transmits air and fibre-optic bundles. A small mirror is attached to this membrane so that the position of the membrane can be determined by measuring the intensity of light reflected back along two fibre-optic bundles (Fig. 24.18). When the membrane is moved towards the interior of the transducer by the intracranial pressure, the intensity of light reflected along one of the bundles is reduced while the intensity along the other bundle is increased.

Air under pressure is then applied to the interior of the transducer to return the membrane to its

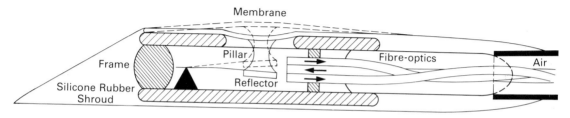

Fig. 24.18. Ladd fibre-optic transducer. The membrane is placed on the dura. The position of the membrane is detected by measuring the intensity of reflected light transmitted down the two outer fibre-optic bundles. Air is then pumped into the chamber until the membrane is restored to its original position. The air pressure can be measured remotely and indicates pressure in the epidural space. (After Levin, 1977.)

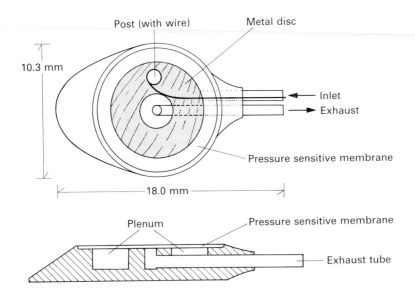

Fig. 24.19. Disposable epidural sensor. Air flows continuously through the sensor at a rate of 40 ml·min^{-1}. An increase in intracranial pressure will cause the membrane to move closer to the gas exhaust port thus decreasing the exhaust gas flow until the pressure inside the sensor equals intracranial pressure. The changes in pressure inside the sensor can be detected by a remote transducer.

resting position, at which point the air pressure and intracranial pressure are equal. Since the air pressure is sensed by a transducer in the control box, intracranial pressure can be measured continuously (Levin, 1977).

The third type of extradural transducer utilizes a disposable sensor with a thin metal membrane which is placed in contact with the dura. A continuous flow of air (40 ml·min^{-1}) is pumped into the transducer through one tube and exits through a second tube, the open end of which is situated just below the membrane (Fig. 24.19). The pressure under the membrane is exactly balanced by the pressure outside as any increase in ICP will move the membrane nearer to the orifice of the outlet so increasing the pressure in the chamber. Thus, by sensing the pressure in the chamber remotely, it is possible to measure ICP.

An extradural transducer is easy to insert and any infection which occurs remains extradural. However, the signal tends to be damped, it is difficult to recalibrate the transducer when it is *in situ* and it is not possible to aspirate CSF in an acute emergency. In patients with an acute increase in ICP the measurement tends to underestimate the true change in ICP (Powell & Crockard, 1985).

Catheter-tip transducers

Recently, a 4 French gauge fibre-optic catheter-tip transducer has been used to monitor pressure in the ventricles, brain tissues or sub-dural space. The catheter tip is covered with an elastic membrane and the distortion of the membrane is sensed by the intensity of light reflected from the back of the membrane. The light is transmitted to and from the membrane through two narrow fibre-optic bundles. The catheter is inserted through a sheath which is inserted through a small hole bored in the skull. After this has been inserted it can be locked in position with a retaining screw (Ostrup *et al.* 1987). The correlation with other methods of measurement is high but the transducer cannot be recalibrated *in situ* and needs to be replaced every 4–5 days to minimize errors due to drift (Crutchfield *et al.* 1990).

INTERPRETATION

The pressure tracing should show arterial pulsations superimposed on cyclic respiratory changes with a mean pressure of less than 15 mmHg. However, in disease states mean pressure may be increased and there may be slower variations in pressure of 10–20 mmHg with a frequency of 1–3 per minute (B-waves). In patients with severe injury, marked increases in pressure of 50–100 mmHg lasting 5–10 min may be seen (A- waves). These are usually of severe prognostic import.

Although some centres use ICP monitoring routinely in the treatment of head injury there is a relatively high incidence of infection (15–20%) and it is difficult to achieve reliable recordings over a period of days. Furthermore, the shape of the pressure–volume curve renders interpretation difficult. An ICP of 10 mmHg is within the normal range whereas a pressure of more than 30 mmHg is certainly elevated. There is some evidence that lowering the ICP at which treatment is commenced from 25 to 20 mmHg increases both the number and condition of survivors (Saul & Ducker, 1982), whilst improved survival appears to occur if the ICP is kept at normal levels during treatment (Lundberg, 1960). For a further consideration of the pros and cons of monitoring see Narayan *et al.* (1982), Greenbaum, (1987) and Hoff and Betz (1989).

References

Aitkenhead, A.R. & Thomas, D.I.L. (1987) Lower oesophageal contractility as an indicator of brain death in paralysed and mechanically ventilated patients with head injury. *British Medical Journal* **294**, 1287.

Ali, H.H., & Savarese, J.J. (1976) Monitoring of neuromuscular function. *Anesthesiology* **45**, 216–249.

Ali, H.H., Utting, J.E. & Gray, T.C. (1971) Quantitative assessment of residual antidepolarizing block (part II) *British Journal of Anaesthesia* **43**, 478–485.

Ali, H.H., Wilson, R.S., Savarese, J.J. & Kitz, R.J. (1975) The effect of tubocurarine on indirectly elicited train-of-four muscle response and respiratory measurements in humans. *British Journal of Anaesthesia* **47**, 570–574.

Arden, J.R., Holley, F.O. & Stanski, D.R. (1986) Increased sensitivity to etomidate in the elderly: initial distribution versus altered brain response. *Anesthesiology* **65**, 19–27.

Bradshaw, K., Webb, J.K. & Fraser, A.M. (1984) Clinical evaluation of spinal cord monitoring in scoliosis surgery. *Spine* **9**, 636–643.

Carter, J.A., Arnold, R., Yate, P.M. & Flynn, P.J. (1986) Assessment of the Datex Relaxograph during anaesthesia and atracurium-induced neuromuscular blockade. *British Journal of Anaesthesia* **58**, 1447–1452.

Chauvin, M., Lebrault, C. & Duvadestin, P. (1987) The neuromuscular blocking effect of vecuronium on the human diaphragm. *Anesthesia and Analgesia* **66**, 117–122.

Crutchfield, J.S., Narayan, R.K., Robertson, C.S. & Michael, L.H. (1990) Evaluation of a fibre-optic intracranial pressure monitor. *Journal of Neurosurgery* **72**, 482–487.

Doenicke, A., Löffler, B., Kugler, J., Stuttmann, H. & Crote, B. (1982) Plasma concentration and the EEG after various regimens of etomidate. *British Journal of Anaesthesia* **54**, 393–400.

Evans, J.M., Fraser, A., Wise, C.C. & Davies, W.L. (1983) Computer controlled anaesthesia. In Prakash, O. (ed.), *Computing in anaesthesia and intensive care*, pp. 279–291. Martinus Nijhoff, Boston.

Fink, B.R. (1960) A method of monitoring muscular relaxation by the integrated abdominal electromyogram. *Anesthesiology* **21**, 178.

Finlay, B., Couchie, D., Boyce, L. & Spencer, E. (1974) Electrosurgery burns resulting from use of miniature ECG electrodes. *Anesthesiology* **41**, 263–269.

Greenbaum, R. (1987) A practical approach to head injuries, including intracranial pressure monitoring and protection of damaged tissue. In Jewkes, D.A. (ed.) *Baillière's Clinical Anaesthesiology*, vol. 1. *Anaesthesia for Neurosurgery*, pp. 365–385. Ballière Tindall, London.

Guedel, A.E. (1937) *Inhalational anesthesia — a fundamental guide.* Macmillan, New York.

Herregods, L. & Rolly, G. (1987) The EMG, the EEG crossing frequency and mean integrated voltage analysis during sleep and anaesthesia. In Rosen, M.J. & Lunn, J.S. (eds) *Conciousness, awareness and pain in general anaesthesia*, pp. 3–8. Butterworth, London.

Hoff, J.T. & Betz, A.L. (eds) (1989) In *Transcranial pressure VII. Rate of infection and cost containment in transcranial pressure recording.* Springer-Verlag, Berlin.

Hudson, R.J, Stanski, D.R., Saidman, L.J. & Meathe, E. (1983) A model for studying depth of anesthesia and acute tolerance to thiopental. *Anesthesiology* **59**, 301–308.

Hug, C.C. (1986) Monitoring. In Miller, R.D. (ed.) *Anesthesia*, 2nd edn., pp. 412–463.

Isaac, P.A. & Rosen, M. (1988) Lower oesophageal contractions and depth of anaesthesia and awareness. *British Journal of Anaesthesia* **60**, 338.

Jones, J.G. (1987) Use of evoked responses in the EEG to measure depth of anaesthesia. In Rosen, M. & Lunn, J.N. (eds), *Consciousness, awareness and pain in general anaesthesia*, pp. 99–111. Butterworths, London.

Jones, J.G. (ed.) (1989) Depth of anaesthesia. *Baillière's Clinical Anaesthesiology*, Vol. **3.1**.

Kalli, I. (1989) Effect of surface electrode positioning on the compound action potential evoked by ulnar nerve stimulation in anaesthetized infants and children. *British Journal of Anaesthesia* **62**, 188–193.

Koster, W.C. & Kuypers, M.H. (1980) Intracranial pressure and its epidural measurement. *Medical Progress through Technology* **7**, 21–27.

Lee, C.M. (1975) Dose relationships of phase II, tachyphylaxis and train-of-four fade in suxamethonium-induced dual neuromuscular block in man. *British Journal of Anaesthesia* **47**, 841–845.

Levin, A.B. (1977) The use of fibre-optic intracranial pressure monitor in clinical practice. *Neurosurgery* **1**, 226–271.

Lippmann, M. & Fields, W.A. (1974) Burns of the skin caused by a peripheral nerve stimulator. *Anesthesiology* **40**, 82–84.

Lundberg, N. (1960) Continuous recording and control of ventricular pressure in neurosurgical practice. *Acta Psychiatrica Scandinavica* **36** (Suppl. 149), 1–193.

Maroon, J.C. & Albin, M.S. (1974) Air embolus diagnosed by Doppler ultrasound. *Anesthesia and Analgesia* **53**, 399–402.

Martin, J.T. (1970) Neuroanaesthetic adjuncts for patients in the sitting position. III. Intravascular electrocardiography. *Anesthesia and Analgesia* **49**, 793–805.

Michenfelder, J.D, Martin, J.T., Altenberg, B.M. & Rehder, K. (1969) Air embolism during neurosurgery. An evaluation of right-atrial catheters for diagnosis and treatment. *Journal of the American Medical Association* **208**, 1353–1358.

Mylrea, K.C., Hameroff, S.R., Calkins, J.M., Blitt, C.D. & Humphrey, L.L. (1984) Evaluation of peripheral nerve stimulators and relationship to possible errors in assessing neuromuscular blockade. *Anesthesiology* **60**, 464–466.

Narayan, R.K., Kishore, P.R., Becker, D.P. *et al.* (1982) Intracranial pressure: to monitor or not to monitor? *Journal of Neurosurgery* **56**, 650–659.

Ostrup, R.C., Luerssen, T.G., Marshall, L.F. & Zornow, M.H. (1987) Continuous monitoring of intracranial pressure with a miniaturized fibre optic device. *Journal of Neurosurgery* **67**, 206–209.

Powell, M.P. & Crockard, H.A. (1985) Behaviour of an extradural pressure monitor in clinical use. Comparison of extradural with intraventricular pressure in patients with acute and chronic raised intracranial pressure. *Journal of Neurosurgery* **63**, 745–749.

Prior, P.F. (1987) The EEG and detection of responsiveness during anaesthesia and coma. In Rosen, M. & Lunn, J.N. (eds) *Consciousness, awareness and pain in general anaesthesia*, pp. 34–45. Butterworths, London.

Rampil, I.J. (1987) Elements of EEG signal processing. *International Journal of Clinical Monitoring and Computing* **4**, 85–98.

Rampil, I.J., Holzer, J.A., Quest, D.O., Rosenbaum, S.H., & Correll, J.W. (1983) Prognostic value of computerized EEG analysis during carotid endarterectomy. *Anesthesia and Analgesia* **62**, 186–192.

Saul, T.C. & Ducker, T.B. (1982) Effect of intracranial pressure monitoring and aggressive treatment on mortality in severe head injury. *Journal of Neurosurgery* **56**, 498–503.

Schüttler, J., Schwilden, H., & Stoeckel, H. (1985) Pharmacokinetic and pharmacodynamic modelling of propofol ('Diprivan') in volunteers and surgical patients. *Postgraduate Medical Journal* **61**, 53–54.

Schüttler, J., Stanski, D.R., White, P.F., Trevor, A.J. & Horai, Y. (1987) Pharmacodynamic modelling of the EEG effects of ketamine and its enantiomers in man. *Journal of Pharmacokinetics and Biopharmacology* **15**, 241–253.

Schwilden, H., Schüttler, J. & Stoeckel, H. (1985) Quantitation of the EEG and pharmacodynamic modelling of hypnotic drugs: etomidate as an example. *European Journal of Anaesthesiology* **2**, 121–131.

Schwilden, H., Schüttler, J. & Stoeckel, H. (1987) Closed-loop feedback control of methohexital anesthesia by quantitative EEG analysis in man. *Anesthesiology* **67**, 341–347.

Sebel, P.S. (1989) Somatosensory, visual and motor evoked potentials in anaesthetized patients. In Jones, J.G. (ed.) *Baillière's Clinical Anaesthesiology*, Vol. **3.3**, *Depth of Anaesthesia* pp. 587–602. Baillière Tindall, London.

Sinclair, M.E. & Suter, P.M. (1987) Lower oesophageal contractility as an indicator of brain death in paralysed and mechanically ventilated patients with head injury. *British Medical Journal* **294**, 935–936.

Stoeckel, H. & Schwilden, H. (1987) Median EEG frequency. In Rosen, M. & Lunn, J.N. (eds), *Consciousness, awareness and pain in general anaesthesia*, pp. 53–60. Butterworth, London.

Teasdale, E., Cardoso, E., Galbraith, S. & Teasdale, G. (1984) CT scan in severe, diffuse, head injury: physiological and clinical correlations. *Journal of Neurology, Neurosurgery and Psychiatry* **47**, 600–603.

Thornton, C., Catley, D.M., Jordan, C., Lethane, J.R., Royston, D. & Jones, J.G. (1983) Enflurane anaesthesia causes graded changes in the brain-stem and early cortical auditory evoked response in man. *British Journal of Anaesthesia* **55**, 479–86.

Thornton, C., & Newton, D.E.F. (1989) The auditory evoked response: a measure of depth of anaesthesia In Jones, J.G. (ed.) *Baillière's clinical anaesthesiology*, Vol. **3.3**, *Depth of Anaesthesia.* pp. 559–585. Baillière Tindall, London.

25: Monitoring in Obstetrics

For many years monitoring in obstetrics was restricted to the measurement of maternal blood pressure, examination of the urine and determination of the fetal heart rate by the use of the fetal stethoscope. In the 1960s and 1970s electronic monitoring of fetal heart rate and uterine activity and fetal acid–base measurements, were introduced. However, some of these measurements were invasive and led to complications, and their value is now being questioned by both patients and medical practitioners.

The use of fetal heart rate monitoring in a low risk obstetric population appears to have little effect on fetal outcome though it may increase the intervention rate (Wood *et al.* 1981). Although ante-partum and intra-partum risk prediction may identify a large proportion of patients with a fetus at risk of damage, about 25% of occurrences causing fetal morbidity and mortality are not predicted and it is therefore difficult to identify which patients might benefit from monitoring. However, it is generally accepted that a high level of monitoring during labour is required in patients with a complicated obstetric history (patients over 35 and those with diabetes, hypertension, cardiac disease, or previous Caesarean section), and in those in whom there is an untoward event during labour, such as an abnormal fetal heart rate, meconium-stained fluid, abnormal presentation, vaginal bleeding or a prolonged second stage.

Routine maternal monitoring

The blood pressure should be measured at least every 30 min during labour. If the patient develops hypertension the frequency of measurement must be increased since life-threatening hypertension can develop rapidly. Body temperature should be measured on admission, and then 2-hourly if the membranes have ruptured, since infection is an ever-present risk. The urine should be checked for protein at every voiding and fetal heart rate measured at regular intervals.

The use of epidural analgesia requires a higher level of monitoring. Arterial pressure should be measured at 5-min intervals after every top-up and the spread of analgesia and motor power observed regularly. Constant supervision by a midwife is required to ensure maternal hypotension is quickly recognized and treated. Supine hypotension is common during epidural analgesia and should be avoided by appropriate positioning and fluid loading. The plethysmograph tracing provided by a pulse oximeter often gives early warning of inferior vena caval obstruction. Close observation of the conscious level and respiratory pattern and frequency is required, particularly if epidural opioids are used during the post-natal period. Facilities for cardiac and respiratory resuscitation must be immediately available. Maternal monitoring must also be augmented if anticonvulsant or antihypertensive therapy is required. Continuous observation of the patient and the use of pulse oximetry are essential if the conscious level is depressed.

If a general anaesthetic is given appropriate monitoring is essential (see Chapter 21). A capnograph should be used routinely immediately after intubation to check the position of the tracheal tube and to monitor the adequacy of ventilation, and the monitoring of inspired oxygen concentration should be supplemented by the use of a pulse oximeter to ensure that the anaesthetic is not complicated by hypoxia. A means of checking the pH of tracheal aspirate after suspected gastric juice aspiration should be readily available.

Uterine activity can be monitored non-invasively by applying a tocodynamometer to the abdominal wall. This senses the frequency and duration of uterine contractions by means of a strain gauge but does not provide an indication of intra-uterine pressure. Artifacts arise from fetal and maternal movement so the patient must remain still while recordings are made.

Direct measurement of intra-uterine pressure can be made by inserting a saline-filled catheter into the uterine cavity after the membranes have ruptured. The catheter is attached to a transducer situated at the level of the uterus. Unfortunately, measurements may be rendered inaccurate by compression of the catheter during contractions and major complications, such as perforation of the uterus by the catheter have occurred (Madanes *et al.* 1982).

Monitoring the fetus

The traditional signs of fetal distress are slowing of the fetal heart rate immediately after contractions (late decelerations) and the presence of meconium-stained fluid. However, it is now generally agreed that the traditional method of counting heart rate with a stethoscope provides inadequate information. Auscultation is subject to large errors in counting, particularly when the fetal heart rate is high, and the measurement averages the heart rate over a period of, say, 30 s. Traditionally fetal heart rate is only measured between contractions and, therefore, the information available during the contractions is ignored.

Fetal heart rate may be recorded non-invasively by placing a sensor on the mother's abdomen. The sensor may consist of a microphone which picks up the heart sounds; these are then processed to display the rate. Such a device is sensitive to other sounds and motion, and may produce inaccurate readings. Ultrasound or Doppler transducers are also used. The Doppler transducer is placed so that the pulse is reflected from the fetal heart or heart valves but it may also pick up pulsations from

the mother's abdominal aorta or common iliac arteries. Precise placement of the probe is therefore essential. The third technique utilizes abdominal wall electrocardiography (ECG). Electrodes on the abdominal wall yield both fetal and maternal ECGs which are separated by judicious filtering. Errors occasionally arise because the maternal ECG is mistaken for the fetal ECG and electronic noise may be difficult to eliminate, particularly if the mother moves. The technique is therefore rarely used nowadays. A better fetal ECG is obtained by placing a sterile spiral metal electrode on the fetal scalp. This provides a much stronger signal and fewer artefacts and is frequently used. However, it is possible to record the maternal ECG from this site in a dead fetus and to mistake maternal heart rate variability for that of the fetus. The development of a haematoma or bleeding from the scalp are possible complications.

Attempts are being made to use mass spectrometry and pulse oximetry on the fetal scalp, but with limited success.

Patterns of fetal heart rate change

The normal fetal heart rate is 120–160 beats per minute (bpm) and there is usually a beat to beat variability of 5–10 bpm (Fig. 25.1). A lack of variability often signals fetal distress, disease or depression by narcotics or sedatives (Gaziano *et al.* 1980). Tachycardia (>160 bpm) may occur in the recovery phase after a period of fetal asphyxia, but is usually not of serious import if the normal variability is present. Tachycardia may also be associated with infection in mother or fetus, thyrotoxicosis, and the administration of drugs such as catecholamines or parasympathetic blockers.

Bradycardia (<120 bpm) is the normal response of the fetus to asphyxia and, again, is usually unimportant if transient or accompanied by variability. However, a rate of less than 80 bpm is associated with a marked reduction in fetal cardiac output which, if sustained, will result in severe fetal asphyxia requiring resuscitation at birth.

There are four main patterns of fetal heart rate change associated with uterine contractions, namely acceleration and early, variable and late decelera-

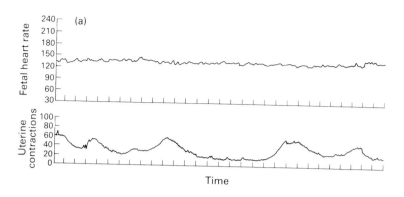

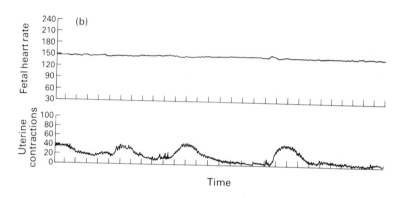

Fig. 25.1. (a) Normal fetal heart rate tracing (upper trace) showing good beat-to-beat variability and no changes with uterine contractions (lower trace). (b) Decreased beat-to-beat variability.

tions (Fig. 25.2). *Accelerations* of fetal heart rate usually have little prognostic significance.

Early decelerations occur simultaneously with the onset of uterine contraction and the heart rate then returns to the baseline level, the changes thus following the uterine contraction pattern. The slowing of heart rate is usually less than 20 bpm. It is believed that these decelerations are due to compression of the fetal head and that they are mediated through a vagal reflex. They have no prognostic significance.

Variable decelerations are probably also of vagal origin but due to reduced blood flow through the umbilical artery. They are characterized by a variation in the time relationship between the uterine contraction and the time of onset, duration and pattern of slowing of fetal heart rate and are not consistently related to fetal asphyxia (Fig. 25.2).

Late decelerations begin 10–30 s after a uterine contraction has started, the fetal heart rate reaching a minimum at the end of the uterine contraction.

This pattern of deceleration is often associated with fetal hypoxia secondary to an inadequate uteroplacental circulation, although the correlation is not strong. However, the combination of late decelerations with decreased variability in rate strongly suggests that the fetus is at risk.

FETAL pH

Whilst the abnormal patterns of fetal heart rate change do provide grounds for concern, it is often difficult to predict the magnitude of fetal distress (Council of Scientific affairs, 1981; Low *et al.* 1981). To provide further information a fetal scalp blood sample may be taken and analysed with a pH electrode. Ideally a maternal sample should be taken at the same time as changes in maternal acid–base balance may affect the fetus. The normal fetal scalp pH is between 7.25 and 7.35. Values below 7.25 are an indication for repeated measurements and possible intervention. A pH less than

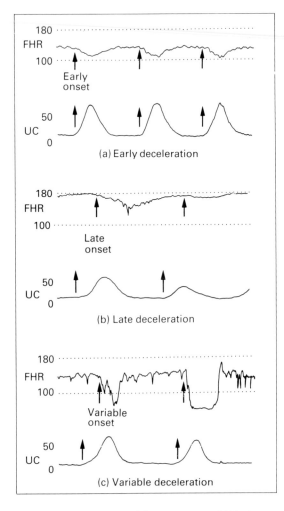

Fig. 25.2. Decelerations of fetal heart rate. (a) Early deceleration. (b) Late deceleration. (c) Variable deceleration. Note variability of onset, shape and duration in (c).

7.2 indicates fetal distress and is often associated with a low Apgar score after delivery.

THE APGAR SCORE

When the baby is born its physical status is usually assessed during the first minute and again at 5 min by means of an Apgar scoring system. This is shown in Table 25.1. A robust baby would have an Apgar score of 8–10, a blue baby without obvious heart beat, unresponsive, limp and without respiratory effort would score 0.

Table 25.1. Apgar scoring system

Index	Score	Observation
Skin colour	0	Blue, pale
	1	Body pink, extremities blue
	2	Completely pink
Heart rate	0	Absent
	1	Below 100
	2	Above 100
Reflex irritability	0	No response
	1	Grimace
	2	Cough, sneeze or cry
Muscle tone	0	Limp
	1	Some movement
	2	Active movement
Respiratory activity	0	Absent
	1	Slow, Irregular
	2	Regular, crying

Other conditions requiring monitoring during labour

PREGNANCY INDUCED HYPERTENSION

Hypertension observed before the 20th week of gestation is usually classified as chronic hypertension to differentiate it from pre-eclampsia. Pre-eclampsia may be defined as an increase in systolic pressure of more than 30 mmHg or diastolic pressure of more than 15 mmHg occurring after the 20th week of gestation and accompanied by proteinuria of >5 g·L^{-1} over 24 hours (equivalent to $>1+$ urine protein). The condition is usually considered mild if the diastolic pressure is less than 100 mmHg, moderate if it is between 100–110 mmHg and severe if the diastolic pressure exceeds 110 mmHg. The accurate measurement of the true diastolic pressure is critical. With the majority of automated non-invasive blood pressure monitors the accuracy of the diastolic measurement is poor (p. 182). Whilst such machines may be used to monitor trends it is important to verify the readings by auscultation of Phase IV of the Korotkoff sounds at intervals of 0.5–1 h or to use direct arterial measurements.

In pre-eclampsia there is a reversible arteriolar vasoconstriction with a contracted intravascular volume and a potential for impaired perfusion in various tissues, including the placenta. The condition is frequently associated with coagulation disorders and, if untreated, may progress to eclampsia with its associated convulsions, cerebral oedema, cerebral infarction and haemorrhage (Lindheimer & Katz, 1985).

Many studies of the haemodynamic changes during pre-eclampsia are confused by previous drug therapy. However, in untreated patients it appears that the increased systemic vascular resistance is associated with a cardiac index which is significantly lower than the value for normal pregnant patients of the same stage of gestation. Pulmonary capillary wedge pressure (PCWP) is low and expansion of intravascular volume results in an increased cardiac output and reduced systemic vascular resistance. The circulation may be further improved by vasodilator therapy and additional fluid loading (Groenendijk et al. 1984; Clark et al. 1986; Cotton et al. 1986). Catecholamine levels are higher than normal and reduced by epidural anaesthesia (Abboud et al. 1982).

The repeated accurate measurement of arterial pressure is essential and central venous pressure (CVP) monitoring is indicated in the severe case. In some patients there is a marked difference between CVP and PCWP (Cotton et al. 1985). In such patients, the use of a Swan–Ganz catheter may prove helpful if aggressive treatment is to be adopted or pulmonary oedema is present (Wasserstrum & Cotton, 1986). Urine output and protein concentration must be measured (Lee et al. 1987) and coagulation defects investigated by the appropriate tests. This is particularly important when a regional block is to be performed. Continuous observation in an intensive care unit is recommended if eclampsia is uncontrolled or pulmonary oedema has occurred and invasive monitoring is indicated.

MATERNAL HEART DISEASE

During pregnancy maternal blood volume is increased by 30–40% and there is a decrease in haematocrit to 35–40%. The reduction in oxygen carrying capacity is compensated by a 30% increase in stroke volume and a 15% increase in heart rate, so that cardiac output is increased by 40–50%. There is also an increase in 2,3-diphosphoglycerate in the red cell which produces a right shift of the oxygen dissociation curve and an increase in P_{50} from about 3.6 kPa (27 mmHg) to 4.0 kPa (30 mmHg) thus making more oxygen available to the tissues. However, as the uterus enlarges there is an increased risk of a reduced venous return due to vena caval occlusion in the supine position and this may lead to severe hypotension in some individuals. It is, therefore, important to ensure that the patient is maintained in the lateral position.

In a normal pregnancy, the increased cardiac output is accommodated by a decreased systemic vascular resistance (largely due to increased flow to the low resistance uterine circulation) so that systolic pressure is reduced by about 5 mmHg and diastolic by about 15 mmHg. Central venous pressure and PCWP are little changed during normal pregnancy although venous pressure in the lower extremities is increased by inferior vena caval obstruction. Total body water is increased by about 7.5 L during pregnancy and colloid osmotic pressure decreases by about 5 mmHg, thus decreasing the colloid osmotic pressure–pulmonary capillary gradient and increasing the risk of pulmonary oedema.

Since most of the increase in cardiac output occurs before the 24th week of pregnancy some patients with cardiac disease may develop cardiac failure during the second trimester. However, the period of greatest risk is during labour, delivery and the early puerperium. Uterine contractions increase central blood volume by 15–25% and in patients with severe mitral stenosis PCWP may be increased by 10–15 mmHg when the uterus contracts after delivery (Clark et al. 1985). Tachycardia associated with the pain of uterine contractions shortens the period available for left ventricular filling in patients with mitral stenosis and decreases coronary blood flow in patients with coronary artery disease. Acute changes in venous return or systemic vascular resistance associated with the induction of general or regional anaesthesia, or the administration of vasopressor agents, may also compromise the circulation in patients with heart disease. Patients with severe aortic stenosis are particularly at risk when major regional blocks are performed. Furthermore, the restoration of vascular tone during recovery from an epidural block or general anaesthetic may impose an additional load on the circulation. High level monitoring should, therefore, be continued for at least 12 h after delivery.

The frequent or continuous measurement of arterial pressure is essential in patients with heart disease and direct intra-arterial recording is indicated if a regional or general anaesthetic is to be administered to a patient who has been in heart failure or who has severe congenital or acquired heart disease. Electrocardiograph and CVP monitoring are also essential. The use of a flow-directed pulmonary artery catheter often proves helpful but is not without risk and the measurements obtained must be interpreted with caution (Hemmings *et al.* 1987; Nadeau & Noble, 1986). The major problem with the measurement of PCWP is that it may not provide a reliable guide to left ventricular filling in patients with mitral valve disease. As with CVP single measurements are less informative than trends in response to therapy.

In patients with potential or active right-to-left shunts changes in systemic or pulmonary vascular resistance may result in marked changes in shunt. In such patients the use of pulse oximetry is essential. Pulse oximetry is also useful for the early detection of pulmonary oedema and for the prevention of the hypoxic complications of anaesthesia.

HAEMORRHAGE

Haemorrhage is still a major cause of maternal death (Confidential Enquiry into Maternal Deaths, 1985–1987). There are three major reasons for the failure to reduce the mortality from haemorrhage. The first is that haemorrhage is often unexpected so that therapy may have to be carried out by junior and inexperienced staff. Secondly, the true extent and cause of the haemorrhage is often not apparent. Thirdly, many obstetric units are situated at a distance from the blood transfusion laboratory so that there is a delay in the provision of blood

products and difficulty in obtaining expert help in the elucidation of clotting defects.

A study of cases reported in the Confidential Enquiry (1985–1987) reveals that in the majority of deaths monitoring was inadequate or not used at all. When abnormal haemorrhage occurs a CVP line should be inserted and if there is any doubt about the adequacy of non-invasive blood pressure monitoring an arterial line should be inserted and direct recording instituted. It is important to recognize that a reduction in arterial pressure represents a late stage of hypovolaemia since it indicates that compensatory mechanisms (such as tachycardia and vasoconstriction) are inadequate. Constriction of superficial veins, a reduction in the amplitude of the pulse plethysmogram and tachycardia are useful signs of concealed blood loss and are an indication for treatment by the infusion of colloids using the increase in central venous pressure as a guide to the adequacy of intravascular volume (p. 323). If there is a blood loss of more than 1–2 L repeated clotting tests should be performed and platelets and other clotting factors replaced as appropriate. All transfused fluids should be warmed and oesophageal temperature and ECG monitored continuously.

References

Abboud, T., Artal, R., Sarkis, F., Henriksen, E.H. & Kammula, R.K. (1982) Sympathoadrenal activity, maternal, fetal and neonatal response after epidural anesthesia in the pre-eclamptic patient. *American Journal of Obstetrics and Gynecology* **144**, 915–918.

Clark, S.L., Phelan, J.P., Greenspoon, J., Aldahl, D. & Horenstein, J. (1985) Labor and delivery in the presence of mitral stenosis: central hemodynamic observations. *American Journal of Obstetrics and Gynecology* **152**, 984–988.

Clark, S.L., Greenspoon, J.S., Aldahl, D. & Phelan, J.P. (1986) Severe pre-eclampsia with persistent oliguria: management of hemodynamic subsets. *American Journal of Obstetrics and Gynecology* **154**, 490–494.

Confidential Enquiry into Maternal Deaths (1985–1987), HMSO, London.

Cotton, D.B., Gonik, B., Dorman, K. & Harrist, R. (1985) Cardiovascular alterations in severe pregnancy-induced hypertension: relationship of central venous pressure to pulmonary capillary wedge pressure. *American Journal of Obstetrics and Gynecology* 151, 762–764.

Cotton, D.B., Longmire, S., Jones, M.M., Dorman, K.F., Tessem, J. & Joyce, T.H. (1986) Cardiovascular alterations in severe pregnancy-induced hypertension: effects of intravenous nitroglycerin coupled with blood volume expansion. *American Journal of Obstetrics and Gynecology* 154, 1053–1059.

Council on Scientific affairs. American Medical Association (1981) Electronic fetal monitoring. *Journal of the American Medical Association* 246, 2370–2373.

Gaziano, E.P., Freeman, D.W. & Bendel, R.P. (1980) FHR variability and other heart rate observations during second stage labor. *Obstetrics and Gynecology* 56, 42–47.

Groenendijk, R., Trimbos, J.B.M.J. & Wallenburg, H.C.S. (1984) Hemodynamic measurements in pre-eclampsia: preliminary observations. *American Journal of Obstetrics and Gynecology* 150, 232–236.

Hemmings, G.T., Whalley, D.G., O'Connor, P.J. & Dunn, C. (1987) Invasive monitoring and anesthetic management of a patient with mitral stenosis. *Canadian Journal of Anaesthesia* 34, 182–185.

Lee, W., Gonik, B. & Cotton, D.B. (1987) Urinary diagnostic indices in pre-eclampsia-associated oliguria: correlation with invasive hemodynamic monitoring. *American Journal of Obstetrics & Gynecology* 156, 100–103.

Lindheimer, M.D. & Katz, A.I. (1985) Current concepts: hypertension in pregnancy. *New England Journal of Medicine* 313, 675–680.

Low, J.A., Cox, M.J., Karchmar, E.J., McGrath, M.J., Pancham, S.R., Piercy, W.N. (1981) The prediction of intrapartum fetal metabolic acidosis by fetal heart rate monitoring. *American Journal of Obstetrics and Gynecology* 139, 299–305.

Madanes, A.E., David, D. & Cetrulo, C. (1982) Major complications associated with intrauterine pressure recording. *Obstetrics and Gynecology* 59, 389–391.

Nadeau, S. & Noble, W.H. (1986) Misinterpretation of pressure measurements from the pulmonary artery catheter. *Canadian Anaesthetists' Society Journal* 33, 352–363.

Wasserstrum, N. & Cotton, D.B. (1986) Hemodynamic monitoring in severe pregnancy induced hypertension. *Clinical Perinatology* 13, 781–799.

Wood, C., Renou, P., Oats, J., Farrell, E., Beischer, N. & Anderson, L. (1981) A controlled trial of fetal heart rate monitoring in a low-risk obstetric population. *American Journal of Obstetrics and Gynecology* 141, 527–534.

Index